Primary Aldosteronism

Per Hellman
Editor

Primary Aldosteronism

Molecular Genetics, Endocrinology, and Translational Medicine

Springer

Editor
Per Hellman
Department of Surgery
University Hospital
Uppsala, Sweden

ISBN 978-1-4939-4622-8 ISBN 978-1-4939-0509-6 (eBook)
DOI 10.1007/978-1-4939-0509-6
Springer New York Heidelberg Dordrecht London

Printed on acid-free paper

Springer is part of Springer Science+Business Media (www.springer.com)

Preface

Primary aldosteronism (PA) may be the best treatable risk factor for cardiovascular disease besides to quit smoking. The discovery of the disease is described in Prof. Gordon's chapter in this book, and the understanding of its prevalence and the epidemiology behind it as well. Thus, PA is common, and millions and millions of individuals worldwide most likely suffer from undiagnosed PA as an underlying reason for their hypertension. To improve the diagnose of PA, understand the derangements and what consequence untreated PA lead to is crucial for development of care of individuals with PA.

Consequences of PA are bearing the risk factor not only for cardiovascular disease but also on life quality. Drs. Stowasser and Ahmed describe the important QoL assessments that have been done until now in one section of this book. It is clear that improvement of QoL is the effect of medical as well as surgical treatment, with a more rapid effect after surgical treatment. Besides the positive effects seen by the reduced blood pressure per se, also less need of medication with reduced negative side-effects with benefits surgery. Reversal of PA also leads to positive effects on various psychological measures, caused by so far unknown mechanisms. Aldosterone is a risk factor for cardiovascular disease, which may be reduced by proper treatment of PA. Thus, there is a higher incidence of cardiovascular events in PA-associated hypertension than in age- and sex-matched populations with essential hypertension.

The diagnostic procedures for PA are discussed in several chapters in this book, commenting on the aldosterone–renin ratio (ARR), confirmatory testings, and the adrenal venous sampling. In clear cases the diagnosis is easy, but in the majority these methods may certainly be beyond the sensitivity level. Thus, a major issue is identification and treatment of early or "subclinical" PA, among patients with essential hypertension. Indeed, there seems to be a continuum of this disease into the entity denoted low-renin hypertension, which in many cases is a mild form of early or subclinical PA. Indices state that this form of the disease is also associated with increased risk for cardiovascular complications and possibly reduced QoL. Today, the method of choice to identify PA is the aldosterone/renin ratio, which has been used also for screening of populations with essential hypertension. However, this method has a number of drawbacks as being sensitive for ongoing medications, posture, diet, etc. In addition, assays of aldosterone and, especially, renin have been unsensitive. Although the ARR still is the most available method to possibly identify also early PA, a continuous search for alternative diagnostic methods to increase the possibility to identify also early "subclinical" PA is needed.

If performing the ARR is a problem, also the confirmatory testings are sometimes difficult with far less than 100 % sensitivity and specificity. Moreover, lateralization may be determined by adrenal venous sampling, but it also has its well-known technical difficulties. Recent development in using positron emission tomography (PET) by, for instance, ^{11}C-metomidate as tracer after Dexamethasone suppression is promising in distinguishing aldosterone-producing from hormonally inactive adenomas.

The recent developments in understanding the genetics behind sporadic PA may lead to novel methods to diagnose the disease in the future. Although no success has been described yet in identifying, for instance, mutated KCNJ5 in plasma samples, further investigations are needed. The identification of mutations in KCNJ5, ATP1A, ATP2B3, and CACNA1D has also made understanding of the pathophysiology of the zona glomerulosa cells more clear. The importance of the membrane potential and depolarization for release of aldosterone is obvious.

Treatment of PA is either medical or surgical. The medical treatment of PA is limited to spironolactone and eplerenone, where the latter has considerably less side effects. This is recommended especially in idiopathic hyperaldosteronism (IHA) where surgery has limited effect due to its bilateral cause. However, in certain cases with assymetrical nodular hyperplasia, a unilateral adrenalectomy may still be beneficial. Interestingly, Dr. Takeda and coworkers comment on the possible epigenetic factors influencing the disease, by proposing that the methylation of CpG islands in the CYP11B2 promoter region may regulate the activity of transcription of this gene, and consequently the amount of aldosterone produced and the level of PA. Long-term treatment with, for instance, spironolactone has in some cases induced, or being associated with, remission of the PA, possibly due to a changed methylation status.

While medical treatment in cases with IHA or milder forms may be successful, surgical treatment has an excellent outcome, and today the laparo- or retroperitoneoscopic approach is an easy procedure for the patient who may leave the hospital the following day. Reversal of PA is instant after surgery, with a dramatic reduction of the number of hypertensive drugs and no need for potassium supplementation, as well as improved QOL and reduction of risk for cardiovascular complications.

The present book presents the disease of primary aldosteronism from pathophysiology to quality-of-life aspects, covering genetics, diagnostics, and different treatments in a truly translational manner.

Uppsala, Sweden — Per Hellman, M.D., Ph.D.

Contents

Contributors

Ashraf H. Ahmed, M.B.B.S., M.Sc., Ph.D. Endocrine Hypertension Research Centre, University of Queensland School of Medicine, Princess Alexandra Hospital, Brisbane, QLD, Australia

Tobias Åkerström Department of Surgical Sciences, Uppsala University, Uppsala, Sweden

Peyman Björklund Department of Surgical Sciences, Clinical Research Department, Uppsala University, Uppsala, Sweden

Sheerazed Boulkroun INSERM, UMRS_970, Paris Cardiovascular Research Center, Paris, France

University Paris Descartes, Sorbonne Paris Cité, Paris, France

Assistance Publique-Hôpitaux de Paris, Hôpital Européen Georges Pompidou, Service de Génétique, Paris, France

Masashi Demura, M.D. Division of Endocrinology and Hypertension, Department of Internal Medicine, Graduate School of Medical Science, Kanazawa University, Kanazawa, Japan

Xing Gao Department of Nephrology, Medical Faculty, Heinrich-Heine University, Duesseldorf, Germany

Richard Douglas Gordon, M.B.B.S., F.R.A.C.P., M.D., Ph.D. Endocrine Hypertension Research Centre, University of Queensland School of Medicine, Greenslopes Hospital, Brisbane, QLD 4120, Australia

Matthias Gruber Department of Medicine III, Technical University, Dresden, Germany

Matthias Haase Department of Endocrinology and Diabetes, Heinrich-Heine University, Duesseldorf, Germany

Department of Medicine III, Technical University, Dresden, Germany

Emil Hagström Departments of Medical Sciences, Uppsala University, Uppsala, Sweden

Per Hellman, M.D., Ph.D. Departments of Surgical Sciences, Uppsala University, Uppsala, Sweden

Livia Lenzini, Ph.D. Department of Medicine – DIMED, University Hospital, University of Padova, Padua, Italy

Silvia Monticone Division of Internal Medicine and Hypertension, Department of Medical Sciences, University of Torino, Torino, Italy

Paolo Mulatero, M.D. Division of Internal Medicine and Hypertension, Department of Medical Sciences, University of Torino, Torino, Italy

Stefan Pilz, M.D., Ph.D. Division of Endocrinology and Metabolism, Department of Internal Medicine, Medical University of Graz, Graz, Austria

Gian Paolo Rossi, M.D., F.A.C.C., F.A.H.A. Clinica Medica 4, Policlinico Universitario, Padova, Italy

Department of Medicine – DIMED, University Hospital, University of Padova, Padua, Italy

Peter Stålberg, M.D., Ph.D. Department of Surgical Sciences, Uppsala University, Uppsala, Sweden

Michael Stowasser, M.B.B.S., F.R.A.C.P., Ph.D. Endocrine Hypertension Research Centre, University of Queensland School of Medicine, Princess Alexandra Hospital, Brisbane, QLD, Australia

Anders Sundin Department of Radiology, Oncology and Radiation Science, Uppsala University, Uppsala, Sweden

Yoshiyu Takeda, M.D. Division of Endocrinology and Hypertension, Department of Internal Medicine, Graduate School of Medical Science, Kanazawa University, Kanazawa, Japan

Andreas Tomasschitz, M.D. Department of Cardiology, Medical University of Graz, Graz, Austria

Specialist Clinic for Rehabilitation PV Bad Aussee, Bad Aussee, Austria

Franco Veglio Division of Internal Medicine and Hypertension, Department of Medical Sciences, University of Torino, Torino, Italy

Oliver Vonend Department of Nephrology, German Clinic of Diagnostics, Wiesbaden, Germany

Holger S. Willenberg, M.D., Ph.D. Division of Endocrinology and Metabolism, University of Rostock, Rostock, Germany

Department of Endocrinology and Diabetes, University Hospital Duesseldorf, Düsseldorf, Germany

Tracy Ann Williams, Ph.D. Division of Internal Medicine and Hypertension, Department of Medical Sciences, University of Torino, Torino, Italy

Takashi Yoneda, M.D. Division of Endocrinology and Hypertension, Department of Internal Medicine, Graduate School of Medical Science, Kanazawa University, Kanazawa, Japan

Maria-Christina Zennaro INSERM, UMRS_970, Paris Cardiovascular Research Center, Paris, France

University Paris Descartes, Sorbonne Paris Cité, Paris, France

Assistance Publique-Hôpitaux de Paris, Hôpital Européen Georges Pompidou, Service de Génétique, Paris, France

Chapter 1
Primary Aldosteronism: Molecular Mechanisms and Diagnosis

Gian Paolo Rossi and Livia Lenzini

Abstract Primary aldosteronism (PA) is the most common endocrine form of high blood pressure (BP) and causes excessive organ damage to the heart, vessels, and kidneys, which translates into an excess of cardiovascular events.

When the diagnosis is made early on and an appropriate therapy is timely instituted, the hyperaldosteronism and the hypokalemia can be cured in practically all the cases, while the arterial hypertension is cured in about 40 % of the cases and BP control markedly ameliorated in the rest. Thus, an aggressive diagnostic approach in hypertensive patients is justified.

The recent discoveries with molecular biology techniques have led to the identification of some mechanisms that can explain the persistent hyperaldosteronism in spite of the high BP, the hypokalemia, and the suppression of renin, all factors that would be expected to shut down aldosterone secretion.

The purpose of this chapter is to provide updated information on molecular genetics of PA and the diagnostic strategy for case detection and subtype differentiation of PA. While a cost effective strategy for the screening of patients with PA can be exploited at most centers, the identification of its subtypes involves adrenal vein sampling, which is a procedure technically difficult to perform and interpret. Therefore, it should be undertaken at tertiary referral centers with experience in performing and interpreting this test.

Keywords Arterial hypertension • Aldosterone • Primary aldosteronism • Diagnosis

---

G.P. Rossi, M.D., F.A.C.C., F.A.H.A. (✉)
Clinica Medica 4, Policlinico Universitario, Via Giustiniani 2, Padova 35126, Italy

Department of Medicine – DIMED, University Hospital, University of Padova, Padua, Italy
e-mail: gianpaolo.rossi@unipd.it

L. Lenzini, Ph.D.
Department of Medicine – DIMED, University Hospital, University of Padova, Padua, Italy

P. Hellman (ed.), *Primary Aldosteronism: Molecular Genetics, Endocrinology, and Translational Medicine*, DOI 10.1007/978-1-4939-0509-6_1,

Introduction

Primary aldosteronism (PA) is a common, albeit markedly under diagnosed, cause of curable arterial hypertension, which is characterized by an increased secretion of aldosterone that is apparently autonomous of the renin–angiotensin system (RAS), because renin is suppressed. This translates into sodium and water retention and potassium loss with hypokalemia. In the presence of a high-to-normal sodium intake, the hyperaldosteronism exerts several detrimental effects [1–19] on the cardiovascular system, which ultimately translate into an excess rate of atrial fibrillation, ischemic stroke [19–21], and cerebral hemorrhage [22], "flash" pulmonary edema, and myocardial infarction [21]. The early identification PA followed by diagnosis of its subtypes, which entail surgically curable and surgically incurable causes (Table 1.1) [23], is key since in the former adrenalectomy cures PA and in the latter institution of specific drug treatment can avoid the ominous consequences of PA, including prominent target organ damage and cardiovascular events.

Molecular Mechanisms of PA

Aldosterone is synthesized from cholesterol in the mitochondria of the adrenocortical zona glomerulosa (ZG) cells. The regulation of this biosynthesis occurs acutely through the increase of cholesterol entry into the mitochondria and chronically by changing the expression of enzymes involved in ZG steroidogenesis, such as the aldosterone synthase, which is responsible for the final step of aldosterone biosynthesis and is encoded by the CYP11B2 gene. When systematically investigated in

Table 1.1 Forms of primary aldosteronism

Surgically curable
Aldosterone-producing adenoma (aldosteronoma)
Unilateral
Bilateral
Primary unilateral adrenal hyperplasia
Multinodular unilateral adrenocortical hyperplasia
Ovary aldosterone-secreting tumor
Familial type II hyperaldosteronism
Familial type III hyperaldosteronism (requiring bilateral adrenalectomy)
Aldosterone-producing adenoma or bilateral adrenal hyperplasia with concomitant pheochromocytoma
Aldosterone-producing carcinoma
Surgically not curable
Bilateral adrenal hyperplasia
Unilateral aldosterone-producing adenoma with bilateral adrenal hyperplasia
Familial type I hyperaldosteronism (also known as glucocorticoid-remediable aldosteronism)

aldosterone-producing adenoma (APA), unexpectedly this gene was not found to be consistently overexpressed as these tumors exhibited heterogeneous levels of the CYP11B2 transcript, indicating a high degree of complexity in the regulation of aldosterone production in PA [24].

It is well established that the major regulators of aldosterone production are angiotensin II, ACTH, endothelin-1, and the extracellular level of potassium (K^+). The former three stimuli were not found to be activated in human PA and therefore are unlikely to play a key role in maintaining the hyperaldosteronism in PA. At variance, the role of K^+ has been emphasized by recent findings: K^+ is a key modulator of aldosterone secretion as small elevations in its serum levels even within the physiological range increase the sensitivity of ZG cells to angiotensin (Ang) II and other secretagogue stimuli. These K^+ oscillations are held to depolarize the cell leading to opening of T-type-low-voltage-activated calcium channels, and thereby to Ca^{2+}-triggered aldosterone synthesis and cell growth. Recently, molecular variants of K^+ Channels genes have been associated with phenotypes mimicking PA in animal models and in humans [25–47].

Moreover, a germinal mutation in the KCNJ5 gene coding for the Kir3.4 potassium channel has recently been described to cause a rare familial form of PA featuring severe drug-resistant high BP and massive bilateral hyperplasia that required bilateral adrenalectomy (Familial Hyperaldosteronism type III) [29, 34, 38, 42]. Besides this exceedingly rare germinal variant, several somatic KCNJ5 mutations were found to occur in approximately one-third of the APA [25, 27, 28, 31–33, 39–42]. All of these variants are located in the selectivity filter of the channel, e.g., the region that confers selectivity for K^+. They were found to be functional in that they cause loss of ion specificity of the channel leading to Na^+ entry and thus to cell depolarization with subsequent opening of T-type Ca^{2+} Channels [35–37, 42]. Besides these mutations, exome sequencing recently revealed additional mutations in the ATP1A1 and ATP2B3 [48] and in the calcium channel CACNA1D [49, 50]. The common denominator of all these changes would be enhanced Ca^{2+} entry with ensuing stimulation of steroidogenesis. However, the reasons for the occurrence of these mutations remain unknown although at this stage it would seem that they represent a mechanism whereby hyperaldosteronism once developed is maintained rather than the initial trigger of the disease. It remains unclear if these mutations are responsible also for enhanced cell proliferation leading to APA development or only for persistent aldosterone excess, as in vitro experiments in transfected cells would support the latter but not the former contention [35, 37, 42].

Overall available data allow the conclusion that molecular alterations of cell handling of K^+ are instrumental in maintaining overproduction of aldosterone in a subset of APA, in spite of the high BP, the suppression of Angiotensin II and the hypokalemia, all factors that occur in PA and by themselves would be expected to blunt aldosterone production. This contention is supported by findings in different animal models in which inactivation of other K^+ channels, the Twik Related Acid Sensitive K^+ (TASK) 1 and/or 3 created a phenotype similar to human PA featuring hyperaldosteronism, sodium-dependent high blood pressure, low plasma renin and low K^+ [45]. These channels generate background, or "leak," K^+ currents that are essential for maintaining a negative resting membrane potential. The homozygous knockout of only one of these channels generated two distinct forms of hyperaldosteronism: the inactivation of TASK-1 caused a severe hyperaldosteronism with low-renin hypertension and a defective adrenocortical zonation, which were glucocorticoid-remediable, albeit only in females [46]. At variance, the knockout of TASK-3 in mice caused a low-renin and salt-sensitive form of hypertension [44, 47].

Recent discoveries, however, have drawn attention also to other molecular mechanisms that can drive aldosterone overproduction in APA. An elevated serum titer of angiotensin-II type-1 receptor auto-antibodies (AT1AA) in patients with an APA, and not with bilateral adrenal hyperplasia was discovered [51]. The peculiar increase of AT1AA in APA patients could have both functional and clinical consequences. In fact, these tumors were found to express functional AT1 receptors and moreover, a considerable proportion of them are responsive to Ang-II. Hence, it might be that these agonistic autoantibodies against type-1 angiotensin-II receptor stimulate aldosterone secretion and trigger the development of hyperplastic changes in the ZG of PA patients. From the clinical standpoint the unique increase in APA and not in IHA can be helpful in selecting the patients to be submitted to adrenal vein sampling.

Another recent study from our group showed that patients with APA have a 31 % higher parathormone (PTH) levels than demographically comparable primary (essential) hypertension patients with similarly elevated blood pressure values [52]. A mild increase of PTH can therefore be a further, albeit hitherto unappreciated, feature of APA that can be useful in pinpointing the patients with these tumors [52]. Moreover, the increase of PTH could be a factor contributing to the persistent hyperaldosteronism in that PTH was shown to concentration-dependently increase aldosterone secretion from human ZG and APA cells in primary culture [53].

In summary, the past 5 years have witnessed unprecedented progresses in the understanding of the molecular mechanisms responsible of human PA. The impact of this novel knowledge in terms of prevention and treatment of this common cause of human hypertension is yet to be fully deployed.

Implications for Case Detection of the High Prevalence of PA

Notwithstanding the fact that normokalemic PA was described in 1965 [54–56], most doctors still believe that hypokalemia is a *conditio sine qua non* of the disease. Hence, they are alerted to search for PA only if hypertensive patients are hypokalemic, which implies that many patients who can have PA, but are not hypokalemic, are not subjected to any investigations to detect PA. This can explain why PA has been markedly under diagnosed and therefore its prevalence has been underestimated among hypertensive patients.

The first large prospective survey designed to furnish solid data on PA prevalence, the PAPY (*P*rimary *A*ldosteronism *P*revalence in h*Y*pertensives) Study, was eventually reported in 2006 [57].

Table 1.2 Cohorts of patients with increased chance of primary aldosteronism

• Resistant hypertension
• Grade 2 or 3 hypertension
• Spontaneous or diuretic-induced hypokalemia
• Incidentally discovered apparently nonfunctioning adrenal mass (incidentaloma)
• Early onset (juvenile) hypertension and/or stroke (<50 years)

Patients with hypertension who also have one or more of these conditions have an increased pretest probability of primary aldosteronism

Using a thorough diagnostic workup and a rigorous set of criteria aimed at establishing the presence of PA, and of its subtype [58], this study evidenced that PA involves 11.2 % of consecutive newly diagnosed hypertensive patients referred to hypertension centers. More importantly, it showed that 4.8 % of the 1,125 patients that were recruited had a surgically curable subtype, which led, the investigators to conclude that PA is the most common endocrine form of hypertension and can be curable in almost half of the cases.

Knowledge of the exact prevalence rate of a disease is fundamental for estimating, along with clinical assessment, the prior probability of PA in individual patients, which in turn is key for deciding whether to proceed with further diagnostic tests. The incremental gain of a diagnostic test is in fact maximized when the patient's prior probability of a disease is between 10 and 30 %. Hence, with a documented high prevalence of PA of 11.2 % in hypertensive patients [57, 59–73] by selecting the categories of patients to be screened (Table 1.2) [74], one could enrich the PA prevalence and therefore make the screening cost-effective.

Screening Strategy

The Endocrine Society guidelines [74] suggested a case detection strategy, which is based on the aforementioned considerations (reviewed in [75]), according to which the screening tests should be performed only in patients with a higher pretest probability of PA (Table 1.2).

However, considering the high prevalence rate of PA [57], and the possibility of preventing cardiovascular complications with an early diagnosis and specific treatment [76], other experts favor a wider strategy, e.g., screening of all newly presenting hypertensive patients. Implementation of this strategy could be too challenging on the health care system of many countries and therefore the decision on what to do depends on several aspects, some of which related to the patient's features and some to the level of health care that a given country can provide.

Nonetheless, the screening is mandatory in the categories of patients listed in Table 1.2, particularly if the patients are reasonable candidate for adrenalectomy and/or have resistant hypertension. Some additional categories of patients could be included in this list, because of a higher risk of PA, including those with evidence of target organ disproportionate to their blood pressure levels, those with obstructive sleep apnea syndrome and patients with hypertension and overweight/obesity [77, 78].

Biochemical Diagnosis

In all these patients the first step for the diagnosis of PA requires the demonstration of a hyperaldosteronism that is autonomous from the RAS. The aldosterone-to-renin ratio (ARR) represents a simplified approach to this goal [79], but its proper use requires consideration to several issues that are discussed in depth elsewhere [80]. Since the ARR value depends on plasma aldosterone concentration (PAC) and on renin, a suppressed renin value will increase the ARR even when PAC is normal. Therefore, a high ARR should be considered as diagnostic for PA only if the PAC is elevated, e.g., ≥15 ng/dL.

Currently available assays for plasma renin activity (PRA) and for direct active renin (DRA) lose their precision in the low range. Therefore, to avoid overinflating the ratio ARR when renin is very low, it is common to fix the lowest renin value at a minimum (which is 0.2 ng/mL/h for PRA and 0.6 mIU/dL (0.36 ng/mL) for DRA) [57, 58]. These precautions are fundamental in the elderly and the population of African origin who usually have low PRA values. Thus, the ARR should not be used in a purely arithmetic manner, but rather interpreted as indicative of PA if a combination of increased ARR and a PAC > 15 ng/dL is found. It has indeed to be acknowledged that the ARR is a crude bivariate analysis. Based on strong theoretical considerations multivariate discriminant analysis strategies can achieve a more accurate identification of PA [63]. They have the additional advantage of furnishing an estimate of the individual patient's probability of PA, which enables clinicians to decide on whether to proceed with further testing [57].

It is worth reckoning that the ARR was shown to be reproducible when repeated under carefully standardized conditions [57, 81], and carries quantitative information. Therefore, an ARR value that was properly determined and resulted to be markedly elevated represents a strong indication of the presence of PA. An ARR value that is not markedly elevated, particularly when a carryover effect of drug treatment cannot be ruled out, should be confirmed at retesting under proper conditions, before being considered as an indication to proceed to AVS [81].

Finally, some important points must to be made concerning the assay to be used for renin measurement. The DRA assay is gaining popularity because it requires handling the samples at room temperature (for review [75]) [82, 83]. On the other hand, when using the PRA assay, handling plasma at room temperature can lead to angiotensin I generation and angiotensinogen consumption, and thus to underestimation of renin. If the samples are properly collected for each assay, the DRA and PRA values show a good correlation; which is and stronger when renin is stimulated weaker in the low range values [84], where the PA patients typically are, because the precision of either assay diminishes in this low range [84]. Moreover, it has, however, to be acknowledged that only one study has prospectively documented the feasibility of using the ARR based on the DRA for identifying APA to date [84], and therefore further experience should be gained before replacement of the PRA could be advised.

Conditions for Testing

A careful preparation of the patient is a key step in the screening because several factors and most antihypertensive drugs affect either PAC or renin values or both, and thereby the ARR (Table 1.3). Treatment must therefore be modified before measuring these hormones.

Importantly, some agents have negligible effects on the ARR: the alpha$_1$-receptor blocker doxazosin minimally affect the renin–angiotensin–aldosterone system, while the long-acting calcium channel blockers (CCB) have a small blunting effect on aldosterone secretion [57, 85, 86]. These agents can therefore be used, alone or in combination, to control blood pressure at screening if withdrawal of the antihypertensive treatment is harmful [57]. If the patient needs a more complex treatment, knowledge of the effect of the different drugs on the ARR and its components (Table 1.4) can assist in interpreting the ARR and making the correct diagnosis: a high PAC in a patient on drugs that should lower aldosterone, and/or a blunted renin value on agents that are expected to raise renin secretion are strong clues to the presence of PA.

Table 1.3 Suggestions for the correct use of the ARR as a screening test

Factors affecting ARR	Suggestion
Serum levels of potassium	Correct hypokalemia, if present, before performing the test to avoid false negative ARR values
PAC	Be aware that high PAC might originate from low salt intake or use of diuretics
	Prepare patient with adequate salt intake, measure 24 h urinary sodium excretion
	Withdraw diuretics at least 3–4 weeks before testing; mineralocorticoid receptor antagonists at least 6 weeks before testing
Renin assay	Because of low precision of the PRA or DRA assay for low renin values, fix the lowest level of renin to be used in the ARR
Patient position and blood sampling	Standardize the position of the patient and sampling conditions at your center
Handling of the samples	Be aware that handling and storage of plasma samples differ for PRA and DRA assays
Drugs	α_1-receptor blocker doxazosin and long-acting calcium channel blockers are allowed
ARR accuracy	The cutoff value that provides the best combination of sensitivity and specificity should be identified at each center by ROC curves
	Be aware that the ARR is a crude bivariate analysis and that multivariate logistic discriminant analysis might provide better diagnostic accuracy

ARR aldosterone–renin ratio, *PAC* plasma aldosterone concentration, *PRA* plasma renin activity, *DRA* direct active renin, *ROC* receiver operating characteristic

Table 1.4 Effects of drugs and conditions

Factor	PAC	Renin	ARR	False positive rate	False negative rate
Medications					
β blockers	↓	↓↓	↑	↑↑	↓
Central α-$_2$ agonists	↓	↓↓	↑	↑	↓
NSAIDs	↓	↓↓	↑	↑	↓
K^+ losing diuretics	↑	↑↑	↓	↓	↑
K^+ sparing diuretics	↑	↑↑	↓	↓	↑
Angiotensin-converting enzyme inhibitors	↓	↑↑	↓	↓	↑
Angiotensin II receptor blockers	↓	↑↑	↓	↓	↑
Long acting calcium channel blockers	→↓	→	↓	→↓	→↑
Renin inhibitors	↓	↓↑[a]	↓[a]↑[a]	↓[a]↑[a]	↓[a]↑[a]
Potassium status					
Hypokalemia	↓	→↑	↓	↓	↑
Potassium loading	↑	→↑	↑	↑	↓
Sodium status					
Sodium depletion	↑	↑↑	↓	↓	↑
Sodium loading	↓	↓↓	↑	↑	↓
Aging	↓	↓↓	↑	↑	
Other conditions					
Renal impairment	→	↓	↑	↑	↓
Pregnancy	↑	↑↑	↓	↓	↓
Renovascular	↑	↑↑	↓	↓	↑
Malignant	↑	↑↑	↓	↓	↑

β Blockers reduce levels of renin but affect PAC relatively less, thus raising the ARR, therefore they increase the false positive rate. Drugs that raise the PRA more than PAC, such as diuretics and mineralocorticoid receptor antagonists increase the rate of false negative diagnoses. Angiotensin-converting enzyme inhibitors, angiotensin II receptor blockers, and renin inhibitors raise renin and reduce aldosterone secretion and therefore they reduce the ARR and markedly increase the false negative rate

[a]Renin inhibitors lower PRA but raise DRA. This effect would be expected to increase false positives when renin is measured as PRA, and false negatives when renin is measured as DRA. Abbreviations: *ARR* aldosterone–renin ratio, *DRA* direct active renin, *PAC* plasma aldosterone concentration, *PRA* plasma renin activity

Exclusion of PA

By definition the screening tests must be highly sensitive to avoid missing any PA case. This implies that they usually carry false positive cases that must be identified and excluded, before selecting the patient for adrenal vein sampling (AVS). The oral sodium loading test, the saline infusion test, the fludrocortisone with salt loading test, and the captopril challenge tests are available to this goal [59, 63, 87, 88]. They are aimed at demonstrating that excess aldosterone secretion is autonomous from the RAS. Unfortunately, this is not often the case since many cases of PA are angiotensin-dependent [89, 90]. Hence, relying on these tests can lead to missing several curable APAs that show suppressible aldosterone excess after blunting renin. Thus, once a markedly elevated ARR, e.g., above 50 or 100, has been found there is no need, in our view, to perform any exclusion test. Whenever the ARR is borderline elevated, e.g., between 26 and 50, but this has been confirmed at a second ARR, at our institution we proceed directly with AVS [81].

Imaging of PA

High-resolution CT with 2–3 mm cuts is the best available technique for identifying adrenal nodules [86, 91, 92], that can be an APA, PAH [93], or BAH. Magnetic resonance is more susceptible to motion artifacts and less acceptable to patients [94]. Both CT and MR are useful to identify the rare aldosterone-producing carcinomas that are large [95, 96]. By contrast, half of the currently identified APA are smaller than 20 mm and up to 42 % less than 6 mm [69, 97]. PAH and MUAN are also most often smaller than 10 mm, which makes them hardly detectable with these imaging technologies.

A CT-evident non-functioning adrenal mass can concur in a hypertensive patient with PA with a tiny CT-undetectable APA; moreover, in a patient with PA an adrenal nodule can be an APA, a macronodule of hyperplasia due to IHA [98, 99], or to PAH [93, 97], but also a non-functioning adenoma ("incidentaloma"), which is common at autopsy regardless of the presence of hypertension [100]. Hence, adrenal imaging is inadequate to achieve discrimination between APA and IHA. In fact CT mistakenly suggested an APA in one quarter of the patients; identified correctly a unilateral or bilateral aldosterone excess only in half; falsely suggested a BAH in one fifth of patients with a unilateral source of aldosterone excess and showed the presence of an APA in the wrong adrenal in some patients [101]. Overall, CT results are confounding in about half of the patients: they can lead to useless and/or inappropriate adrenalectomy in one quarter of the cases and to exclusion from adrenalectomy of another quarter of the patients who are potentially curable with this procedure [101, 102].

Subtype Differentiation by Adrenal Vein Sampling (AVS)

Given the fallacies of imaging tests, the cornerstone for diagnosing unilateral production of aldosterone remains AVS [103]. The patients should be carefully selected for AVS, which is expensive, technically demanding and carries a tiny risk of adrenal vein rupture [104, 105].

Since AVS is aimed at posing the indication for adrenalectomy, it should be offered to all patients before adrenalectomy. Surgery should not be undertaken without evidence of lateralized aldosterone secretion, it should be reserved only to the patients in whom there is a strong biochemical evidence of PA and in whom rarer forms of mineralocorticoid excess have been excluded [23, 58]. Moreover, these patients should be candidates for general anesthesia and surgery and should be willing to undergo adrenalectomy.

Conversely, AVS should not be offered to the patients in whom surgery is already indicated because of the large size of the adrenal mass and/or a likely diagnosis of adrenocortical carcinoma, which, however, only rarely secrete only aldosterone [95, 96]. In contrast, some centers reserve AVS only for those who are older than 40 years, based on the premise that the prevalence of non-functioning adenoma ("incidentaloma") increases with age and therefore an adrenal mass in a patients younger than 40 with PA "must be an APA" [101, 106, 107]. However, as PA can be due to BAH or to a small CT-invisible APA contralateral to the identified node we do not support this view.

AVS should be performed only after correction of the hypokalemia, if present, and, if feasible, after withdrawal of confounding drugs (Table 1.4). Both the performance and the interpretation of AVS require considerable experience; hence, this test should be reserved to third level referral centers [108].

The measurement of plasma cortisol concentration (PCC), besides that of PAC, in adrenal vein blood is essential for calculation of the selectivity index to confirm catheter placement and correct for dilution during sampling [103]. Values of this index >2.0 under unstimulated conditions, or >3.0 after cosyntropin stimulation allows to establish that the study was bilaterally selective, which is held to be a prerequisite for use of AVS data for diagnostic purposes at many centers. ACTH (cosyntropin) stimulation, which is being used to abolish stress-related differences between sides, increases markedly the selectivity index [101, 104, 108, 109]. Without stimulation, which is being used to abolish stress-related differences between sides [101, 104, 108–110]. This stimulation is unnecessary when bilateral simultaneous AVS [108] is used and moreover exerts a confounding effect on the lateralization index. Therefore, we and others do not support its use [103, 108–111].

A major source of variation in interpretation of AVS results depends on the difficulty in catheterization of the right adrenal vein, which is short and sometimes shares an egress with inferior accessory hepatic veins resulting in mixing of adrenal blood from liver blood. This dilutes the PCC and PAC, which can result to be even lower than peripheral values due to liver metabolism of the steroids [111]. Superselective catheterization of the right adrenal vein after identifying the hepatic vein (by CT or phlebography) [111], can allow to this problem [112, 113].

Bilaterally selective AVS results should be assessed by calculating the lateralization index [103], which usually provides an accurate diagnosis [114]. Although consensus on the cutoff values to be used lacks and variable cutoffs have also been proposed based on the concomitant assessment of contralateral suppression (see later) [115–117], common cutoffs to differentiate unilateral production from bilateral aldosterone excess are between 2.0 and 5.0 [101, 118, 119]. Undoubtedly use of high cutoff values allows selecting patients that are most likely to benefit from adrenalectomy, but it can preclude curative surgery to many patients who show lower values. Results of studies that have formally assessed the performance of different cutoff values showed that a low lateralization index of 2.0 was associated with strong evidence of cure post-adrenalectomy [103, 114]; moreover, 20.5 % of the patients in a recent study were cured even despite having a lateralization index below 2.0 [103]. These observations, along with the report that even patients with bilateral aldosterone excess can benefit from adrenalectomy [120], collectively indicate that use of the higher (restrictive) cutoffs lead to denying beneficial adrenalectomy to many patients, thus supporting adoption of a low cutoff value for the lateralization index.

To address the several issues that remain controversial and/or unresolved in the interpretation of AVS [121], an international multicentre study, the Adrenal Vein sampling International Study (AVIS, http://clinicaltrials.gov/ct2/show/NCT0 1234220) was recently completed [105]. It showed that even despite the guidelines recommendations, many patients with PA still undergo adrenalectomy without AVS. Moreover, it showed that AVS is a safe procedure with a rate of adrenal vein rupture of 0.6 % [105].

C^{11}methomidate positron emission tomography could be an alternative approach to the demonstration of lateralized aldosterone excess, but it requires a positron facility for the preparation of the tracer and therefore could be used only at large tertiary referral centers. Whether it could identify the majority of APAs that are tiny remains to be proven.

Treatment

In patients who are candidate for general anesthesia and wish to achieve long term cure a lateralized aldosterone secretion should be demonstrated before undertaking surgery. Laparoscopic adrenalectomy is currently the best treatment, which can be performed with a short hospital stay at a very low operative risk [122–124]. When adrenalectomy is performed after demonstration of lateralized aldosterone excess the cure rate of PA is close to 100 % and the long-term cure of hypertension is about 42 %. Moreover, adrenalectomy was shown to induce regression of left ventricular hypertrophy [20], and to improve diastolic dysfunction when present [8].

Lower rates of cure of hypertension [125, 126] can be due to performance of adrenalectomy on the basis of imaging alone that, as mentioned above, can be misleading in a substantial proportion of the cases. Even when antihypertensive treatment cannot be withdrawn, a marked improvement is usually seen in that the number and/or the doses of antihypertensive drugs can be markedly decreased and/or resistant can be resolved [76]. As the blood pressure outcome was predicted by a short known duration of hypertension [127], and the presence of vascular remodelling [76], overall these data support the concept that the sooner the diagnosis is made and adrenalectomy is performed, the better in terms of outcome.

Failure to cure can derive from an inaccurate diagnosis, that is the lack of performing or correctly interpreting AVS results, the development of bilateral APA over time or, more commonly to the concurrence of primary hypertension. Given the high prevalence of PA and primary (essential) hypertension up to 40 % of the patients with PA can also have concurrent primary hypertension [128], which indicates that adrenalectomy can only cure hormonal alterations, but not hypertension, in these cases.

MR receptor antagonists, as spironolactone, canrenone, potassium canrenoate, and the more selective, but more expensive, shorter acting eplerenone are a reasonable alternative to adrenalectomy for the patients who either are not candidates for surgery, or do not show lateralized aldosterone excess. Additional potent and specific MR antagonists are also being developed [3]. Pilot studies suggest that they can effectively control blood pressure in PA patients and decrease left ventricular mass, but whether they are as effective as adrenalectomy in providing regression of target organ damage remain to be conclusively proven. The occurrence of gynecomastia and impotence, which can occur with the oldest MR receptor antagonists, is dose-dependent, which suggests the use of lower doses in combination, if necessary, with other agents such as long-acting CCB, some of which also have MR antagonistic properties [129], ACE inhibitors or ARBs. Both the latter drugs can be particularly useful as they effectively control the stimulation of the RAS provoked by the diuretic action of the MR antagonists. Since the MR antagonists, while being effective in controlling the hyperaldosteronism, do not correct it, aldosterone synthase inhibitors are also being developed and tested in phase 3 trials.

Conclusions

Many so-called "essential" hypertensive patients whose high blood pressure is caused by PA can successfully be identified by following few simple rules. Hyperaldosteronism and hypokalemia can be cured with adrenalectomy in practically all these patients; blood pressure can also be normalized or markedly lowered in a substantial proportion if a unilateral cause of PA is discovered. Hence, screening for PA can be particularly rewarding, when hypertension is severe and/or resistant to treatment because removal of an APA can bring blood pressure under control even despite withdrawal or a prominent reduction of the number and doses of antihypertensive medications.

Acknowledgments The studies reported in this chapter were supported by research grants from FORICA (The FOundation for advanced Research in Hypertension and CArdiovascular diseases), from the Young Research Program of the Italy's Health Minister Project GR-2009–1524351 and the Società Italiana dell'Ipertensione Arteriosa.

References

1. Fritsch Neves M, Schiffrin EL (2003) Aldosterone: a risk factor for vascular disease. Curr Hypertens Rep 5:59–65
2. Pu Q, Neves MF, Virdis A, Touyz RM, Schiffrin EL (2003) Endothelin antagonism on aldosterone-induced oxidative stress and vascular remodeling. Hypertension 42:49–55
3. Schupp N, Queisser N, Wolf M, Kolkhof P, Barfacker L, Schafer S, Heidland A, Stopper H (2010) Aldosterone causes DNA strand breaks and chromosomal damage in renal cells,

which are prevented by mineralocorticoid receptor antagonists. Horm Metab Res 42: 458–465
4. Rocha R, Rudolph AE, Frierdich GE, Nachowiak DA, Kekec BK, Blomme EA, McMahon EG, Delyani JA (2002) Aldosterone induces a vascular inflammatory phenotype in the rat heart. Am J Physiol Heart Circ Physiol 283:H1802–H1810
5. Brilla CG, Maisch B, Weber KT (1992) Myocardial collagen matrix remodelling in arterial hypertension. Eur Heart J 13(Suppl D):24–32
6. Brilla CG, Pick R, Tan LB, Janicki JS, Weber KT (1990) Remodeling of the rat right and left ventricles in experimental hypertension. Circ Res 67:1355–1364
7. Rossi GP, Sacchetto A, Pavan E, Scognamiglio R, Pietra M, Pessina AC (1997) Left ventricular systolic function in primary aldosteronism and hypertension. J Hypertens 19(Suppl 8): S147–S151
8. Rossi GP, Sacchetto A, Pavan E, Palatini P, Graniero GR, Canali C, Pessina AC (1997) Remodeling of the left ventricle in primary aldosteronism due to Conn's adenoma. Circulation 95:1471–1478
9. Rossi GP, Di Bello V, Ganzaroli C, Sacchetto A, Cesari M, Bertini A, Giorgi D, Scognamiglio R, Mariani M, Pessina AC (2002) Excess aldosterone is associated with alterations of myocardial texture in primary aldosteronism. Hypertension 40:23–27
10. Farquharson CA, Struthers AD (2002) Aldosterone induces acute endothelial dysfunction in vivo in humans: evidence for an aldosterone-induced vasculopathy. Clin Sci (Lond) 103:425–431
11. Nishizaka MK, Zaman MA, Green SA, Renfroe KY, Calhoun DA (2004) Impaired endothelium-dependent flow-mediated vasodilation in hypertensive subjects with hyperaldosteronism. Circulation 109:2857–2861
12. Taddei S, Virdis A, Mattei P, Salvetti A (1993) Vasodilation to acetylcholine in primary and secondary forms of human hypertension. Hypertension 21:929–933
13. Muiesan ML, Rizzoni D, Salvetti M, Porteri E, Monteduro C, Guelfi D, Castellano M, Garavelli G, Agabiti-Rosei E (2002) Structural changes in small resistance arteries and left ventricular geometry in patients with primary and secondary hypertension. J Hypertens 20:1439–1444
14. Rizzoni D, Muiesan ML, Porteri E, Salvetti M, Castellano M, Bettoni G, Tiberio G, Giulini SM, Monteduro C, Garavelli G, Agabiti-Rosei E (1998) Relations between cardiac and vascular structure in patients with primary and secondary hypertension. J Am Coll Cardiol 32:985–992
15. Halimi JM, Mimran A (1995) Albuminuria in untreated patients with primary aldosteronism or essential hypertension. J Hypertens 13:1801–1802
16. Rossi GP, Bernini G, Desideri G, Fabris B, Ferri C, Giacchetti G, Letizia C, Maccario M, Mannelli M, Matterello MJ, Montemurro D, Palumbo G, Rizzoni D, Rossi E, Pessina AC, Mantero F, PAPY Study Participants (2006) Renal damage in primary aldosteronism: results of the PAPY Study. Hypertension 48:232–238
17. Rossi GP, Sechi LA, Giacchetti G, Ronconi V, Strazzullo P, Funder JW (2008) Primary aldosteronism: cardiovascular, renal and metabolic implications. Trends Endocrinol Metab 19:88–90
18. Sechi LA, Novello M, Lapenna R, Baroselli S, Nadalini E, Colussi GL, Catena C (2006) Long-term renal outcomes in patients with primary aldosteronism. JAMA 295:2638–2645
19. Nishimura M, Uzu T, Fujii T, Kuroda S, Nakamura S, Inenaga T, Kimura G (1999) Cardiovascular complications in patients with primary aldosteronism. Am J Kidney Dis 33: 261–266
20. Rossi GP, Cesari M, Cuspidi C, Maiolino G, Cicala MV, Bisogni V, Mantero F, Pessina AC (2013) Long-term control of arterial hypertension and regression of left ventricular hypertrophy with treatment of primary aldosteronism. Hypertension 62:62–69
21. Milliez P, Girerd X, Plouin PF, Blacher J, Safar ME, Mourad JJ (2005) Evidence for an increased rate of cardiovascular events in patients with primary aldosteronism. J Am Coll Cardiol 45:1243–1248
22. Takeda R, Matsubara T, Miyamori I, Hatakeyama H, Morise T (1995) Vascular complications in patients with aldosterone producing adenoma in Japan: comparative study with essential hyper-

tension. The Research Committee of Disorders of Adrenal Hormones in Japan. J Endocrinol Invest 18:370–373
23. Rossi GP (2006) Surgically correctable hypertension caused by primary aldosteronism. Best Pract Res Clin Endocrinol Metab 20:385–400
24. Lenzini L, Seccia TM, Aldighieri E, Belloni AS, Bernante P, Giuliani L, Nussdorfer GG, Pessina AC, Rossi GP (2007) Heterogeneity of aldosterone-producing adenomas revealed by a whole transcriptome analysis. Hypertension 50:1106–1113
25. Arnesen T, Glomnes N, Stromsoy S, Knappskog S, Heie A, Akslen LA, Grytaas M, Varhaug JE, Gimm O, Brauckhoff M (2013) Outcome after surgery for primary hyperaldosteronism may depend on KCNJ5 tumor mutation status: a population-based study from Western Norway. Langenbecks Arch Surg 398:869–874
26. Beuschlein F (2013) Regulation of aldosterone secretion: from physiology to disease. Eur J Endocrinol 168:R85–R93
27. Boulkroun S, Golib Dzib JF, Samson-Couterie B, Rosa FL, Rickard AJ, Meatchi T, Amar L, Benecke A, Zennaro MC (2013) KCNJ5 mutations in aldosterone producing adenoma and relationship with adrenal cortex remodeling. Mol Cell Endocrinol 371:221–227
28. Li NF, Li HJ, Zhang DL, Zhang JH, Yao XG, Wang HM, Abulikemu S, Zhou KM, Zhang XY (2013) Genetic variations in the KCNJ5 gene in primary aldosteronism patients from Xinjiang, China. PLoS One 8:e54051
29. Scholl UI, Lifton RP (2013) New insights into aldosterone-producing adenomas and hereditary aldosteronism: mutations in the K+ channel KCNJ5. Curr Opin Nephrol Hypertens 22:141–147
30. Stowasser M (2013) Primary aldosteronism and potassium channel mutations. Curr Opin Endocrinol Diabetes Obes 20:170–179
31. Akerstrom T, Crona J, Delgado Verdugo A, Starker LF, Cupisti K, Willenberg HS, Knoefel WT, Saeger W, Feller A, Ip J, Soon P, Anlauf M, Alesina PF, Schmid KW, Decaussin M, Levillain P, Wangberg B, Peix JL, Robinson B, Zedenius J, Backdahl M, Caramuta S, Iwen KA, Botling J, Stalberg P, Kraimps JL, Dralle H, Hellman P, Sidhu S, Westin G, Lehnert H, Walz MK, Akerstrom G, Carling T, Choi M, Lifton RP, Bjorklund P (2012) Comprehensive re-sequencing of adrenal aldosterone producing lesions reveal three somatic mutations near the KCNJ5 potassium channel selectivity filter. PLoS One 7:e41926
32. Azizan EA, Murthy M, Stowasser M, Gordon R, Kowalski B, Xu S, Brown MJ, O'Shaughnessy KM (2012) Somatic mutations affecting the selectivity filter of KCNJ5 are frequent in 2 large unselected collections of adrenal aldosteronomas. Hypertension 59:587–591
33. Boulkroun S, Beuschlein F, Rossi GP, Golib-Dzib JF, Fischer E, Amar L, Mulatero P, Samson-Couterie B, Hahner S, Quinkler M, Fallo F, Letizia C, Allolio B, Ceolotto G, Cicala MV, Lang K, Lefebvre H, Lenzini L, Maniero C, Monticone S, Perrocheau M, Pilon C, Plouin PF, Rayes N, Seccia TM, Veglio F, Williams TA, Zinnamosca L, Mantero F, Benecke A, Jeunemaitre X, Reincke M, Zennaro MC (2012) Prevalence, clinical, and molecular correlates of KCNJ5 mutations in primary aldosteronism. Hypertension 59:592–598
34. Mulatero P, Tauber P, Zennaro MC, Monticone S, Lang K, Beuschlein F, Fischer E, Tizzani D, Pallauf A, Viola A, Amar L, Williams TA, Strom TM, Graf E, Bandulik S, Penton D, Plouin PF, Warth R, Allolio B, Jeunemaitre X, Veglio F, Reincke M (2012) KCNJ5 mutations in European families with nonglucocorticoid remediable familial hyperaldosteronism. Hypertension 59:235–240
35. Murthy M, Azizan EA, Brown MJ, O'Shaughnessy KM (2012) Characterization of a novel somatic KCNJ5 mutation delI157 in an aldosterone-producing adenoma. J Hypertens 30: 1827–1833
36. Oki K, Plonczynski MW, Lam ML, Gomez-Sanchez EP, Gomez-Sanchez CE (2012) The potassium channel, Kir3.4 participates in angiotensin II-stimulated aldosterone production by a human adrenocortical cell line. Endocrinology 153:4328–4335
37. Oki K, Plonczynski MW, Luis Lam M, Gomez-Sanchez EP, Gomez-Sanchez CE (2012) Potassium channel mutant KCNJ5 T158A expression in HAC-15 cells increases aldosterone synthesis. Endocrinology 153:1774–1782

38. Scholl UI, Nelson-Williams C, Yue P, Grekin R, Wyatt RJ, Dillon MJ, Couch R, Hammer LK, Harley FL, Farhi A, Wang WH, Lifton RP (2012) Hypertension with or without adrenal hyperplasia due to different inherited mutations in the potassium channel KCNJ5. Proc Natl Acad Sci U S A 109:2533–2538
39. Seccia TM, Mantero F, Letizia C, Kuppusamy M, Caroccia B, Barisa M, Cicala MV, Miotto D, Rossi GP (2012) Somatic mutations in the KCNJ5 gene raise the lateralization index: implications for the diagnosis of primary aldosteronism by adrenal vein sampling. J Clin Endocrinol Metab 97:E2307–E2313
40. Taguchi R, Yamada M, Nakajima Y, Satoh T, Hashimoto K, Shibusawa N, Ozawa A, Okada S, Rokutanda N, Takata D, Koibuchi Y, Horiguchi J, Oyama T, Takeyoshi I, Mori M (2012) Expression and mutations of KCNJ5 mRNA in Japanese patients with aldosterone-producing adenomas. J Clin Endocrinol Metab 97:1311–1319
41. Yamada M, Nakajima Y, Taguchi R, Okamura T, Ishii S, Tomaru T, Ozawa A, Shibusawa N, Yoshino S, Toki A, Ishida E, Hashimoto K, Satoh T, Mori M (2012) KCNJ5 mutations in aldosterone- and cortisol-co-secreting adrenal adenomas. Endocr J 59:735–741
42. Choi M, Scholl UI, Yue P, Bjorklund P, Zhao B, Nelson-Williams C, Ji W, Cho Y, Patel A, Men CJ, Lolis E, Wisgerhof MV, Geller DS, Mane S, Hellman P, Westin G, Akerstrom G, Wang W, Carling T, Lifton RP (2011) K+ channel mutations in adrenal aldosterone-producing adenomas and hereditary hypertension. Science 331:768–772
43. Zennaro MC, Jeunemaitre X (2011) Mutations in KCNJ5 gene cause hyperaldosteronism. Circ Res 108:1417–1418
44. Penton D, Bandulik S, Schweda F, Haubs S, Tauber P, Reichold M, Cong LD, El Wakil A, Budde T, Lesage F, Lalli E, Zennaro MC, Warth R, Barhanin J (2012) Task3 potassium channel gene invalidation causes low renin and salt-sensitive arterial hypertension. Endocrinology 153:4740–4748
45. Davies LA, Hu C, Guagliardo NA, Sen N, Chen X, Talley EM, Carey RM, Bayliss DA, Barrett PQ (2008) TASK channel deletion in mice causes primary hyperaldosteronism. Proc Natl Acad Sci U S A 105:2203–2208
46. Heitzmann D, Derand R, Jungbauer S, Bandulik S, Sterner C, Schweda F, El Wakil A, Lalli E, Guy N, Mengual R, Reichold M, Tegtmeier I, Bendahhou S, Gomez-Sanchez CE, Aller MI, Wisden W, Weber A, Lesage F, Warth R, Barhanin J (2008) Invalidation of TASK1 potassium channels disrupts adrenal gland zonation and mineralocorticoid homeostasis. EMBO J 27:179–187
47. Guagliardo NA, Yao J, Hu C, Schertz EM, Tyson DA, Carey RM, Bayliss DA, Barrett PQ (2012) TASK-3 channel deletion in mice recapitulates low-renin essential hypertension. Hypertension 59:999–1005
48. Beuschlein F, Boulkroun S, Osswald A, Wieland T, Nielsen HN, Lichtenauer UD, Penton D, Schack VR, Amar L, Fischer E, Walther A, Tauber P, Schwarzmayr T, Diener S, Graf E, Allolio B, Samson-Couterie B, Benecke A, Quinkler M, Fallo F, Plouin PF, Mantero F, Meitinger T, Mulatero P, Jeunemaitre X, Warth R, Vilsen B, Zennaro MC, Strom TM, Reincke M (2013) Somatic mutations in ATP1A1 and ATP2B3 lead to aldosterone-producing adenomas and secondary hypertension. Nat Genet 45:440–444, 444e1–2
49. Scholl UI, Goh G, Stölting G, de Oliveira RC, Choi M, Overton JD, Fonseca AL, Korah R, Starker LF, Kunstman JW, Prasad ML, Hartung EA, Mauras N, Benson MR, Brady T, Shapiro JR, Loring E, Nelson-Williams C, Libutti SK, Mane S, Hellman P, Westin G, Åkerström G, Björklund P, Carling T, Fahlke C, Hidalgo P, Lifton RP (2013) Somatic and germline CACNA1D calcium channel mutations in aldosterone-producing adenomas and primary aldosteronism. Nat Genet 45:1050–1054
50. Azizan EA, Poulsen H, Tuluc P, Zhou J, Clausen MV, Lieb A, Maniero C, Garg S, Bochukova EG, Zhao W, Shaikh LH, Brighton CA, Teo AE, Davenport AP, Dekkers T, Tops B, Küsters B, Ceral J, Yeo GS, Neogi SG, McFarlane I, Rosenfeld N, Marass F, Hadfield J, Margas W, Chaggar K, Solar M, Deinum J, Dolphin AC, Farooqi IS, Striessnig J, Nissen P, Brown MJ. (2013) Somatic mutations in ATP1A1 and CACNA1D underlie a common subtype of adrenal hypertension. Nat Genet 45:1055–1060

51. Rossitto G, Regolisti G, Rossi E, Negro A, Nicoli D, Casali B, Toniato A, Caroccia B, Seccia TM, Walther T, Rossi GP (2013) Elevation of angiotensin-II type-1-receptor autoantibodies titer in primary aldosteronism as a result of aldosterone-producing adenoma. Hypertension 61:526–533
52. Rossi GP, Ragazzo F, Seccia TM, Maniero C, Barisa M, Calo LA, Frigo AC, Fassina A, Pessina AC (2012) Hyperparathyroidism can be useful in the identification of primary aldosteronism due to aldosterone-producing adenoma. Hypertension 60:431–436
53. Mazzocchi G, Aragona F, Malendowicz LK, Nussdorfer GG (2001) PTH and PTH-related peptide enhance steroid secretion from human adrenocortical cells. Am J Physiol Endocrinol Metab 280:E209–E213
54. Conn JW (1977) Primary aldosteronism. In: Genest J, Koiw E, Kuchel O (eds) Hypertension: pathophysiology and treatment, vol 1. McGraw-Hill, New York, pp 768–780
55. Conn JW (1990) Part I. Painting background. Part II. Primary aldosteronism, a new clinical syndrome. J Lab Clin Med 116:253–267
56. Conn JW (1964) Plasma renin activity in primary aldosteronism. JAMA 190:222–225
57. Rossi GP, Bernini G, Caliumi C, Desideri G, Fabris B, Ferri C, Ganzaroli C, Giacchetti G, Letizia C, Maccario M, Mallamaci F, Mannelli M, Mattarello MJ, Moretti A, Palumbo G, Parenti G, Porteri E, Semplicini A, Rizzoni D, Rossi E, Boscaro M, Pessina AC, Mantero F, PAPY Study Investigators (2006) A prospective study of the prevalence of primary aldosteronism in 1,125 hypertensive patients. J Am Coll Cardiol 48:2293–2300
58. Rossi GP, Pessina AC, Heagerty AM (2008) Primary aldosteronism: an update on screening, diagnosis and treatment. J Hypertens 26:613–621
59. Gordon RD, Ziesak MD, Tunny TJ, Stowasser M, Klemm SA (1993) Evidence that primary aldosteronism may not be uncommon: 12 % incidence among antihypertensive drug trial volunteers 1. Clin Exp Pharmacol Physiol 20:296–298
60. Gordon RD, Stowasser M, Tunny TJ, Klemm SA, Rutherford JC (1994) High incidence of primary aldosteronism in 199 patients referred with hypertension. Clin Exp Pharmacol Physiol 21:315–318
61. Abdelhamid S, Muller-Lobeck H, Pahl S, Remberger K, Bonhof JA, Walb D, Rockel A (1996) Prevalence of adrenal and extra-adrenal Conn syndrome in hypertensive patients. Arch Intern Med 156:1190–1195
62. Brown MA, Cramp HA, Zammit VC, Whitworth JA (1996) Primary hyperaldosteronism: a missed diagnosis in 'essential hypertensives'? Aust N Z J Med 26:533–538
63. Rossi GP, Rossi E, Pavan E, Rosati N, Zecchel R, Semplicini A, Perazzoli F, Pessina AC (1998) Screening for primary aldosteronism with a logistic multivariate discriminant analysis. Clin Endocrinol (Oxf) 49:713–723
64. Mosso L, Fardella C, Montero J, Rojas P, Sanchez O, Rojas V, Rojas A, Huete A, Soto J, Foradori A (1999) [High prevalence of undiagnosed primary hyperaldosteronism among patients with essential hypertension]. Rev Med Chil 127:800–806
65. Rayner BL, Opie LH, Davidson JS (2000) The aldosterone/renin ratio as a screening test for primary aldosteronism. S Afr Med J 90:394–400
66. Loh KC, Koay ES, Khaw MC, Emmanuel SC, Young WF Jr (2000) Prevalence of primary aldosteronism among Asian hypertensive patients in Singapore. J Clin Endocrinol Metab 85:2854–2859
67. Denolle T, Hanon O, Mounier-Vehier C, Marquand A, Fauvel JP, Laurent P, Tison E, Equine O, Ducloux D, Girerd X (2000) [What tests should be conducted for secondary arterial hypertension in hypertensive patients resistant to treatment?]. Arch Mal Coeur Vaiss 93: 1037–1039
68. Cortes P, Fardella C, Oestreicher E, Gac H, Mosso L, Soto J, Foradori A, Claverie X, Ahuad J, Montero J (2000) [Excess of mineralocorticoids in essential hypertension: clinical-diagnostic approach]. Rev Med Chil 128:955–961
69. Nishikawa T, Omura M (2000) Clinical characteristics of primary aldosteronism: its prevalence and comparative studies on various causes of primary aldosteronism in Yokohama Rosai Hospital. Biomed Pharmacother 54(Suppl 1):83s–85s

70. Lim PO, Dow E, Brennan G, Jung RT, MacDonald TM (2000) High prevalence of primary aldosteronism in the Tayside hypertension clinic population. J Hum Hypertens 14:311–315
71. Calhoun DA, Nishizaka MK, Zaman MA, Thakkar RB, Weissmann P (2002) Hyperaldosteronism among black and white subjects with resistant hypertension. Hypertension 40:892–896
72. Schwartz GL, Turner ST (2005) Screening for primary aldosteronism in essential hypertension: diagnostic accuracy of the ratio of plasma aldosterone concentration to plasma renin activity. Clin Chem 51:386–394
73. Rossi E, Regolisti G, Negro A, Sani C, Davoli S, Perazzoli F (2002) High prevalence of primary aldosteronism using postcaptopril plasma aldosterone to renin ratio as a screening test among Italian hypertensives. Am J Hypertens 15:896–902
74. Funder JW, Carey RM, Fardella C, Gomez-Sanchez CE, Mantero F, Stowasser M, Young WF Jr, Montori VM (2008) Case detection, diagnosis, and treatment of patients with primary aldosteronism: an endocrine society clinical practice guideline. J Clin Endocrinol Metab 93:3266–3281
75. Rossi GP, Seccia TM, Pessina AC (2007) Clinical use of laboratory tests for the identification of secondary forms of arterial hypertension. Crit Rev Clin Lab Sci 44:1–85
76. Rossi GP, Bolognesi M, Rizzoni D, Seccia TM, Piva A, Porteri E, Tiberio GA, Giulini SM, Agabiti-Rosei E, Pessina AC (2008) Vascular remodeling and duration of hypertension predict outcome of adrenalectomy in primary aldosteronism patients. Hypertension 51: 1366–1371
77. Goodfriend TL, Calhoun DA (2004) Resistant hypertension, obesity, sleep apnea, and aldosterone: theory and therapy. Hypertension 43:518–524
78. Rossi GP, Belfiore A, Bernini G, Fabris B, Caridi G, Ferri C, Giacchetti G, Letizia C, Maccario M, Mannelli M, Palumbo G, Patalano A, Rizzoni D, Rossi E, Pessina AC, Mantero F, Primary Aldosteronism Prevalence in hYpertension Study Investigators (2008) Body mass index predicts plasma aldosterone concentrations in overweight-obese primary hypertensive patients. J Clin Endocrinol Metab 93:2566–2571
79. Hiramatsu K, Yamada T, Yukimura Y, Komiya I, Ichikawa K, Ishihara M, Nagata H, Izumiyama T (1981) A screening test to identify aldosterone-producing adenoma by measuring plasma renin activity. results in hypertensive patients. Arch Intern Med 141:1589–1593
80. Rossi GP (2011) A comprehensive review of the clinical aspects of primary aldosteronism. Nat Rev Endocrinol 7:485–495
81. Rossi GP, Seccia TM, Palumbo G, Belfiore A, Bernini G, Caridi G, Desideri G, Fabris B, Ferri C, Giacchetti G, Letizia C, Maccario M, Mallamaci F, Mannelli M, Patalano A, Rizzoni D, Rossi E, Pessina AC, Mantero F, Primary Aldosteronism in the Prevalence in hYpertension (PAPY) Study Investigators (2010) Within-patient reproducibility of the aldosterone: renin ratio in primary aldosteronism. Hypertension 55:83–89
82. Sealey JE, Gordon RD, Mantero F (2005) Plasma renin and aldosterone measurements in low renin hypertensive states. Trends Endocrinol Metab 16:86–91
83. Roding JH, Weterings T, van der Heiden C (1997) Plasma renin activity: temperature optimum at approximately 45 degrees C. Clin Chem 43:1243–1244
84. Rossi GP, Barisa M, Belfiore A, Desideri G, Ferri C, Letizia C, Maccario M, Morganti A, Palumbo G, Patalano A, Roman E, Seccia TM, Pessina AC, Mantero F, PAPY Study Investigators (2010) The aldosterone-renin ratio based on the plasma renin activity and the direct renin assay for diagnosing aldosterone-producing adenoma. J Hypertens 28: 1892–1899
85. Mulatero P, Rabbia F, Milan A, Paglieri C, Morello F, Chiandussi L, Veglio F (2002) Drug effects on aldosterone/plasma renin activity ratio in primary aldosteronism. Hypertension 40:897–902
86. Stowasser M, Gordon RD, Rutherford JC, Nikwan NZ, Daunt N, Slater GJ (2001) Diagnosis and management of primary aldosteronism. J Renin Angiotensin Aldosterone Syst 2: 156–169
87. Agharazii M, Douville P, Grose JH, Lebel M (2001) Captopril suppression versus salt loading in confirming primary aldosteronism. Hypertension 37:1440–1443

88. Castro OL, Yu X, Kem DC (2002) Diagnostic value of the post-captopril test in primary aldosteronism. Hypertension 39:935–938
89. Irony I, Kater CE, Biglieri EG, Shackleton CH (1990) Correctable subsets of primary aldosteronism. Primary adrenal hyperplasia and renin responsive adenoma. Am J Hypertens 3:576–582
90. Gordon RD, Gomez-Sanchez CE, Hamlet SM, Tunny TJ, Klemm SA (1987) Angiotensin-responsive aldosterone-producing adenoma masquerades as idiopathic hyperaldosteronism (iha:Adrenal hyperplasia) or low-renin hypertension. J Hypertens Suppl 5(suppl 5):S103–S106
91. Gordon RD (1995) Primary aldosteronism. J Endocrinol Invest 18:495–511
92. Mulatero P, Stowasser M, Loh KC, Fardella CE, Gordon RD, Mosso L, Gomez-Sanchez CE, Veglio F, Young WF Jr (2004) Increased diagnosis of primary aldosteronism, including surgically correctable forms, in centers from five continents. J Clin Endocrinol Metab 89: 1045–1050
93. Goh BK, Tan YH, Chang KT, Eng PH, Yip SK, Cheng CW (2007) Primary hyperaldosteronism secondary to unilateral adrenal hyperplasia: an unusual cause of surgically correctable hypertension. A review of 30 cases. World J Surg 31:72–79
94. Rossi GP, Chiesura-Corona M, Tregnaghi A, Zanin L, Perale R, Soattin S, Pelizzo MR, Feltrin GP, Pessina AC (1993) Imaging of aldosterone-secreting adenomas: a prospective comparison of computed tomography and magnetic resonance imaging in 27 patients with suspected primary aldosteronism 9. J Hum Hypertens 7:357–363
95. Rossi GP, Vendraminelli R, Cesari M, Pessina AC (2000) A thoracic mass with hypertension and hypokalaemia. Lancet 356:1570
96. Seccia TM, Fassina A, Nussdorfer GG, Pessina AC, Rossi GP (2005) Aldosterone-producing adrenocortical carcinoma: an unusual cause of Conn's syndrome with an ominous clinical course. Endocr Relat Cancer 12:149–159
97. Omura M, Sasano H, Fujiwara T, Yamaguchi K, Nishikawa T (2002) Unique cases of unilateral hyperaldosteronemia due to multiple adrenocortical micronodules, which can only be detected by selective adrenal venous sampling. Metabolism 51:350–355
98. Fallo F, Pilon C, Williams TA, Sonino N, Morra DC, Veglio F, De Iasio R, Montanari P, Mulatero P (2004) Coexistence of different phenotypes in a family with glucocorticoid-remediable aldosteronism. J Hum Hypertens 18:47–51
99. Magill SB, Raff H, Shaker JL, Brickner RC, Knechtges TE, Kehoe ME, Findling JW (2001) Comparison of adrenal vein sampling and computed tomography in the differentiation of primary aldosteronism. J Clin Endocrinol Metab 86:1066–1071
100. Mantero F, Terzolo M, Arnaldi G, Osella G, Masini AM, Ali A, Giovagnetti M, Opocher G, Angeli A (2000) A survey on adrenal incidentaloma in Italy. Study Group on Adrenal Tumors of the Italian Society of Endocrinology. J Clin Endocrinol Metab 85:637–644
101. Young WF, Stanson AW, Thompson GB, Grant CS, Farley DR, van Heerden JA (2004) Role for adrenal venous sampling in primary aldosteronism. Surgery 136:1227–1235
102. Kempers MJ, Lenders JW, van Outheusden L, van der Wilt GJ, Schultze Kool LJ, Hermus AR, Deinum J (2009) Systematic review: diagnostic procedures to differentiate unilateral from bilateral adrenal abnormality in primary aldosteronism. Ann Intern Med 151:329–337
103. Rossi GP, Pitter G, Bernante P, Motta R, Feltrin G, Miotto D (2008) Adrenal vein sampling for primary aldosteronism: the assessment of selectivity and lateralization of aldosterone excess baseline and after adrenocorticotropic hormone (ACTH) stimulation. J Hypertens 26: 989–997
104. Daunt N (2005) Adrenal vein sampling: how to make it quick, easy, and successful. Radiographics 25(Suppl 1):S143–S158
105. Rossi GP, Barisa M, Allolio B, Auchus RJ, Amar L, Cohen D, Degenhart C, Deinum J, Fischer E, Gordon R, Kickuth R, Kline G, Lacroix A, Magill S, Miotto D, Naruse M, Nishikawa T, Omura M, Pimenta E, Plouin PF, Quinkler M, Reincke M, Rossi E, Rump LC, Satoh F, Schultze Kool L, Seccia TM, Stowasser M, Tanabe A, Trerotola S, Vonend O,

Widimsky J Jr, Wu KD, Wu VC, Pessina AC (2012) The Adrenal Vein Sampling International Study (AVIS) for identifying the major subtypes of primary aldosteronism. J Clin Endocrinol Metab 97:1606–1614
106. Mulatero P, Milan A, Fallo F, Regolisti G, Pizzolo F, Fardella C, Mosso L, Marafetti L, Veglio F, Maccario M (2006) Comparison of confirmatory tests for the diagnosis of primary aldosteronism. J Clin Endocrinol Metab 91:2618–2623
107. Kupers EM, Amar L, Raynaud A, Plouin PF, Steichen O (2012) A clinical prediction score to diagnose unilateral primary aldosteronism. J Clin Endocrinol Metab 97:3530–3537
108. Rossi GP, Ganzaroli C, Miotto D, De Toni R, Palumbo G, Feltrin GP, Mantero F, Pessina AC (2006) Dynamic testing with high-dose adrenocorticotrophic hormone does not improve lateralization of aldosterone oversecretion in primary aldosteronism patients. J Hypertens 24:371–379
109. Seccia TM, Miotto D, De Toni R, Pitter G, Mantero F, Pessina AC, Rossi GP (2009) Adrenocorticotropic hormone stimulation during adrenal vein sampling for identifying surgically curable subtypes of primary aldosteronism. Comparison of 3 different protocols. Hypertension 53:761–766
110. Rossi GP, Pitter G, Miotto D (2007) To stimulate or not to stimulate: is adrenocorticotrophic hormone testing necessary, or not? J Hypertens 25:481–484
111. Miotto D, De Toni R, Pitter G, Seccia TM, Motta R, Vincenzi M, Feltrin G, Rossi GP (2009) Impact of accessory hepatic veins on adrenal vein sampling for identification of surgically curable primary aldosteronism. Hypertension 54:885–889
112. Mengozzi G, Rossato D, Bertello C, Garrone C, Milan A, Pagni R, Veglio F, Mulatero P (2007) Rapid cortisol assay during adrenal vein sampling in patients with primary aldosteronism. Clin Chem 53:1968–1971
113. Auchus RJ, Michaelis C, Wians FH Jr, Dolmatch BL, Josephs SC, Trimmer CK, Anderson ME, Nwariaku FE (2009) Rapid cortisol assays improve the success rate of adrenal vein sampling for primary aldosteronism. Ann Surg 249:318–321
114. Rossi GP, Sacchetto A, Chiesura-Corona M, De Toni R, Gallina M, Feltrin GP, Pessina AC (2001) Identification of the etiology of primary aldosteronism with adrenal vein sampling in patients with equivocal computed tomography and magnetic resonance findings: results in 104 consecutive cases. J Clin Endocrinol Metab 86:1083–1090
115. Mulatero P, Bertello C, Rossato D, Mengozzi G, Milan A, Garrone C, Giraudo G, Passarino G, Garabello D, Verhovez A, Rabbia F, Veglio F (2008) Roles of clinical criteria, computed tomography scan, and adrenal vein sampling in differential diagnosis of primary aldosteronism subtypes. J Clin Endocrinol Metab 93:1366–1371
116. Mulatero P, Bertello C, Sukor N, Gordon R, Rossato D, Daunt N, Leggett D, Mengozzi G, Veglio F, Stowasser M (2010) Impact of different diagnostic criteria during adrenal vein sampling on reproducibility of subtype diagnosis in patients with primary aldosteronism. Hypertension 55:667–673
117. Rossi GP (2007) New concepts in adrenal vein sampling for aldosterone in the diagnosis of primary aldosteronism. Curr Hypertens Rep 9:90–97
118. Young WF, Stanson AW (2009) What are the keys to successful adrenal venous sampling (AVS) in patients with primary aldosteronism? Clin Endocrinol (Oxf) 70:14–17
119. Letavernier E, Peyrard S, Amar L, Zinzindohoue F, Fiquet B, Plouin PF (2008) Blood pressure outcome of adrenalectomy in patients with primary hyperaldosteronism with or without unilateral adenoma. J Hypertens 26:1816–1823
120. Sukor N, Gordon RD, Ku YK, Jones M, Stowasser M (2009) Role of unilateral adrenalectomy in bilateral primary aldosteronism: a 22-year single center experience. J Clin Endocrinol Metab 94:2437–2445
121. Auchus RJ, Wians FH Jr, Anderson ME, Dolmatch BL, Trimmer CK, Josephs SC, Chan D, Toomay S, Nwariaku FE (2010) What we still do not know about adrenal vein sampling for primary aldosteronism. Horm Metab Res 42:411–415
122. Toniato A, Bernante P, Rossi GP, Piotto A, Pelizzo MR (2000) Laparoscopic versus open adrenalectomy: outcome in 35 consecutive patients. Int J Surg Investig 1:503–507

123. Jeschke K, Janetschek G, Peschel R, Schellander L, Bartsch G, Henning K (2003) Laparoscopic partial adrenalectomy in patients with aldosterone-producing adenomas: indications, technique, and results. Urology 61:69–72
124. Meria P, Kempf BF, Hermieu JF, Plouin PF, Duclos JM (2003) Laparoscopic management of primary hyperaldosteronism: clinical experience with 212 cases. J Urol 169:32–35
125. Sawka AM, Young WF, Thompson GB, Grant CS, Farley DR, Leibson C, van Heerden JA (2001) Primary aldosteronism: factors associated with normalization of blood pressure after surgery. Ann Intern Med 135:258–261
126. Lumachi F, Ermani M, Basso SM, Armanini D, Iacobone M, Favia G (2005) Long-term results of adrenalectomy in patients with aldosterone-producing adenomas: multivariate analysis of factors affecting unresolved hypertension and review of the literature. Am Surg 71:864–869
127. Obara T, Ito Y, Okamoto T, Kanaji Y, Yamashita T, Aiba M, Fujimoto Y (1992) Risk factors associated with postoperative persistent hypertension in patients with primary aldosteronism. Surgery 112:987–993
128. Proye CA, Mulliez EA, Carnaille BM, Lecomte-Houcke M, Decoulx M, Wemeau JL, Lefebvre J, Racadot A, Ernst O, Huglo D, Carre A (1998) Essential hypertension: first reason for persistent hypertension after unilateral adrenalectomy for primary aldosteronism? Surgery 124:1128–1133
129. Dietz JD, Du S, Bolten CW, Payne MA, Xia C, Blinn JR, Funder JW, Hu X (2008) A number of marketed dihydropyridine calcium channel blockers have mineralocorticoid receptor antagonist activity. Hypertension 51:742–748

Chapter 2
Epidemiology and the Need for Screening

Richard Douglas Gordon

Abstract Because of change in the accepted meaning of the term "primary aldosteronism" (PA), and in the methods used to screen for and diagnose it, the "perceived" prevalence of PA (and hence the epidemiology of PA) has undergone and is still undergoing progressive change since the first description of PA. As well, methodology for measuring renin and aldosterone has always been not only variable from centre to centre but often suboptimal. Hence in 2013 there existed an understandable, healthy, scientific and clinical lack of complete agreement on the definition of PA, its prevalence and how it is best identified, by screening and definitive tests, and managed. Nevertheless, the prevailing view among clinicians diagnosing and treating significant numbers of PA patients is that it is a common enough cause of hypertension, associated with unusually high morbidity if not treated early, for (1) early detection to be vigorously pursued by screening, with appropriate education of doctors and the community regarding the need to do so; for (2) identification of unilateral disease to have very high priority because surgery yields best patient outcomes and that (3) a recently proposed, "public health" approach involving the addition of "low-dose" aldosterone "antagonists" to first-line treatment of all hypertensive patients is not an appropriate alternative. It would (1) make diagnosis of unilateral PA difficult or impossible, reducing the quality of outcome for up to one-third of patients; (2) make prevalence permanently unknowable; (3) make deciding the appropriate dosage of aldosterone antagonist impossible when interfering medications are also being taken and (4) carry significant hyperkalemic risk. An increasing understanding of the genetic bases of PA holds promise that one day it may be possible to identify not only most PA patients but also a predisposition to PA early enough to prevent or significantly modify its development. In this chapter perceived prevalence is traced chronologically before attempting any estimates of true prevalence in primary and secondary care.

R.D. Gordon, M.B.B.S., M.D., Ph.D., F.R.A.C.P., F.R.C.P. (✉)
Endocrine Hypertension Research Centre, University of Queensland School of Medicine, Greenslopes Hospital, Brisbane, QLD 4120, Australia

P. Hellman (ed.), *Primary Aldosteronism: Molecular Genetics, Endocrinology, and Translational Medicine*, DOI 10.1007/978-1-4939-0509-6_2,

Keywords Hypertension • Curable hypertension • Aldosterone • Potassium • Primary aldosteronism • Renin • Screening • Prevalence • Incidence • Epidemiology • Genetics

Introduction

Primary aldosteronism (PA) is currently the commonest specifically treatable and potentially curable form of hypertension. Recognition and appropriate treatment can be life changing and life saving [75, 86]. Only one obvious clinical characteristic distinguishes PA from hypertension without a recognised cause, the so-called essential hypertension. This is unprovoked hypokalaemia. Unfortunately, hypokalaemia is usually a late development in PA, and, in most recently reported series, more than 50 % of patients are normokalemic. By the time hypokalaemia develops, and independently of blood pressure level, aldosterone excess may have caused atrial fibrillation, heart failure, stroke or renal impairment. It is therefore mandatory to screen for, and diagnose, PA as early as possible, preferably before hypokalaemia develops. Currently available screening tests for PA, though fraught with problems, are therefore undoubtedly worthwhile. Through more vigorous education of primary care doctors, specialists and the general community, screening should gradually be more widely applied to the large hypertensive population. The precise prevalence and incidence of PA, in general and in defined hypertensive populations, respectively, are unknown, with widely varying estimates depending on the extent of testing and the interpretation of the screening and diagnostic tests [87]. An impediment to obtaining definitive information on prevalence is difficulty establishing a certain diagnosis of PA in all patients included in the survey. After removing an adrenal in unilateral PA and finding an adenoma, ideally, immunohistochemical evidence of appropriate biosynthetic capacity would be established, together with biochemical evidence of disappearance of un-suppressible (autonomous) aldosterone secretion postoperatively [41]. The great hope for future understanding of the prevalence of PA, and for precise diagnostic testing, is an understanding of the genetic bases of PA. This commenced in 1992 [55] with elucidation of the genetic basis of a rare familial form, leading to a specific genetic test, and has recently progressed with identification of several other genetic mutations which cause PA [5, 6, 8, 62, 64], in one case being not uncommon as a somatic mutation in certain aldosterone-producing adenomas (APAs). Evidence so far suggests that there may be geographic and ethnic differences (1) in the frequency of occurrence of APAs in comparison with diffuse or nodular bilateral adrenocortical hyperplasia (BAH); (2) in the currently known inherited forms of PA and in the frequency of a particular genetic mutation and thus, finally, (3) in the overall prevalence of PA. These problems associated with establishing a reliable estimate of the prevalence of PA have led to vigorous controversy, with a minority view that it is sufficiently uncommon not to warrant screening [7, 19, 49–52, 54, 69, 70]. The origins, basis and elements of this controversy have already been described in great detail [34], including many of the issues requiring discussion here. In fact, little has changed since 2004, apart from growing support for screening and diagnosis of PA, based on the evidence that untreated, potentially curable PA is associated with a significantly higher risk of atrial fibrillation, stroke, heart failure and renal impairment [58, 79, 82] than other forms of hypertension of equal severity in terms of blood pressure (BP) level. A recent proposal that screening be abandoned in favour of including treatment suitable for patients with PA in the first-line treatment of "all" hypertensives will be discussed later.

First Recognition and Clinical Description of PA; Early Recognition of Its Normokalemic Form and of the Importance of Suppressed Plasma Renin Activity in Its Diagnosis; and First Suggestion of High Prevalence in the General Hypertensive Population

In a brilliant example of deductive logic, made possible by wartime experience studying adaptation to tropical climates [9], Jerome Conn in 1954 was the first to recognise and successfully treat a patient with PA due to an APA. Based on that one patient, he described the clinical and biochemical features of the condition [10], which became known as "Conn's syndrome", with severe hypokalaemia initially a salient feature. Not surprisingly, with the prevalence of PA presumably as high then as it is today, and hence an untouched population ripe for the picking, Conn was referred many hypokalemic hypertensive patients. By 1964 he could report analysis of 145 cases [16] and come to the reasonable conclusion that it was not uncommon. During the 10-year period following his description of the index case, Conn published a number of seminal observations on PA. These included that suppressed plasma renin activity (PRA) was the hallmark of the condition and not hypokalaemia, having recognised normokalemic PA and correctly deduced that it was an early form [12, 13, 15, 17, 18]. Realising that normokalemic PA could masquerade as essential hypertension [18] and hence go unrecognised, and being aware of a 20 % incidence of adrenal adenomas in an autopsy series in which hypertensives were compared with normotensives [80], Conn came up with the idea that as many as 20 % of hypertensives might have PA. This provoked alarm and even hostility among his colleagues. He later revised this estimate down to 10 % and then to about 7 % of "referred" hypertensive patients [11, 14], the latter figure being probably as close to the mark as anyone's guess today. His Harvey Lecture [14] is well worth reading. Conn's initial high estimate stimulated investigation by colleagues with an interest in hypertension ([21, 49, 50, 53]), recognising that if Conn was correct in suggesting that potentially curable PA was common, it would be necessary to look for it in all hypertensive patients [21]. A positive answer to this question was capable of dramatically changing accepted medical practice. Grant Liddle's group at Vanderbilt University studied 90 consecutive hypertensive referrals who had never had unprovoked hypokalaemia, measuring aldosterone secretion or excretion by the tedious double-isotope dilution/derivative technique in all and PRA by bio-assay in the nephrectomised rat in some [21]. The then current assumption was accepted that aldosterone production had to be above the normal range and that PRA had to be suppressed for PA to be present. Using these criteria, 87 patients had either normal aldosterone or unsuppressed PRA or both, leading by exclusion to a suggested maximal incidence for PA of 3.3 %. Two with raised aldosterone had PRA near the lower limit of normal and were thought to merit further observation. Five of 24 with aldosterone within the normal range had markedly suppressed PRA, and these days would be considered possible PA patients and subjected to a suppression test. Thus the incidence of PA in these 90 referred normokalemic hypertensives remains unclear. It might have been higher than 3.3 % and possibly as high as 11 %. It is fair to say that almost as large a degree of difficulty in deciding on the prevalence of PA based on clinical studies and biochemical changes remains to this day. This and other studies considered "negative" led to a quoted textbook prevalence of PA in the hypertensive population [7, 54] of less than 1 % and advised to look for PA only if hypokalaemia is present. This view persisted for a remarkable 20 years.

Early Diagnostic Methodology for PA and Observed Microscopic Features of APA

During a lull in further information forthcoming on the prevalence (or incidence in discrete populations) of PA, attention was paid to methods of screening and diagnostic testing [92]. Up to a week of dietary salt restriction in order to demonstrate chronically suppressed PRA was often employed as a screening test, followed by a salt loading test to demonstrate lack of suppressibility (autonomous secretion) of aldosterone as a definitive test. Interest was taken in the gross and microscopic features of APAs, many of them paradoxically composed of predominantly zona fasciculata-type cells which in the normal adrenal are responsible for cortisol, not aldosterone, production. It was noted that in many patients with APAs plasma aldosterone (which circulates in 1,000th the concentration of cortisol and is therefore much more difficult to measure accurately) fell with upright posture following overnight recumbency (instead of rising, as in normals), and this was proposed as a diagnostic test to aid in diagnosis of APA and its separation from bilateral adrenal hyperplasia (BHA), in which aldosterone also rose with upright posture [28]. It was appreciated that there were exceptions to this rule, but they were thought to be rare. The University of Queensland Endocrine Hypertension Research Unit, Greenslopes Hospital, Brisbane, Australia, began in 1987 to describe the contrasting clinical and biochemical characteristics of patients with posture [and angiotensin, by infusion [23, 94]]-unresponsive APAs (AII-U APAs) and of posture- and angiotensin-responsive APAs (AII-R APAs). The AII-R APAs on posture testing could be mistaken for BHA or essential hypertension [37, 38]. They differed from AII-U APAs in having normal levels of plasma and urinary 18-oxo-steroids, as did patients with BHA [31, 37, 38]. AII-R APAs also showed morphological differences [35, 90, 91], being composed predominantly of zona glomerulosa or hybrid-type cells, in contrast with the AII-U APAs which were composed predominantly of zona fasciculata-type cells. Interestingly, recent genetic studies have revealed another probable difference between the two tumour types, somatic KCNJ5 mutations being more commonly found in AII-U APAs of fasciculata-type morphology [5, 6]. Importantly, in the Greenslopes Hospital series, relying on adrenal venous sampling rather than plasma aldosterone response to posture and organ imaging in order to recognise unilateral aldosterone production suitable for unilateral adrenalectomy, AII-R APAs proved to be just as common as AII-U APAs [30, 41]. This, together with adoption of universal screening for PA by measurement of aldosterone/renin ratio in all new hypertensives (see later), led to the numbers of patients having unilateral adrenalectomy in the Greenslopes Unit increasing from 3–5 per year to 25–30 per year [41]. Clearly, PA was "not uncommon", just as Jerome Conn had suggested [12, 14] 30 years earlier.

The Impact of Application of the Aldosterone/Plasma Renin Activity Ratio to Screening on the Diagnosis and Apparent High Prevalence of PA

The possibility of measuring renin and aldosterone simultaneously and calculating the ratio of aldosterone divided by renin (ARR) permits recognition of early forms of primary aldosteronism before either hormone has moved out of the wide normal range [32, 33, 34, 41, 84]. Hiramatsu and colleagues [47] initiated a resurgence of interest in PA by showing that it could be detected in an unselected population of hypertensives by measuring the aldosterone-to-PRA ratio. It much later became apparent that measuring the concentration of the enzyme renin (PRC or DRC) in order to generate the ratio, rather than PRA which incorporated the effect of substrate levels, gave different and sometimes misleading results, especially in females [3, 4, 71, 85]. Hiramatsu and colleagues screened 348 hypertensives and diagnosed and removed nine APAs. This was an incidence of 2.6 %, much higher than expected in 1981. Furthermore, six of the nine were normokalemic, confirming Conn's predictions and personal findings which had been largely ignored. The incidence of PA would almost certainly have been higher, because small adenomas and all bilateral hyperplasia (BHA) causing PA would have been undetected by the methods available and employed [34]. As well, the effects of antihypertensive medications on the ARR had been unexplored at that time. This promising use of the ARR stimulated the Greenslopes Hospital Unit to study the aldosterone/PRA ratio in 18 patients with known hypokalemic PA (12 APA, 4 BHA, and 2 FH-I) after cessation of aldosterone antagonists and angiotensin-converting enzyme inhibitors [46]. A cut-off point of 25 ng/ml/h for PRA appeared to most likely discriminate PA from normals and other hypertensives. It was concluded that the ratio was very promising, but further study of its consistency and of the effects of sodium and potassium balance and of antihypertensive medications was required. With further experience, significant limitations of the ratio became apparent, as did the need for great care in the collection of samples and the assay methods used [33, 34, 40, 78, 83, 85]. Current guidelines for performing the ARR are set out in detail in other chapters in this book. However, despite significant problems, the carefully applied ARR can produce a very important yield of specifically treatable and sometimes curable hypertension, as is detailed in the following sections.

Initial Denial Followed by Acceptance of the Concept of a Higher Prevalence for PA

After demonstration of the efficacy of ARR as a screening test [47] and a favourable first "in-house" assessment [46], the Greenslopes Hospital Hypertension Unit employed it in the late 1980s to recognise the presence of PA in a surprisingly high percentage of a small cohort of extremely resistant hypertensives [30, 34, 39]. This convinced them to introduce screening of "all" new hypertensive patients for PA. Their rate of diagnosis of PA (fludrocortisone suppression testing) following at least two positive ARRs increased five- to tenfold [41], and it soon became apparent that PA was certainly "not uncommon" among normokalemic hypertensives [30, 39, 41–43, 45] and might even be the commonest specifically treatable and potentially curable cause of hypertension. The Greenslopes Unit's findings and reports, not surprisingly, were greeted with considerable caution by those researching in the area of hypertension. However, William F Young Jr from the Mayo Clinic in 1997 noted an order of magnitude increase in his unit's diagnosis of PA following his application of the ARR as a screening test, and he subsequently enthusiastically advocated its use [60, 95–99]. By 2000, reports supporting the "new higher prevalence" for PA were appearing from Scotland [56], Singapore [57], South Africa [72], Japan [66] and South America [20]. By 2004, Mulatero could draw attention to the "increased incidence of primary aldosteronism, including surgically correctible forms, in centers from five continents" [63]. It is important to point out that it is the incidence of PA confirmed by aldo suppression tests [31, 61] which should be considered in evaluating prevalence, not the incidence of a raised ratio. The observed incidence of raised ARR in a primary care hypertensive population before any suppression testing has been as high as 30 % but falls significantly after suppression testing [29, 76]. It should also be remembered that prevalence of PA is likely to be higher in a specialist hypertension clinic known to be screening for potentially treatable causes than in a general medical clinic and, even more so, in a primary care population. Omura and co-workers [68] reported a surprisingly high incidence of 6 % for PA among Japanese hypertensive patients attending a general medical clinic.

Other Problems with Screening

One of the major problems with screening for PA using the ARR is the fact that most hypertensives have been screened while still taking antihypertensive medications which affect the levels of renin and/or aldosterone and confound interpretation of the ratio, causing false positives and false negatives [2, 3, 33, 34, 85]. False positives are seen in women during the luteal phase of the menstrual cycle when renin is measured as direct renin concentration (DRC), but not when measured as PRA [3, 71]. It is difficult to take patients off interfering medications and even dangerous in some circumstances. Substitution with non-interfering medications is a very worthwhile approach used by the Greenslopes Hospital Unit for many years [85] but time consuming and not always possible. It is therefore highly desirable to screen before treatment is commenced, and this is what the Greenslopes Unit has advocated in presentations and discussions with primary care physicians and specialists. Others also advocate this approach [67], including the Japan Endocrine Society [77]. Therefore, data on prevalence of PA obtained in a primary care setting in "untreated" hypertensives is extremely valuable but rarely available. Such a prospective study was that of Westerdahl et al. [93] in a Swedish primary care setting, finding a prevalence of PA of 5.5 % among 200 patients. This excellent study employed ARR, FST and AVS as investigations and concluded that the diagnosis of PAL should be considered in newly diagnosed hypertensive subjects and that screening is warranted. A much larger, prospective study was performed in 3,000 treated and untreated consecutive hypertensive patients referred between June 1999 and October 2002 to a Hypertension Centre in Pavia, Italy [22]. Interfering medications were painstakingly withdrawn according to a well-reasoned protocol before measuring ARR. A saline infusion test was performed in those with ARR >25 in order to confirm autonomous aldo production. Those with aldo not suppressing with saline went on to have adrenal CT scans and a dexamethasone suppression test, the latter followed by a chimeric gene test if positive, to diagnose or exclude GSH (FH-I). Of these 3,000 hypertensive patients referred to the clinic by general practitioners, as many as 684 (22.8 %) had ARR >25, but only approximately one-quarter of these (177, 5.9 % of the whole hypertensive population) had, as well, a positive saline loading test, leading to a positive diagnosis of primary aldosteronism. Note the big fall in possible incidence when a suppression test is included after a positive ARR. This was a single-centre study and thus avoided the major problem with multi-centre studies of differences in performance criteria, methodology and "cut-off" points for ARR from centre to centre. One such large, prospective, multi-centre Italian study of 1,125 hypertensive patients who were referred to 14 different hypertension clinics [74] also used ARR to screen (after ceasing or changing antihypertensive medications) and yielded an apparent incidence for PA which was higher at 11.2 % (APA 4.8 %, IHA 6.4 %). Thus we began to see glimpses of a possible prevalence for PA of around 5 % in a primary care hypertensive population and 10 % in a specialist hypertension clinic seeing referred patients.

Epidemiology Changes with New Forms and Definitions of Primary Aldosteronism

It can be seen from the above that, at the present time, a precise description of the epidemiology of primary aldosteronism is impossible, but we can describe "trends". The true epidemiology of PA will become known, if ever, only when the genetic bases of all forms of PA have been discovered, genetic tests which provide a definite "yes" or "no" for the presence of a known causative mutation are widely available and the prevalence will probably vary depending on location. This will be to some extent explained by genetic diversity in different ethnic populations. For example, the percentage of APAs which harbour a *KCNJ5* mutation may be higher in Japan than in Brisbane, Australia, or Cambridge, England. The first widely accepted definition of PA was based on patients with hypertension and hypokalaemia, suppressed PRA and "unsuppressible" aldosterone who harboured an adrenal tumour. There are still some clinicians who favour confining use of the term "Conn's syndrome" to a solitary, benign, APA. However, there is general acceptance of less classic forms of PA. This follows acceptance of bilateral diffuse or nodular hyperplasia (unilateral or bilateral) and of adrenal carcinoma as being also capable of causing PA. As soon as Conn recognised normokalemic forms, these needed to be and were included in the definition. When Hiramatsu and colleagues in 1981 popularised the ARR as a screening test for PA, adrenal imaging was very difficult and adrenal morphology did not figure prominently in the diagnosis or the definition of PA, except by examination of a removed adrenal which cured the hypertension and, if present, the hypokalaemia—reasonable proof that primary aldosteronism was the cause of the patient's condition. By the mid-1990s, however, when reliable abdominal organ imaging by computerised tomography (CT) became available, the definition of "possible" PA was expanded to include an adrenal abnormality on CT scanning (typically a hypo-dense nodule) in a hypertensive patient which might be an APA. However, such a nodule could also be an "incidental" finding (during investigation for abdominal pain), and not autonomously producing aldo or any other commonly measured steroid, and sometimes a metastasis. The definition of PA has continued to be challenged by recognition not only of early, less severe, usually normokalemic forms but also by initially rare, but now more commonly diagnosed (including by the Greenslopes Unit), normotensive forms, in which all the other clinical and biochemical (low potassium, low renin, unsuppressible aldo) features of PA may be present. Ito and co-workers [48] looked for and found an incidence of this normotensive form of PA of at least 1.4 % in healthy normotensive subjects. Is it appropriate to call this normotensive PA?

Insights and Questions Arising from Study of Familial Forms

A more recent, completely different challenge to our perceptions of definition and prevalence of PA has arisen. When a normotensive, normokalemic member of a family some of whose members suffer from a form of familial PA such as FH-I is tested and found to have "the hybrid gene", would it be best to say that this patient has PA or alternatively to describe this clinical scenario in terms of "a high risk" of eventually developing PA? We have learned much about the evolution (natural history) of PA by the study of families harbouring genetic mutations capable of causing full-blown or classic PA [35, 44, 81] but also early, less florid phenotype. Increasing knowledge of human genetics and advances in methodology and in the interpretation of findings have altered our perceptions of PA in many ways [39], starting in 1992 with the genetic basis of familial glucocorticoid-remediable PA [55], first described clinically 26 years earlier [88]. Some affected members of FH-I families will develop hypertension early, even presenting with stroke [73]. Many will remain normokalemic. Others, especially women, even if hypokalemic, may not develop hypertension until after the menopause, if at all. Developing knowledge of the diversity of genotype as well as phenotype is an ongoing process which is accelerating, with the recent demonstration of causal mutations in the *KCNJ5* gene [5, 6, 8, 62, 64].

Obtaining a Definitive Diagnosis

In addition to the challenge to current definitions of PA represented by the above development of techniques permitting definitive diagnosis of a genetic predisposition to PA, there remain seemingly insurmountable problems to overcome in order to establish its prevalence. The first step towards resolution, not yet taken, is widespread recognition and acceptance that the problems exist, and the second step will be a collective will to solve them. What are these seemingly insurmountable problems? Up to the present time, the best methods for screening and diagnosing PA remain highly controversial. Accurate, robust methods for measuring renin, "renin activity", angiotensin and aldosterone are still not widely available, 60 years after the clinical description of PAL by Conn, and 50 years after he defined the pathophysiology using a bio-assay in the nephrectomised rat to assess renin activity, and tedious, time-consuming double-isotope derivative dilution techniques to quantify aldosterone. A seminal issue concerns whether measurement of the enzyme renin (present in precursor, inactive and active forms) is helpful or confusing. The end product of the enzyme (renin) reaction with its substrate (angiotensinogen) is angiotensin I (Ang-I) which is rapidly converted to angiotensin-II (Ang-II), and it is this peptide, not renin the enzyme, which is not only the major regulator of aldosterone production but also capable of "feeding back" negatively to suppress renin release. Changes in levels and reactivity of substrate as well as other known and unknown influences on angiotensin generation are ignored if levels of renin in one of its many forms are relied on to assess the activity of the system in terms of its effects on aldosterone levels. More precise and reproducible methods which incorporate mass spectrometry of generated angiotensin I are beginning to appear in the literature, and methods for measuring circulating angiotensin II will almost certainly follow. Methods for measurement of aldo by mass spectrometry are well established [89] but not yet widely available. If the methodological problems can been solved, another significant problem will remain. Importantly and unavoidably, regardless of the methodology, quoted "cut-off" points for ARR which are utilised when screening, and are accepted as delineating "likely" or "unlikely" PA, are always arbitrary and contentious. They represent a "best guess", even when statistically derived, for example using receiver–operator curves. Similarly, definitive tests for PA are necessarily arbitrary in discriminating between normality and abnormality. Neither sets of criteria will be transferable from laboratory to laboratory because of differences, sometimes subtle and sometimes not, in methods of collection of blood samples, detailed handling of the samples and precise conditions utilised in the assays. This is why an element of local preference, based on local experience of outcomes, should always override "guidelines" when there is a clash. Hence at the present time, and into the foreseeable future, somewhat arbitrary assumptions have to be made (quite often after treatment has been commenced) regarding the correctness of the diagnosis of PA. Removal of an adenoma with typical histological features has often been regarded as sufficient to unequivocally establish a firm diagnosis of PA, without appropriate immuno-histochemical evidence of aldosterone secretory capacity. Might it have been an "incidentaloma"? Normokalemia and a normal post-operative aldo suppression test [41] are the best currently available evidence of removal of all abnormal, unsuppressible aldosterone-producing tissue. This provides convincing evidence that PA due to APA was present but is rarely performed. Lack of very strong evidence of a correct diagnosis of PA will always threaten the validity of estimated prevalence or incidence of PA.

"Need for Screening" Depends on Perceived Epidemiology

The following general points regarding epidemiology apply equally to screening and epidemiology of PA. The intensity of need for screening for a clinical condition will depend on factors such as (a) the seriousness of a negative outcome if the condition is not recognised (that is, "missed"); (b) whether it is sufficiently common to make screening worthwhile and (c) that screening methods are sufficiently robust to unequivocally identify those affected. In the case of PA, the first two of these arbitrarily chosen criteria suggesting a "high need for screening" appear to be well satisfied, while the third is doubtful, as already discussed. Epidemiology is always greatly influenced by the intensity and quality of screening. Epidemiology is the historical record of recognised instances of a condition, such as PA, in a community setting which can range from a very small to a very large community. Epidemiology changes not only with place, but with time, especially if it is due to an infective agent. It will at any given time depend on the reliability and precision of the criteria for recognition (that is, for diagnosis) that the condition is or was indeed present, and this will also vary with both place and time, as diagnostic criteria change and are, or are not, taken up and acted upon to confirm or exclude the diagnosis. Critically, it will depend on (a) identification of an infective or genetic cause or, if not infective or genetic, (b) a tight and universally acceptable definition of what the condition is. This has become a real difficulty for PA, as already discussed.

Most importantly of all, however, it will depend on the prevailing attitudes, global or local, regarding the commonness and importance of the condition, and hence the degree of enthusiasm regarding the need to make the diagnosis. Thus the epidemiology of primary aldosteronism in Brisbane, Queensland, Australia, might be vastly different from that in Dallas, TX, USA. Norman Kaplan has argued persuasively that PA is being over-diagnosed in Brisbane and elsewhere and that screening for it is not only unnecessary but also a waste of "the health dollar". These fundamental differences in approach and inevitable outcomes (normokalemic PA will rarely be diagnosed in Kaplan's clinic) illustrate that, most importantly of all, the epidemiology of PA will vary greatly from place to place depending mainly on whether or not it is sought in the local community, illustrating a very important truism—"If you don't look, you certainly won't find".

Such differences of opinion are healthy and form the basis on which science, and certainly biological science, makes its stuttering but seminal advances. It is only problematic if it results in (a) patients who deserve and require specific treatment missing out on such treatment, which is very serious, or (b) health-directed public funds being spent unnecessarily, unproductively and therefore unwisely. This is less serious, but obviously best avoided. In the case of PA, lack of screening is indeed very serious. Dedicated clinicians who follow individual patients closely are strongly moved by unnecessary, permanent morbidity caused by unrecognised and therefore not specifically treated PA, when cerebral, cardiac and renal damage occurs and is irreversible. This is preventable (by screening) and results from failure to recognise PA early in its natural history, and hence make use of the specific and highly effective medical and surgical (in carefully selected cases) treatments available.

Current Recommendations for Screening, Including "The Endocrine Society" Guidelines

Clinical management guidelines issued from time to time by the Endocrine Society (United States) have proved useful to endocrinologists worldwide. Given widely divergent opinions on the prevalence and management of primary aldosteronism over the 50 years since its first description, the Endocrine Society convened a panel of clinicians experienced in the management of primary aldosteronism under the chairmanship of John Funder, of Monash University, Melbourne, Australia. Funder is a medical graduate but not a clinician, with a long and distinguished research record in mineralocorticoid receptors and aldosterone action based predominantly on animal studies. As well, he closely follows clinical studies concerning PA and was very interested in the initial clinical trials in hypertension and heart failure of the aldosterone antagonist, eplerenone, which has negligible interaction with the androgen receptor when compared with spironolactone. The panel addressed the issues of screening (who and how to screen), how to establish a firm diagnosis and subtype differentiation and how to treat PA. A good attempt was made to identify patient groups especially deserving of screening, including those with an expected higher incidence of PA, such as patients with resistant hypertension, with spontaneous hypokalaemia or with a family history of PA [59]. The guidelines were published in J Clin Endocrinol Metab in 2008 [27] and met with a mixed reception, particularly in Europe, especially with regard to the universality of screening and whether adrenal venous sampling is necessary. Resolving these controversial issues depends particularly on to what extent each patient is assessed as a unique individual and to what extent the patient, following very full discussion, is involved in decision-making. Rather than advocating "one size fits all" and seeking a consensus, an alternative point of view which I strongly favour is to ask the clinician to consider local facilities and local expertise as prime determinants of best possible practice in that patient [36]. Recently, John Funder, who considers PA to be common but treats no PA patients, and Norman Kaplan, a clinician who considers PA to be uncommon and admits to seeing few patients with PA, agreed that the best and cheapest way to deal effectively with PA would be to include low-dose aldosterone antagonists such as spironolactone, eplerenone and amiloride as part of first-line treatment of hypertension [24–26, 52]. Clinicians experienced in managing patients with PA as well as other patients with hypertension could find the recent Funder/Kaplan proposal unattractive for several reasons. The incidence of hypertension increases with age, and the majority of hypertensive patients are old enough to be experiencing a decline in renal glomerular function. Administration of either potassium supplements or drugs which reduce potassium excretion has been known for at least 40 years to carry significant risk of hyperkalaemia in those with declining renal function. For example, the approval of amiloride for clinical use was followed by reports of serious hyperkalemic episodes. Despite well thought out, enthusiastic education of doctors regarding the use of eplerenone and spironolactone in heart failure patients, with apparent safety in tightly controlled clinical trial conditions, most hypertensives are treated by busy general practitioners (GPs or primary care doctors) who are unfamiliar with the delayed onset and offset of the antihypertensive and volume-depleting effects of aldosterone blockade. It is highly unlikely that the slow, cautious approach employed by endocrinologists, nephrologists and cardiologists prescribing these medications would be followed by all GPs, who may be following hypertension treatment guidelines which recommend incremental increase of medication until a target (often impossible to reach in older patients) is reached. Ideally, the dosage of spironolactone, eplerenone or amiloride should be adjusted based on serial measurements of plasma levels of renin, aldosterone, creatinine and potassium. For renin levels to be interpretable, medications which affect them would need to be avoided, or at least taken into account, which requires experience and skill and takes time. This is difficult enough in specialist practice and unlikely to be possible in primary care, where many doctors may also not be sufficiently familiar with the renin–angiotensin–aldosterone system in clinical practice. Because of renin becoming unsuppressed, once aldosterone antagonism is introduced into a hypertensive patient's treatment, it will be impossible, without ceasing it, to diagnose unilateral aldosterone production due to an APA by adrenal venous sampling, depriving such patients of the possibility of cure and condemning them to life-long drug therapy, probably in increasing doses. As well, some clinicians and institutions will still be recommending screening of all hypertensive patients for PA, preferably before medications are commenced. These will most likely include the Greenslopes Hospital Hypertension Unit and the Japan Endocrine Society [77] into the foreseeable future.

Conclusions

We have been forced to directly address the question of the definition of PA, not at the beginning of a chapter entitled "Epidemiology and need for screening", as the reader might reasonably expect, but at the end, because it is constantly evolving and inevitably the subject of controversy. PA is certainly not now as Conn described it, hypertension with severe hypokalaemia. It has moved through normokalemic PA to normotensive PA and, perhaps, even to enough unsuppressible aldosterone in the context of falling nephron numbers and a persisting high salt intake to cause hypertension with suppressed renin, as in the Framingham Offspring study of subjects over 50 years of age [65]. Will PA finally be defined by a variety of genetic mutations either in the adrenal only or in the entire genome? Only time will tell. While knowledge of the genetics of PA began 21 years ago with the discovery of mutations causing the rare glucocorticoid-remediable familial form of PA [55], it is only very recently that meaningful breakthroughs have followed, identifying somatic adrenal and genomic mutations causing PA of varying severity (FH-III), the former not uncommon and the latter rare. If the genetic bases of the more common FH-II can be elucidated, then we might be in a position to identify with certainty many subjects with PA, or at least an inherited tendency to develop PA, following a single blood test. That would give us new, clearer definitions for at least some subtypes of PA on a genetic rather than a clinical, biochemical or morphological basis.

In the meantime, agreement on epidemiology depends critically on widely accepted "working" definitions, not yet available. We have therefore considered only the various estimates of prevalence, how these have changed over time and how dependent they are on criteria used to identify hypertension and to identify PA. They have varied widely, from 2 to 30 % for prevalence of PA in primary care and from 5 to 30% in secondary care. A reasonable guess might be at least 2.5 % in primary care and at least 7 % in secondary care. There seems no doubt that PA prevalence in resistant hypertension is very significant, at least 10 % and probably much higher.

References

1. Ahmed AH, Calvird M, Gordon RD, Taylor PJ, Ward G, Pimenta E, Stowasser M (2011) Effects of two selective serotonin reuptake inhibitor antidepressants, sertraline and escitalopram on aldosterone-renin ratio in normotensive, depressed male patients. J Clin Endocrinol Metab 96:1039–1045
2. Ahmed AHA, Gordon RD, Taylor PJ, Ward G, Pimenta E, Stowasser M (2010) Effect of atenolol on aldosterone-renin ratio calculated by both plasma renin activity and direct renin concentration in healthy male volunteers. J Clin Endocrinol Metab 95:3201–3206

3. Ahmed AH, Gordon RD, Taylor PJ, Ward G, Pimenta E, Stowasser M (2011) Are women more at risk of false-positive primary aldosteronism screening and unnecessary suppression testing than men? J Clin Endocrinol Metab 96(2):E340–E346
4. Ahmed AH, Gordon RD, Taylor PJ, Ward G, Pimenta E, Stowasser M (2011) Effects of contraceptives on aldosterone-renin ratio may vary according to components of contraceptives, renin assay method and possibly route of administration. J Clin Endocrinol Metab 96:1797–1804
5. Azizan EAB, Lam BYH, Newhouse SJ, Zhou J, Kuc RE et al (2012) Microarray, qPCR, and KCNJ5 sequencing of aldosterone-producing adenomas reveal differences in genotype and phenotype between zona glomerulosa- and zona fasciculata-like tumors. J Clin Endocrinol Metab 97(5):E819–E829
6. Azizan EAB, Murthy M, Stowasser M, Gordon RD, Kowalski B, Xu S, Brown MJ, O'Shaughnessy KM (2012) Somatic mutations affecting the selectivity filter of KCNJ5 are frequent in two large unselected collections of adrenal aldosteronomas. Hypertension 59:587–591
7. Biglieri EG, Kater CE (1991) Disorders of the adrenal cortex. In: Stein JH (ed) Internal medicine, 3rd edn. Boston, MA, Little, Brown, pp 2188–2207
8. Choi M, Ul S, Yue P, Bjorklund P, Zhao B, Nelson-Williams C, Ji W, Cho Y, Patel A, Men CJ, Lolis E, Wisgerhof MV, Geller DS, Mane S, Hellman P, Westin G, Akerstrom G, Wang W, Carling T, Lifton RP (2011) K channel mutations in adrenal aldosterone-producing adenomas and hereditary hypertension. Science 331:768–772
9. Conn JW (1949) Electrolyte composition of sweat: clinical implications as an index of adrenal cortical function. Arch Intern Med 83:416–428
10. Conn JW (1955) Primary aldosteronism, a new clinical syndrome. J Lab Clin Med 45:3–7
11. Conn JW (1959) A concluding response. Arch Intern Med 123:154–155
12. Conn JW (1960) Evolution of primary aldosteronism as a highly specific clinical entity. JAMA 172:1650–1653
13. Conn JW (1964) Plasma renin activity in primary aldosteronism: importance in differential diagnosis and in research of essential hypertension. JAMA 190:222–225
14. Conn JW (1968) The evolution of primary aldosteronism: 1954–1967. Harvey Lect 62: 257–291
15. Conn JW, Cohen EL, Rovner DR (1964) Suppression of plasma renin activity in primary aldosteronism: distinguishing primary from secondary aldosteronism in hypertensive disease. JAMA 190:213–221
16. Conn JW, Knopf RF, Nesbit RM (1964) Clinical characteristics of primary aldosteronism from an analysis of 145 cases. Am J Surg 107:159–172
17. Conn JW, Cohen EL, Rovner DR, Nesbit RM (1965) Normokalemic primary aldosteronism: a detectable cause of curable "essential" hypertension. JAMA 193:200–206
18. Conn JW, Rovner DR, Cohen EL, Nesbit RM (1966) Normokalemic primary aldosteronism: its masquerade as "essential" hypertension. JAMA 195:21–26
19. Connell JM (2002) Is there an epidemic of primary aldosteronism. J Hum Hypertens 16: 151–152
20. Fardella CE, Mosso L, Gomez-Sanchez CE, Cortez P, Soto J, Gomez L et al (2000) Primary aldosteronism in essential hypertensives; prevalence, biochemical profile and molecular biology. J Clin Endocrinol Metab 85:1863–1867
21. Fishman LM, Kuchel O, Liddle GW, Michelakis AM, Gordon RD, Chick WT (1968) Incidence of primary aldosteronism in uncomplicated "essential" hypertension. A prospective study with elevated aldosterone secretion and suppressed plasma renin activity used as diagnostic criteria. JAMA 205(7):497–502
22. Fogari R, Preti P, Zoppi A, Rinaldi A, Fogari E, Mugellini A (2007) Prevalence of primary aldosteronism among unselected hypertensive patients: a prospective study based on the use of an aldosterone/renin ratio above 25 as a screening test. Hypertens Res 30(2):111–117
23. Fraser R, Beretta-Piccoli C, Brown JJ, Cumming AM, Lever AF, Mason PA, Morton JJ, Roberstson JI (1981) Response of aldosterone and 18-hydroxycorticosterone to angiotensin II in normal subjects, and patients with essential hypertension, Conn's syndrome, and nontumorous hyperaldosteronism. Hypertension 3(Suppl I):I-87–I-92

24. Funder JW (2011) Envoi. Rev Endoc Metab Disord 12:53–54
25. Funder JW (2012) Primary aldosteronism: clinical lateralisation and costs. J Clin Endocrinol Metab 97(10):3450–3457
26. Funder JW (2012) Ultimately we are in furious agreement. J Hypertens 30:1903–1905
27. Funder J, Carey R, Fardella C, Gomez-Sanchez C, Mantero P, Stowasser M, Young W, Montori VM (2008) Case detection, diagnosis and treatment of patients with primary aldosteronism: an Endocrine Society clinical practice guideline. J Clin Endocrinol Metab 93:3266–3281
28. Ganguly A, Dowdy AJ, Luetscher JA, Melada GA (1973) Anomalous postural response of plasma aldosterone concentration in patients with aldosterone-producing adrenal adenoma. J Clin Endocrinol Metab 36:401
29. Giachetti G, Ronconi V, Lucarelli G et al (2006) Analysis of screening and confirmatory tests in the diagnosis of primary aldosteronism: need for a standardised protocol. J Hypertens 24:737–745
30. Gordon RD (1993) Primary aldosteronism: a new understanding. Med J Aust 158(Jun 7): 729–731
31. Gordon RD (1995) Primary aldosteronism. J Endocrinol Invest 18(7):495–511
32. Gordon RD (1997) Primary aldosteronism: a new understanding. In: Proceedings of the first Franco-Australian meeting on hypertension. Lokhandwala MF (ed). Clin Exper Hypertens 19(5,6):857–870
33. Gordon RD (2004) The challenge of more robust and reproducible methodology in screening for primary aldosteronism. J Hypertens 22(2):251–255
34. Gordon RD (2004) Primary aldosteronism—actual epidemics or false alarm. Arq Bras Endocrinol Metabol 48(5):666–673
35. Gordon RD, Stowasser M (1998) Familial forms broaden horizons for primary aldosteronism. Trends Endocrinol Metab 9:220–227
36. Gordon RD, Stowasser M (2007) Primary aldosteronism: the case for screening. Nat Clin Pract Nephrol 8:582–583
37. Gordon RD, Gomez-Sanchez CE, Hamlet SM, Tunny TJ, Klemm SA (1987) Angiotensin-responsive aldosterone-producing adenoma masquerades as idiopathic hyperaldosteronism (IHA: adrenal hyperplasia) or low renin essential hypertension. J Hypertens 5(Suppl 5): s103–s106
38. Gordon RD, Hamlet SM, Tunny TJ, Klemm SA (1987) Aldosterone-producing adenomas responsive to angiotensin pose problems in diagnosis. Clin Exp Pharmacol Physiol 14: 175–179
39. Gordon RD, Klemm SA, Tunny TJ, Stowasser M (1992) Primary aldosteronism: hypertension with a genetic basis. Lancet 340(8812):159–161
40. Gordon RD, Laragh JH, Funder JW (2005) Low renin hypertensive states: perspectives, unsolved problems, future research. Trends Endocrinol Metab 16(3):108–113
41. Gordon RD, Rutherford JC, Stowasser M (2001) Primary aldosteronism: are we diagnosing and operating on too few patients? World J Surg 25(7):941–947
42. Gordon RD, Stowasser M, Klemm SA, Tunny TJ (1994) Primary aldosteronism and other forms of mineralocorticoid hypertension. In: Swales JD (ed) Textbook of hypertension. Blackwell, London
43. Gordon RD, Stowasser M, Tunny TJ, Klemm SA, Rutherford JC (1994) High incidence of primary aldosteronism in 199 patients referred with hypertension. Clin Exp Pharmacol Physiol 21:315–318
44. Gordon RD, Stowasser M, Klemm SA, Tunny TJ (1995) Primary aldosteronism—some genetic, morphological and biochemical aspects of subtypes. Steroids 60:35–41
45. Gordon RD, Ziesak MD, Tunny TJ, Stowasser M, Klemm SA (1993) Evidence that primary aldosteronism may not be uncommon: 12% incidence among antihypertensive drug trial volunteers. Clin Exp Pharmacol Physiol 20:296–298
46. Hamlet SM, Tunny TJ, Woodland E, Gordon RD (1985) Is aldosterone/renin ratio useful to screen a hypertensive population for primary aldosteronism? Clin Exp Pharmacol Physiol 12:249–252

47. Hiramatsu K, Yamada T, Yukimura Y, Komiya I, Ichikawa K, Ichihara M et al (1981) A screening test to identify aldosterone-producing adenoma by measuring plasma renin activity. Results in hypertensive patients. Arch Intern Med 141:1589–1593
48. Ito Y, Takeda R, Karashima S, Yamamaoto Y, Yoneda T, Takeda Y (2011) Prevalence of primary aldosteronism among prehypertensive and stage 1 hypertensive subjects. Hypertens Res 34:98–102
49. Kaplan NM (1967) The steroid content of adrenal adenomas and measurements of aldosterone production in patients with essential hypertension and primary aldosteronism. J Clin Invest 46:728–734
50. Kaplan NM (1969) Commentary on the incidence of primary aldosteronism. Current estimations based on objective data. Arch Intern Med 123:152–155
51. Kaplan NM (2001) Cautions over the current epidemic of primary aldosteronism. Lancet 357:953–954
52. Kaplan NM (2012) Primary aldosteronism: evidence against a second epidemic. J Hypertens 30(10):1899–1902
53. Laragh JH, Sealey JE, Sommers SC (1966) Patterns of adrenal secretion and urinary excretion of aldosterone and plasma renin activity in normal and hypertensive subjects. Circ Res 18(Suppl 1):158–174
54. Ledingham JGC (1987) Secondary hypertension. In: Weatherall DJ, Ledingham JGC, Warrell DA (eds) Oxford textbook of medicine. Oxford University Press, Oxford, pp 13.382–13.387
55. Lifton RP, Dluhy RG, Powers M, Rich GM, Cook S, Ulick S, Lalouel JM (1992) A chimaeric 11B-hydroxylase/aldosterone synthase gene causes glucocorticoid-remediable aldosteronism and human hypertension. Nature 355:262–265
56. Lim PO, Dow E, Brennan G, Jung RT, MacDonald TM (2000) High prevalence of primary aldosteronism in the Tayside hypertension clinic population. J Hum Hypertens 14:311–315
57. Loh KC, Koay ES, Khaw MC, Emmanuel SC, Young WF Jr (2000) Prevalence of primary aldosteronism among Asian hypertensive patients in Singapore. J Clin Endocrinol Metab 85:2854–2859
58. Milliez P, Girerd X, Plouin PF, Blacher J, Safar ME, Mourad JJ (2005) Evidence for an increased rate of cardiovascular events in patients with primary aldosteronism. J Am Coll Cardiol 45:1243–1248
59. Monticone S, Viola A, Tizzani D, Crudo V, Burrello J, Calmozzi M, Veglio F, Mulatero P (2012) Primary aldosteronism: who should be screened? Horm Metab Res 44(3):163–169
60. Montori VM, Young WF Jr (2002) Use of plasma aldosterone concentration-to-plasma renin activity ratio as a screening test for primary aldosteronism. A systematic review of the literature. Endocrinol Metab Clin North Am 31:619–632
61. Mulatero P, Milan A, Fallo F, Regolisti G, Pizzolo F, Fardella C, Mosso L, Marafetti L, Veglio F, Maccario M (2006) Comparison of confirmatory tests for the diagnosis of primary aldosteronism. J Clin Endocrinol Metab 91:2618–2623
62. Mulatero P, Monticone S, Rainey WE, Veglio F, Williams TA (2012) Role of KCNJ5 in familial and sporadic primary aldosteronism. Nat Rev Endocrinol 9:104–112. doi:10.1038/nrendo.2012.230
63. Mulatero P, Stowasser M, Loh KC, Fardella CE, Gordon RD, Mosso L, Gomez-Sanchez CE, Veglio Y, Young WF Jr (2004) Increased diagnosis of primary aldosteronism, including surgically correctible forms, in centers from five continents. J Clin Endocrinol Metab 89:1045–1050
64. Mulatero P, Tauber P, Zennaro M-C, Monticone S, Lang K, Beuschlein F, Fischer E et al (2012) KCNJ5 mutations in European families with nonglucocorticoid remediable familial hyperaldosteronism. Hypertension 59(2):235–240
65. Newton-Cheh C, Guo CY, Gona P et al (2008) Clinical and genetic correlates of aldosterone-to-renin ratio and relations to blood pressure in a community sample. Hypertension 49:846–856
66. Nishikawa T, Omura M (2000) Clinical characteristics of primary aldosteronism: its prevalence and comparative studies on various causes of primary aldosteronism in Yokohama Rosai Hospital. Biomed Pharmacother 54(Suppl 1):83–85

67. Nishikawa T, Saito J, Omura M (2007) Prevalence of primary aldosteronism: should we screen for primary aldosteronism before treating hypertensive patients with medication? Endocr J 54(4):487–495
68. Omura M, Saito J, Yamaguchi K, Kakuta Y, Nishikawa T (2004) Prospective study on the prevalence of secondary hypertension among hypertensive patients visiting a general outpatient clinic in Japan. Hypertens Res 27:193–202
69. Padfield PL (2003) Prevalence and role of a raised aldosterone to renin ratio in the diagnosis of primary aldosteronism: a debate on the scientific logic of the use of the ratio in practice. Clin Endocrinol 59:422–426
70. Padfield P (2007) Primary aldosteronism: the case against screening. Nat Clin Pract Nephrol 3:580–581
71. Pizzolo F, Raffaelli R, Memmo A, Chiecchi L, Pavan C, Guarini P, Guidi GC, Franchi M, Corrocher R, Olivieri O (2010) Effects of female sex hormones and contraceptive pill on the diagnostic workup for primary aldosteronism. J Hypertens 28:135–142
72. Rayner BL, Opie LH, Davidson JS (2000) The aldosterone/renin ratio as a screening test for primary aldosteronism. S Afr Med J 90:394–400
73. Rich GM, Ulick S, Cook S, Wang JZ, Lifton RP, Dluhy RG (1992) Glucocorticoid-remediable aldosteronism in a large kindred: clinical spectrum and diagnosis using a characteristic biochemical phenotype. Ann Intern Med 116:813–820
74. Rossi GP, Bernini G, Caliumi C, Desideri G, Fabris B, Ferri C, Ganzaroli C et al (2006) A prospective study of the prevalence of primary aldosteronism in 1125 hypertensive patients. J Am Coll Cardiol 48(11):2293–2300
75. Rutherford JR, Taylor WL, Stowasser M, Gordon RD (1998) Success of surgery for primary aldosteronism judged by residual autonomous aldosterone production. World J Surg 22(12): 1243–1245
76. Salva M, Cicala MV, Mantero F (2012) Primary aldosteronism: the role of confirmatory tests. Horm Metab Res 44:177–180
77. Satoh F, Morimoto R, Iwakura Y, Ono Y, Kudo M, Takase K, Ito S (2011) Primary aldosteronism. A Japanese perspective. Rev Endocr Metab Disord 12:11–14
78. Sealey JE, Gordon RD, Mantero F (2005) Plasma renin and aldosterone measurements in low renin hypertensive states. Trends Endocrinol Metab 16(3):86–91
79. Sechi LA, Di Fabio A, Bazzocchi M, Uzzau A, Catena C (2009) Intrarenal hemodynamics in primary aldosteronism before and after surgery. J Clin Endocrinol Metab 94:1191–1197
80. Shamma AH, Goddard JW, Sommers SC (1958) Study of adrenal status in hypertension. J Chron Dis 8:587–595
81. Stowasser M, Gordon RD (2000) Primary aldosteronism: learning from the study of familial varieties. J Hypertens 18:1165–1176
82. Stowasser M, Gordon RD (2001) Prevalence and diagnostic work-up of primary aldosteronism. Nephrology 6:119–126
83. Stowasser M, Gordon RD (2004) Primary aldosteronism—careful investigation is essential and rewarding. Mol Cell Endocrinol 217(1–2):33–39
84. Stowasser M, Gordon RD (2006) Aldosterone assays: an urgent need for improvement. Clin Chem 52(9):1640–1642
85. Stowasser M, Ahmed AH, Pimenta E, Taylor PJ, Gordon RD (2012) Factors affecting the aldosterone/renin ratio. Horm Metab Res 44:170–176
86. Stowasser M, Gordon RD, Rutherford JC, Nikwan NZ, Daunt N, Slater GJ (2001) Diagnosis and management of primary aldosteronism. J Renin Angiotensin Aldosterone Syst 2(3): 156–169
87. Stowasser M, Gordon RD, Gunasekera TG, Cowley DC, Ward G, Archibald C, Smithers BM (2003) High rate of detection of primary aldosteronism, including surgically treatable forms, after non-selective screening of hypertensive patients. J Hypertens 21(11):2149–2157
88. Sutherland DJ, Ruse JL, Laidlaw JC (1966) Increased aldosterone secretion and low plasma renin activity relieved by dexamethasone. Can Med Assoc J 95:1109–1119

89. Taylor PJ, Cooper DP, Gordon RD, Stowasser M (2009) Measurement of aldosterone in human plasma by semi-automated high performance liquid chromatography-tandem mass spectrometry. Clin Chem 55:1155–1162
90. Tunny TJ, Gordon RD, Klemm SA, Cohn D (1991) Histological and biochemical distinctiveness of atypical aldosterone-producing adenomas responsive to upright posture and angiotensin. Clin Endocrinol 34:363–369
91. Tunny TJ, Klemm SA, Stowasser M, Gordon RD (1993) Angiotensin-responsive aldosterone-producing adenomas: postoperative disappearance of aldosterone response to angiotensin. Clin Exp Pharmacol Physiol 20:306–309
92. Weinberger MH, Grim CE, Holliefield JW, Kem DC, Ganguly A, Kramer NJ, Yune HW, Wellman H, Donohue JP (1979) Primary aldosteronism: diagnosis, localisation and treatment. Ann Intern Med 90:386–395
93. Westerdahl C, Bergenfelz A, Isaksson A, Nerbrand C, Valdemarsson S (2011) Primary aldosteronism among newly diagnosed and untreated hypertensive patients in a Swedish primary care area. Scand J Prim Health Care 29:57–62
94. Wisgerhof M, Brown RD, Hogan MJ, Carpenter PC, Edis AJ (1981) The plasma aldosterone response to angiotensin II infusion in aldosterone-producing adenoma and idiopathic hyperaldosteronism. J Clin Endocrinol Metab 52:195
95. Young WF Jr (1997) Primary aldosteronism: update on diagnosis and treatment. Endocrinologist 7:213–221
96. Young WF Jr (1997) Pheochromocytoma and primary aldosteronism: diagnostic approaches. Endocrinol Metab Clin North Am 26:801–827
97. Young WF Jr (1999) Primary aldosteronism: a common and curable form of hypertension. Cardiol Rev 7(4):207–214
98. Young WF (2003) Minireview: primary aldosteronism—changing concepts in diagnosis and treatment. Endocrinology 144:2208–2213
99. Young WF Jr (2007) Primary aldosteronism: renaissance of a syndrome. Clin Endocrinol (Oxf) 66(5):607–618

Chapter 3
Low-Renin Hypertension

Per Hellman and Emil Hagström

Abstract Low-renin hypertension is a condition that relates to the sodium status, but a similar situation is present in approximately 25 % of individuals with essential hypertension, without having high aldosterone levels. Indeed, the aldosterone–renin ratio may be raised, and among these individuals some suffer from primary aldosteronism. Thus, there is an overlap between essential hypertension, low-renin hypertension, and primary aldosteronism, indicating that similar treatment regimes may be successful.

Keywords Renin • Essential hypertension • Aldosteronism • Aldosterone–renin ratio

One of the key consequences of primary aldosteronism (PA) is the overproduction of aldosterone and the compensatory low renin levels. However, in the literature on hypertension the term "low-renin hypertension," not necessarily caused by an inappropriate secretion of aldosterone as the underlying cause, is present. Moreover, search for patients with primary aldosteronism among patients with low renin often fails [1–3]. The term low-renin hypertension was initially proposed after studies dividing patients into subgroups based renin activity relative to urinary sodium excretion but is in many cases more or less a reflection of the sodium status. The normal physiological response to sodium overload is reduction of both aldosterone

P. Hellman, M.D., Ph.D. (✉)
Departments of Surgical Sciences, Uppsala University,
Akademiska sjukhuset ing 70 1 tr, 751 85 Uppsala, Sweden
e-mail: per.hellman@surgsci.uu.se

E. Hagström
Departments of Medical Sciences, Uppsala University, Uppsala, Sweden

P. Hellman (ed.), *Primary Aldosteronism: Molecular Genetics, Endocrinology, and Translational Medicine*, DOI 10.1007/978-1-4939-0509-6_3,

and renin, and a "low-renin" situation occurs. Another view of the same entity is to refer to the subset of the population with essential hypertension (EH) and low renin levels. This is present in approximately 25 % of all EH patients [3, 4]. In most of these patients plasma aldosterone is normal, but the aldosterone–renin ratio becomes increased. Indeed, in the field of endocrinology there are several similar situations with normal, but still inappropriate, hormone levels seen only in the resulting parameter indicating decreased functional negative feedback. Such examples would be the situation in mild primary hyperparathyroidism (pHPT) with normal levels of parathyroid hormone (PTH) but slightly elevated ionized calcium levels, thus signalling that the calcium sensing of the parathyroid cells is disturbed [5]. Another situation occurs in insulinomas, often seen only by low levels of plasma glucose but still normal, but inappropriately high, serum insulin levels. The same situation may occur in primary aldosteronism—a normal plasma aldosterone—but in case of a disturbed regulation system may be seen as low renin levels and hypertension but described as low-renin hypertension. In many situations with low levels of renin, also aldosterone levels are low, such as in mineralocorticoid excess of other reasons such as cortisol treatment as well as in situations with increased extracellular volume due to sodium retention [6, 7]. Thorough investigations of patients with low renin and normal aldosterone levels nevertheless reveal subsets with primary aldosteronism [8]. Thus, the fraction of patients with hypokalemia, normal aldosterone levels, and low renin levels, not necessarily being hypertensive or only suffering from mild hypertension, is a plausible subgroup of low-renin hypertensive patients, possibly suffering from mechanisms similar to the dysregulation seen in pure PA (summary of cellular mechanisms to be disturbed is seen in Fig. 3.1)

Although Conn in his initial prediction of the frequency of primary aldosteronism among hypertensive populations actually was around the numbers we estimate today, there will always be an overlap between what should be regarded as pathological or merely a normal variant. A recent study identified low renin levels in 93 out of 303 hypertensive subjects in the Framingham Offspring Study, and approximately half of these (approximately 10 % of all hypertensive individuals) also had elevated aldosterone [4], again supporting previous PA prevalence numbers in hypertensive subjects. It is actually suggested that the total share of individuals exhibiting inappropriately elevated aldosterone secretion may be in the order of 30–40 % of all hypertensive individuals [9, 10]. Further support of low-renin hypertension and PA being in the continuum of the same disease is the similar response to treatment with mineralocorticoid antagonists [9, 10].

Genetic variations may be an underlying cause not only for PA itself but also for low-renin EH. Low renin may be more common in certain parts of the world due to normal genetic variation such as polymorphisms in the CYP11B1 and B2 genes [11, 12]. The -344C/T polymorphism in the CYP11B2 gene has been thoroughly investigated in hypertensive individuals, and association with higher blood pressure is present in European as well as Chinese populations [13, 14]. Interestingly, a haplotype of -344C/T and K173 is more common in patients with aldosterone-producing adenomas than in patients with normal adrenals, and the haplotype is associated with increased CYP11B2 expression, higher aldosterone production, and also blood pressure [15].

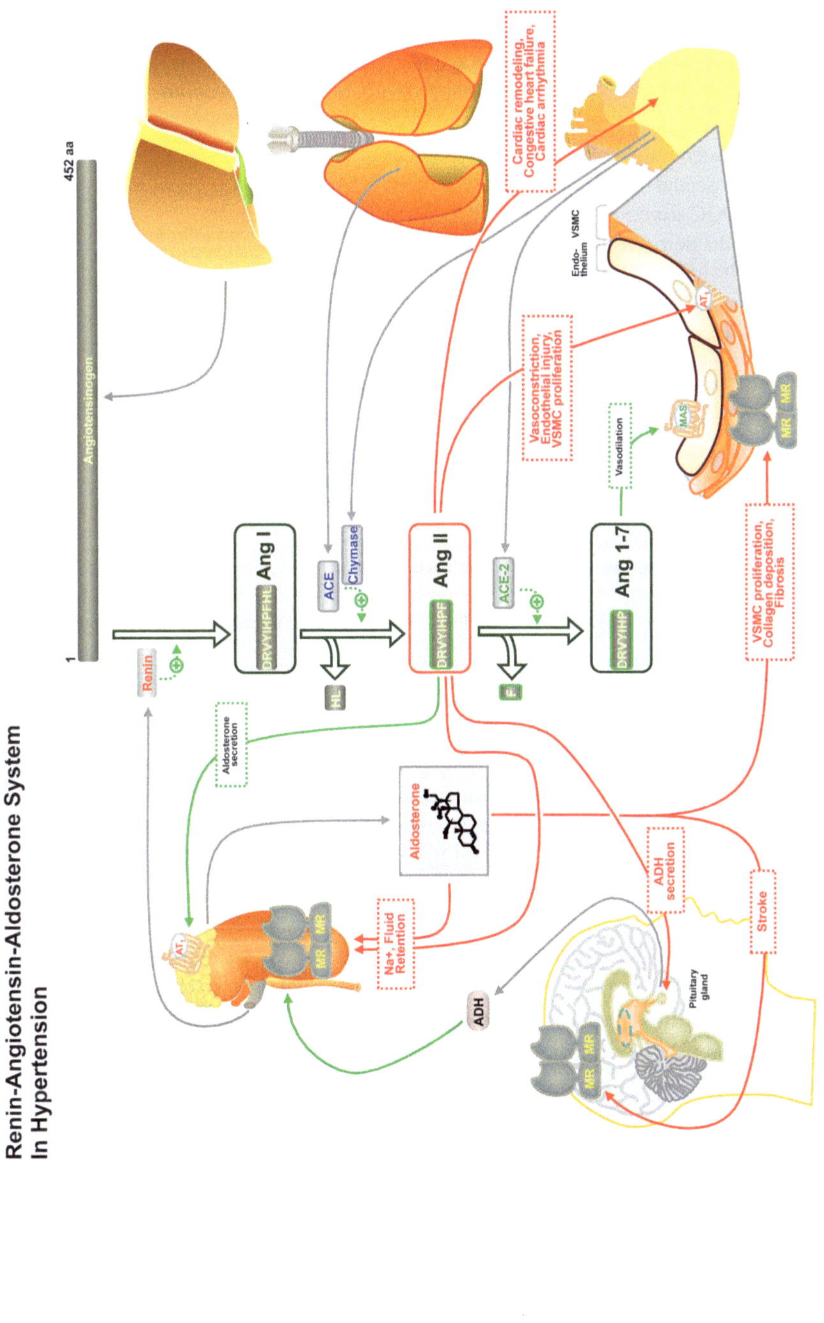

Fig. 3.1 Overview of the renin–angiotensin–aldosterone system. Published with acceptance from VisiScience

Table 3.1 Revised from Gordon et al. TRENDS in Endocrinology and Metabolism, 2005: 16: 108–113

Miscellaneous
1. An unremarkable hypertensive patient taking a very generous salt diet
2. Consistent ingestion of licorice, by inhibition of 11β-hydroxysteroid dehydrogenase (HSD-2)
Intrinsic renal causes
A greatly reduced nephron population caused by, for example, unilateral nephrectomy, congenital solitary kidney, diabetic nephropathy, chronic glomerulonephritis, or aging
Intrinsic mineralocorticoid excess
1. Primary aldosteronism
2. Low-renin essential hypertension
3. Excessive DOC secreted by benign or malignant adrenocortical tumors
4. Ectopic production of ACTH by neoplastic tissue, such as bronchial carcinoids and small-cell tumors of the lung, causing excessive secretion of 11-decoxycorticosterone (DOC)
Familial forms of salt-sensitive hypertension (rare)
1. Familial hyperaldosteronism type I, II, or III
2. Pseudohyperaldosteronism (Liddle's syndrome)
3. Syndrome of hypertension and hyperkalemia with normal glomerular filtration rate (pseudohyperaldosteronism type 2, PHA-2, Gordon's syndrome)
4. Deficiency of HSD-2, leading to "apparent mineralocorticoid excess"
5. Hypertensive forms of congenital adrenal hyperplasia (excess DOC)
11β-hydroxylase deficiency
17α-hydroxylase deficiency
6. Mutations of the mineralocorticoid receptor leading to activation by progesterone and pregnancy hypertension
7. Mutations of the glucocorticoid receptor leading to resistance to cortisol and ACTH-driven DOC-induced hypertension (glucocorticoid resistance syndrome)

A study from China of 1,356 consecutive patients with hypertension identified 235 with potential primary aldosteronism and consequently the remaining 913 as exhibiting essential hypertension. Analyses of SNPs in KCNJ5 revealed a male predominance for one variation of rs2604204 in PA patients, implying that potential underlying prerequisites for PA may occur also in this gene [16].

In the future, findings of similar associations in the recently discovered genes linked to PA, such as KCNJ5, ATP1A1, ATP2B3, or CACNA1D, may also theoretically be associated to hyperplasia of adrenocortical tissue and increased aldosterone secretion leading to suppression of renin as well as hypertension, without obvious findings of nodular hyperplasia or adrenocortical adenomas.

Indeed, there are a number of causes of low renin levels, but most likely the most frequent one is variations in the normal physiological response to sodium intake and plasma levels of sodium and possible polymorphic variations in involved genes or in a rather rare fraction by genetic disturbances in the population (Table 3.1).

One of the key issues when discussing low renin levels is the difficulty in measuring renin in plasma. It may be stated either as plasma renin activity (PRA) as a measure of its capacity to generate angiotensin I from a substrate or as the pure plasma renin level usually by immunochemiluminometric methods [17]. The problem, as is the case in any immunoassay-based method measuring low concentration levels, is the detection level in any of these assays. The development during recent years has resulted in that renin is predominantly measured in plasma rather than indirectly after measuring its activity. As with measurements of plasma aldosterone, many antihypertensive drugs affect the plasma renin level; e.g., β-blockers lower plasma renin levels and ACE inhibitors increase renin levels, the latter being possible to use as a diagnostic tool—cases with low renin despite taking ACE inhibitors or angiotensin receptor antagonists have an increased risk of having PA [1]. Since medication also influences plasma aldosterone levels, the aldosterone–renin ratio will most likely be disturbed, which has to taken into account when interpreting results. For instance, patients with calcium channel blockers, which suppress aldosterone secretion, may still have low renin levels, thus masking a subclinical PA but also indicating not yet fully investigated pathophysiological mechanisms with potential underlying causes for disturbance. Results of several screening programs address the problem with pharmacological treatment affecting the ratio, many reporting that among the patients screened for pathological aldosterone–renin ratios only a very small number have pure adrenocortical aldosterone-producing adenomas. Indeed, the share of patients with adrenocortical hyperplasia may be much higher, but among these also a fraction of patients with low-renin EH may also be present and the distinction difficult to identify due to definition problems and lack of imaging methodology which identifies adrenocortical hyperplasia.

Treatment of low-renin hypertension is, in case of finding an individual in the PA–low renin continuum, aldosterone antagonists, such as spironolactone or eplerenone, while low-renin hypertension with normal aldosterone levels respond well to thiazide therapy, unless hypokalemia is also present. Low-renin EH is typically salt and volume sensitive indicating good response to diuretics and dietary modifications. Most of these patients are likely to have a gain of function in the renal sodium channels but lack of ability to reduce aldosterone levels, even though the renin levels are suppressed. Indeed the concomitant water reabsorption may mask the increased sodium retention until hypokalemia occurs [1]. The monogenic variants listed in Table 3.1 are very rare but have in common retention of sodium and increased blood volume.

As a conclusion—future investigations may have public health implications since identifying patients with low-renin hypertension may be of help in order to both offer proper treatment strategies for overtly hypertensive individuals and identify those with subclinical or lower degree of hypertension in order to reduce the risk of developing manifest hypertension.

References

1. Mackenzie IS, Brown MJ (2009) Molecular and clinical investigations in patients with low-renin hypertension. Clin Exp Nephrol 13(1):1–8, Epub 2008/08/16
2. Gunnells JC Jr, McGuffin WL Jr (1975) Low renin hypertension. Annu Rev Med 26:259–275, Epub 1975/01/11
3. Mulatero P, Verhovez A, Morello F, Veglio F (2007) Diagnosis and treatment of low-renin hypertension. Clin Endocrinol (Oxf) 67(3):324–334, Epub 2007/06/19
4. Adlin EV, Braitman LE, Vasan RS (2013) Bimodal aldosterone distribution in Low-renin hypertension. Am J Hypertens 26(9):1076–1085, Epub 2013/06/13
5. Cusano NE, Silverberg SJ, Bilezikian JP (2013) Normocalcemic primary hyperparathyroidism. J Clin Densitom 16(1):33–39, Epub 2013/02/05
6. Gomez-Sanchez CE (1982) The role of steroids in human essential hypertension. Biochem Pharmacol 31(6):893–897, Epub 1982/03/15
7. Epstein MT, Espiner EA, Donald RA, Hughes H (1977) Effect of eating liquorice on the renin-angiotensin aldosterone axis in normal subjects. Br Med J 1(6059):488–490, Epub 1977/02/19
8. Mulatero P, Stowasser M, Loh KC, Fardella CE, Gordon RD, Mosso L et al (2004) Increased diagnosis of primary aldosteronism, including surgically correctable forms, in centers from five continents. J Clin Endocrinol Metab 89(3):1045–1050, Epub 2004/03/06
9. Ori Y, Chagnac A, Korzets A, Zingerman B, Herman-Edelstein M, Bergman M et al (2013) Regression of left ventricular hypertrophy in patients with primary aldosteronism/low-renin hypertension on low-dose spironolactone. Nephrol Dial Transplant 28(7):1787–93, Epub 2013/02/05
10. Funder JW (2013) Primary aldosteronism and low-renin hypertension: a continuum? Nephrol Dial Transplant 28(7):1625–7, Epub 2013/03/29
11. Tsukada K, Ishimitsu T, Teranishi M, Saitoh M, Yoshii M, Inada H et al (2002) Positive association of CYP11B2 gene polymorphism with genetic predisposition to essential hypertension. J Hum Hypertens 16(11):789–793, Epub 2002/11/22
12. Nicod J, Bruhin D, Auer L, Vogt B, Frey FJ, Ferrari P (2003) A biallelic gene polymorphism of CYP11B2 predicts increased aldosterone to renin ratio in selected hypertensive patients. J Clin Endocrinol Metab 88(6):2495–2500, Epub 2003/06/06
13. Russo P, Loguercio M, Lauria F, Barba G, Arnout J, Cappuccio FP et al (2007) Age- and gender-dependent association of the -344C/T polymorphism of CYP11B2 with blood pressure in European populations. J Hum Hypertens 21(4):333–336, Epub 2007/02/03
14. Li W, Liu C (2012) The -344C/T polymorphism in the CYP11B2 gene is associated with essential hypertension in the Chinese. J Renin Angiotensin Aldosterone Syst. Epub 2012/12/04
15. Tanahashi H, Mune T, Takahashi Y, Isaji M, Suwa T, Morita H et al (2005) Association of Lys173Arg polymorphism with CYP11B2 expression in normal adrenal glands and aldosterone-producing adenomas. J Clin Endocrinol Metab 90(11):6226–6231, Epub 2005/08/25
16. Li NF, Li HJ, Zhang DL, Zhang JH, Yao XG, Wang HM et al (2013) Genetic variations in the KCNJ5 gene in primary aldosteronism patients from Xinjiang, China. PLoS One 8(1):e54051, Epub 2013/02/06
17. Fischer E, Reuschl S, Quinkler M, Rump LC, Hahner S, Bidlingmaier M et al (2013) Assay characteristics influence the aldosterone to renin ratio as a screening tool for primary aldosteronism: results of the German Conn's registry. Horm Metab Res 45(7):526–531, Epub 2013/04/25

Chapter 4
Molecular Derangements in Sporadic Primary Aldosteronism

Per Hellman, Tobias Åkerström, and Peyman Björklund

Abstract Until very recently molecular derangements were merely unknown in primary aldosteronism. New genetic techniques have allowed detailed searches which have led to identification (to date) of a number of mutated genes—KCNJ5, ATP1A1, ATP2B3, and CACNA1D—all encoding for channel proteins which when activated or disturbed cause depolarization of the glomerulosa cell and release of aldosterone. In addition, activation of the beta catenin pathway has also been noticed in these cells. Identification of these genes gives hope for future development of targeted drugs, detailed diagnostic procedures, and individualized medicine.

Keywords KCNJ5 • ATP1A1 • ATP2B3 • CACNA1D • Depolarization • Beta catenin

Introduction: Primary Aldosteronism, a Channelopathy?

KCNJ5

The molecular disturbances causing primary aldosteronism (PA) have been largely unknown until recently. Mutations in only few genes, all detected by next-generation sequencing (NGS), are suggested to account for almost 60 % of all aldosterone-producing adenomas (APA). The first identified mutation was in *KCNJ5*, a gene coding for the potassium channel Kir 3.4 regulating ion flow through the membrane.

P. Hellman, M.D., Ph.D. (✉) • T. Åkerström
Departments of Surgical Sciences, Uppsala University,
Akademiska sjukhuset ing 70 1 tr, 751 85 Uppsala, Sweden
e-mail: per.hellman@surgsci.uu.se

P. Björklund
Department of Surgical Sciences, Clinical Research Department, Uppsala University,
kademiska sjukhuset ing 70 3 tr, 751 85 Uppsala, Sweden

P. Hellman (ed.), *Primary Aldosteronism: Molecular Genetics, Endocrinology, and Translational Medicine*, DOI 10.1007/978-1-4939-0509-6_4,

It was previously known that activation of the angiotensin II type 1 receptor on the surface of the adrenal zona glomerulosa cells trigger depolarization and activation of the voltage-gated calcium channels, which leads to release of aldosterone [1]. Disturbances in this system, leading to aldosterone secretion excess, cause hyperaldosteronism. The identification of mutated KCNJ5 directly involved in this regulatory system was done by whole-exome capture and Illumina sequencing as well as confirmation by Sanger sequencing of initially 4 APAs and corresponding blood samples, and further investigation of 14 samples revealed either of the 2 tumor-specific mutations—G151R and L168R in *KCNJ5* in 8 of 22 tumors [2]. In the selection process samples with low levels of loss of heterozygosity were chosen in order to increase the possibility to identify specific somatic mutations. The mutations led to changes in highly conserved amino acids within the selectivity filter in KCNJ5. Further studies revealed that the mutation led to an increased ion conductance, allowing sodium entering the cell followed by depolarization, opening of voltage-gated calcium channels, increase in intracellular calcium concentration, and thereby stimulated release of aldosterone (Figs. 4.1 and 4.2). It is also speculated that the same mechanism leads to stimulated cell proliferation, although not yet fully proven and in some studies even questioned [3]. A similar and parallel mechanism is seen also in KCNJ11 (Kir 6.2) mutations associated with beta-cell hyperplasia [4].

Further analyses from several groups and different parts of the world demonstrate that altogether slightly less than 50 % of all adenomas exhibit mutations in this gene (Table 4.1). One of the mutations, T158A, was specifically investigated in relation to increased expression of CYP11B2, indicating a more profound and long-standing effect also on synthesis of aldosterone [3]. This is supported by yet another study, showing that *KCNJ5*-mutated APAs had higher CYP11B2 expression than non-*KCNJ5*-mutated APAs [5]. Investigated unilateral primary hyperplasias of adrenal cortex have not shown any mutations, while 40 % of adenomas with surrounding marked hyperplasias harbored a mutation [6]. This suggests that possessing a *KCNJ5* mutation is strongly associated with exhibiting an adenoma, which is most likely to lateralize in adrenal venous sampling. Indeed, this was supported by findings that patients with *KCNJ5*-mutated APAs more likely demonstrated aldosterone excess from the affected adrenal than others without *KCNJ5* mutations [7]. An interesting accessory and hitherto unexplained finding is the female predominance in possessing *KCNJ5* mutations, 49–63 vs. 19–24 % [6, 8].

Interestingly, the finding of *KCNJ5* mutations is in line with earlier mice studies, where the TWIK-related acid-sensitive K (TASK) channels demonstrated crucial influence on aldosterone secretion. They appear to be the complex which sets the membrane potential in the zona glomerulosa cells in mice, thereby regulating aldosterone secretion [9]. Knockout mice verified the causal role of these proteins, leading to primary aldosteronism in mice [10]. However, KCNJ5 and the TASK proteins have important differences, despite the importance of the potassium channels to set the membrane potential and thereby regulate the intracellular calcium concentration [11]. One of the TASK family members, TASK1, is similar to the human KCNJ3, and siRNA knockdown of this protein in human cells leads to activation of CYP11B2 and increased aldosterone production [12]. However, so far no mutations in *KCNJ3* have been reported.

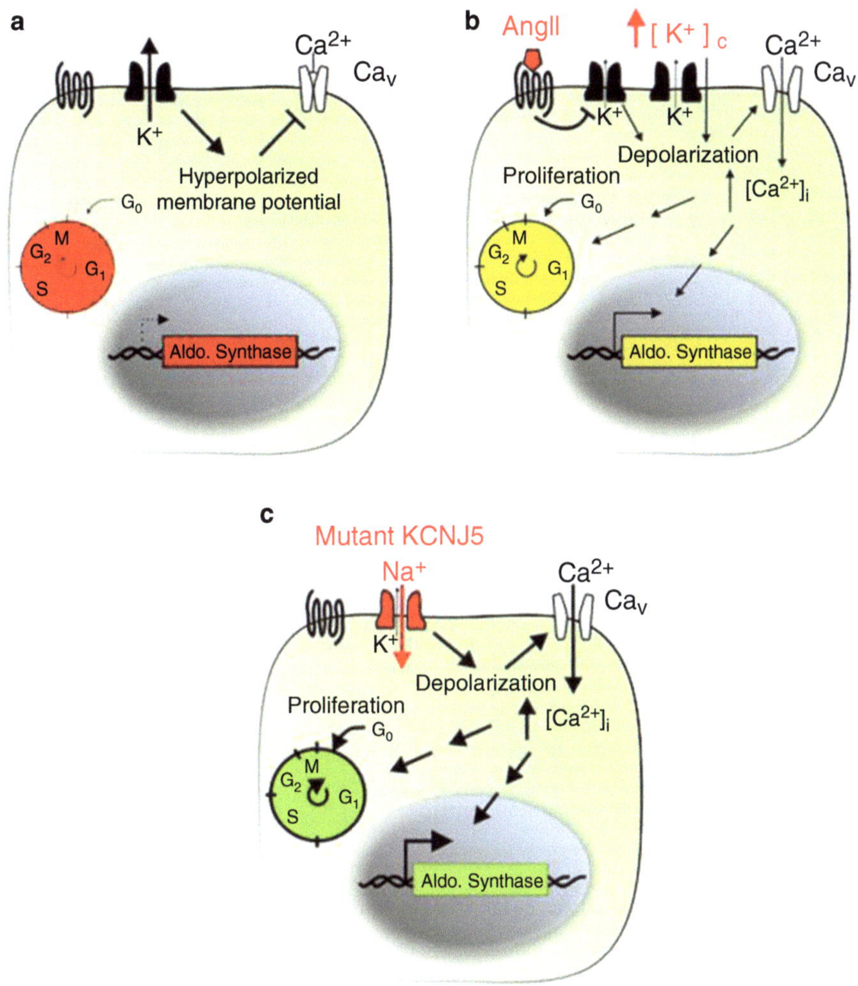

Fig. 4.1 Mechanisms for function of KCNJ5 in normal cells as well as cells with mutations. Reprint from Choi et al. [2]

ATPases

The Na^+/K^+-ATPases regulate the potassium transport over the cell membrane and are thereby important for maintaining the resting potential of the cell. Mutations in genes *ATP1A1* encoding for a subunit in the Na^+/K^+-ATPase and *ATP2B3* encoding a plasma membrane Ca^{2+} ATPase have been recently reported [13, 14]. *ATP1A1* was found mutated in 16 of 308 APAs (5.2 %) and 10 of 152 (6.6 %) in respective study, while *ATP2B3* mutations were found in 5 of 308 APAs (1.6 %) [13]. Mutations found in *ATP1A1* affect L104, V332, or A963, all of which are residues involved in

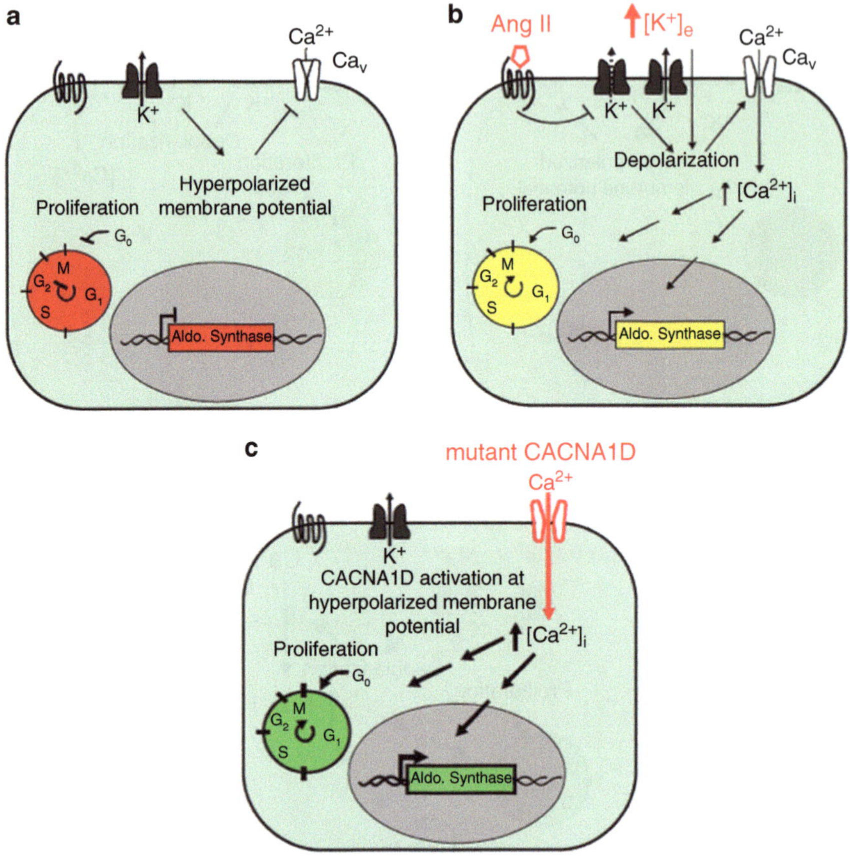

Fig. 4.2 Mechanisms for functional disturbances in normal zona glomerulosa cells as well as in cells with mutated CACNA1D. Reprint from Scholl et al. [19]

pore formation. Interestingly the deletions found in this gene are also affecting these residues. Even mutations found in *ATP2B3* affect pore formation. All these mutations are believed to affect polarization of the cells implicating an important role for the membrane potential in dysregulation of aldosterone secretion and activation of CYP11B2. However implication of the Na^+/K^+-ATPase in regulation of aldosterone secretion [15, 16] and effect of angiotensin II on the Na^+/K^+-ATPase activity [17] are well studied, and higher serum aldosterone concentration in *Atp1a1* knockout mice has been reported [18].

The Na^+/K^+-ATPase can be blocked by ouabain resulting in enhanced aldosterone secretion [15, 16]. This suggests a possibility to identify small-molecule “activators” of this channel as a hypothetic drug in aldosteronism.

Table 4.1 Prevalence of found KCNJ5 mutation in publications 2011–2013

Study	Prevalence	Type of mutation
Choi et al. [2]	8/22 (36 %)	L168R ($n=6$)
		G151R ($n=2$)
Boulkron et al. [8]	129/380 (34 %)	L168R ($n=53$)
		G151R ($n=76$)
Azizan et al. [27]	30/73 (41 %)	L168R ($n=10$)
		G151R ($n=19$)
		delI157 ($n=1$)
Akerstrom et al. [6]	157/348 (47 %)	L168R ($n=71$)
		G151R ($n=84$)
		E145Q ($n=2$)
Monticone et al. [5]	18/47 (38 %)	L168R ($n=10$)
		G151R ($n=8$)
Taguchi et al. [28]	15/23 (65 %)	L168R ($n=3$)
		G151R ($n=12$)
Arnesen et al. [29]	10/28 (36 %)	L168R ($n=4$)
		G151R ($n=6$)
Yamada et al. [30]	2/3 (66 %)	L168R ($n=1$)
		G151R ($n=1$)
Xekouki et al. [31]	2/16 (12 %)	G151R ($n=2$)

Voltage-Gated Calcium Channels

Two recent reports who performed NGS on non-*KCNJ5*-mutated APAs revealed somatic mutations in *CACNA1D*, encoding for a voltage-gated calcium channel in 5 out of 43 specimens (11.6 %) [19] and 7 out of 142 (5 %) [14]. The most common mutation was G403, again in somewhat parallel to *KCNJ5* residing in the channel pore. Exome sequencing was performed in pairs of DNA from tumor and peripheral blood in order to identify tumor-specific DNA changes. *CACNA1D* encodes $Ca_V1.3$, the α_1 subunit of an L-type voltage-gated calcium channel. The found missense mutations, G403R and I750M, were confirmed by Sanger sequencing. The mutation facilitated channel opening as presented in patch-clamp analyses.

Interestingly, in 2 out of 100 individuals with unexplained hypertension and PA early in life the G403D mutation was found in peripheral blood, implicating a new genetic syndrome with gain-of-function mutation in *CACNA1D*, which in these cases were de novo mutations since there was no family history. These individuals did not exhibit adrenal enlargement (hyperplasia) on computed tomography. The mechanism for excess aldosterone secretion mimics that of KCNJ5, ATP1A1, and ATP2B3 regarding increased cytoplasmic calcium concentration, in these cases by increased flux through the mutated L-type calcium channel.

CACNA1D mutations seem to occur in older individuals, equally in male and female, and cause smaller tumors than *KCNJ5* mutations.

Other Possible Derangements

Another molecular derangement possibly involved in subsets of PA is within the APC (adenomatosis polyposis coli)/beta catenin pathway. An initial finding that patients with familial adenomatosis coli have increased prevalence of adrenal masses is in concordance with this hypothesis [20]. Indeed, this may be a consequence of selection bias since adrenal incidentaloma occurs in approximately 10 % of all CT scans. Aberrant activation and accumulation of beta catenin with subsequent translocation to the nucleus and functioning as a transcription factor may occur in several ways, such as inactivating mutations in *APC* or mutation in the third exon of *CTNNB1* leading to uncoupling of phosphorylation possibilities and thereby stabilization of beta catenin which avoids degradation. The Wnt/beta catenin pathway is important for embryological adrenal development and for cell renewal in the adult adrenal cortex [21]. Abnormal immunohistochemical expression of beta catenin is seen in adrenocortical adenomas as well as adrenocortical cancers (ACC), and in PPNAD nuclear accumulation of beta catenin is also seen, implying importance in adrenocortical tumorigenesis [22]. In a mouse model where adrenocortical restricted activation of beta catenin occurs adrenocortical hyperplasia develops, which with time translates into primary aldosteronism as well as ACC [23]. In APAs low frequency of mutations in *CTNNB1* has been noted as well [24]. Indeed, although clearly associated with cortisol excess and ACC, activation of the Wnt/beta catenin pathway is present in APAs as well as in the surrounding adrenal cortex [25, 26].

References

1. Uebele VN, Nuss CE, Renger JJ, Connolly TM (2004) Role of voltage-gated calcium channels in potassium-stimulated aldosterone secretion from rat adrenal zona glomerulosa cells. J Steroid Biochem Mol Biol 92(3):209–218, Epub 2004/11/24
2. Choi M, Scholl UI, Yue P, Bjorklund P, Zhao B, Nelson-Williams C et al (2011) K^+ channel mutations in adrenal aldosterone-producing adenomas and hereditary hypertension. Science 331(6018):768–772, Epub 2011/02/12
3. Oki K, Plonczynski MW, Luis Lam M, Gomez-Sanchez EP, Gomez-Sanchez CE (2012) Potassium channel mutant KCNJ5 T158A expression in HAC-15 cells increases aldosterone synthesis. Endocrinology 153(4):1774–1782, Epub 2012/02/09
4. Flechtner I, de Lonlay P, Polak M (2006) Diabetes and hypoglycaemia in young children and mutations in the Kir6.2 subunit of the potassium channel: therapeutic consequences. Diabetes Metab 32(6):569–580
5. Monticone S, Hattangady NG, Nishimoto K, Mantero F, Rubin B, Cicala MV et al (2012) Effect of KCNJ5 mutations on gene expression in aldosterone-producing adenomas and adrenocortical cells. J Clin Endocrinol Metab 97(8):E1567–E1572, Epub 2012/05/26
6. Akerstrom T, Crona J, Delgado Verdugo A, Starker LF, Cupisti K, Willenberg HS et al (2012) Comprehensive re-sequencing of adrenal aldosterone producing lesions reveal three somatic mutations near the KCNJ5 potassium channel selectivity filter. PloS One 7(7):e41926, Epub 2012/08/01

7. Seccia TM, Mantero F, Letizia C, Kuppusamy M, Caroccia B, Barisa M et al (2012) Somatic mutations in the KCNJ5 gene raise the lateralization index: implications for the diagnosis of primary aldosteronism by adrenal vein sampling. J Clin Endocrinol Metab 97(12): E2307–E2313, Epub 2012/09/27
8. Boulkroun S, Beuschlein F, Rossi GP, Golib-Dzib JF, Fischer E, Amar L et al (2012) Prevalence, clinical, and molecular correlates of KCNJ5 mutations in primary aldosteronism. Hypertension 59(3):592–598, Epub 2012/01/26
9. Bayliss DA, Barrett PQ (2008) Emerging roles for two-pore-domain potassium channels and their potential therapeutic impact. Trends Pharmacol Sci 29(11):566–575, Epub 2008/10/01
10. Davies LA, Hu C, Guagliardo NA, Sen N, Chen X, Talley EM et al (2008) TASK channel deletion in mice causes primary hyperaldosteronism. Proc Natl Acad Sci U S A 105(6):2203–2208, Epub 2008/02/06
11. Spat A (2004) Glomerulosa cell–a unique sensor of extracellular K^+ concentration. Mol Cell Endocrinol 217(1–2):23–26, Epub 2004/05/12
12. Nogueira EF, Gerry D, Mantero F, Mariniello B, Rainey WE (2010) The role of TASK1 in aldosterone production and its expression in normal adrenal and aldosterone-producing adenomas. Clin Endocrinol (Oxf) 73(1):22–29, Epub 2009/11/03
13. Beuschlein F, Boulkroun S, Osswald A, Wieland T, Nielsen HN, Lichtenauer UD et al (2013) Somatic mutations in ATP1A1 and ATP2B3 lead to aldosterone-producing adenomas and secondary hypertension. Nat Genet 45(4):440–444, 4e1-2. Epub 2013/02/19
14. Azizan EA, Poulsen H, Tuluc P, Zhou J, Clausen MV, Lieb A et al (2013) Somatic mutations in ATP1A1 and CACNA1D underlie a common subtype of adrenal hypertension. Nat Genet 45(9):1055–1060, Epub 2013/08/06
15. Yingst DR, Davis J, Krenz S, Schiebinger RJ (1999) Insights into the mechanism by which inhibition of Na, K-ATPase stimulates aldosterone production. Metabolism 48(9):1167–1171, Epub 1999/09/14
16. Neri G, De Toni R, Tortorella C, Rebuffat P, Bova S, Cargnelli G et al (2006) Ouabain chronic infusion enhances the growth and steroidogenic capacity of rat adrenal zona glomerulosa: the possible involvement of the endothelin system. Int J Mol Med 18(2):315–319, Epub 2006/07/06
17. Hajnoczky G, Csordas G, Hunyady L, Kalapos MP, Balla T, Enyedi P et al (1992) Angiotensin-II inhibits Na^+/K^+ pump in rat adrenal glomerulosa cells: possible contribution to stimulation of aldosterone production. Endocrinology 130(3):1637–1644, Epub 1992/03/01
18. Moseley AE, Huddleson JP, Bohanan CS, James PF, Lorenz JN, Aronow BJ et al (2005) Genetic profiling reveals global changes in multiple biological pathways in the hearts of Na, K-ATPase alpha 1 isoform haploinsufficient mice. Cell Physiol Biochem 15(1–4):145–158, Epub 2005/02/15
19. Scholl UI, Goh G, Stolting G, de Oliveira RC, Choi M, Overton JD et al (2013) Somatic and germline CACNA1D calcium channel mutations in aldosterone-producing adenomas and primary aldosteronism. Nat Genet 45(9):1050–1054, Epub 2013/08/06
20. Smith TG, Clark SK, Katz DE, Reznek RH, Phillips RK (2000) Adrenal masses are associated with familial adenomatous polyposis. Dis Colon Rectum 43(12):1739–1742, Epub 2001/01/13
21. Kim AC, Reuter AL, Zubair M, Else T, Serecky K, Bingham NC et al (2008) Targeted disruption of beta-catenin in Sf1-expressing cells impairs development and maintenance of the adrenal cortex. Development 135(15):2593–2602, Epub 2008/07/05
22. Tissier F, Cavard C, Groussin L, Perlemoine K, Fumey G, Hagnere AM et al (2005) Mutations of beta-catenin in adrenocortical tumors: activation of the Wnt signaling pathway is a frequent event in both benign and malignant adrenocortical tumors. Cancer Res 65(17):7622–7627, Epub 2005/09/06
23. Berthon A, Sahut-Barnola I, Lambert-Langlais S, de Joussineau C, Damon-Soubeyrand C, Louiset E et al (2010) Constitutive beta-catenin activation induces adrenal hyperplasia and promotes adrenal cancer development. Hum Mol Genet 19(8):1561–1576, Epub 2010/01/29
24. Tadjine M, Lampron A, Ouadi L, Bourdeau I (2008) Frequent mutations of beta-catenin gene in sporadic secreting adrenocortical adenomas. Clin Endocrinol (Oxf) 68(2):264–270, Epub 2007/09/15

25. Bonnet S, Gaujoux S, Launay P, Baudry C, Chokri I, Ragazzon B et al (2011) Wnt/beta-catenin pathway activation in adrenocortical adenomas is frequently due to somatic CTNNB1-activating mutations, which are associated with larger and nonsecreting tumors: a study in cortisol-secreting and -nonsecreting tumors. J Clin Endocrinol Metab 96(2):E419–E426, Epub 2010/11/19
26. Boulkroun S, Samson-Couterie B, Golib-Dzib JF, Amar L, Plouin PF, Sibony M et al (2011) Aldosterone-producing adenoma formation in the adrenal cortex involves expression of stem/progenitor cell markers. Endocrinology 152(12):4753–4763, Epub 2011/10/06
27. Azizan EA, Murthy M, Stowasser M, Gordon R, Kowalski B, Xu S et al (2012) Somatic mutations affecting the selectivity filter of KCNJ5 are frequent in 2 large unselected collections of adrenal aldosteronomas. Hypertension 59(3):587–591, Epub 2012/01/19
28. Taguchi R, Yamada M, Nakajima Y, Satoh T, Hashimoto K, Shibusawa N et al (2012) Expression and mutations of KCNJ5 mRNA in Japanese patients with aldosterone-producing adenomas. J Clin Endocrinol Metab 97(4):1311–1319, Epub 2012/01/27
29. Arnesen T, Glomnes N, Stromsoy S, Knappskog S, Heie A, Akslen LA et al (2013) Outcome after surgery for primary hyperaldosteronism may depend on KCNJ5 tumor mutation status: a population-based study from Western Norway. Langenbecks Arch Surg 398(6):869–874, Epub 2013/06/20
30. Yamada M, Nakajima Y, Taguchi R, Okamura T, Ishii S, Tomaru T et al (2012) KCNJ5 mutations in aldosterone- and cortisol-co-secreting adrenal adenomas. Endocr J 59(8):735–741, Epub 2012/08/07
31. Xekouki P (2012) KCNJ5 mutations in the National Institutes of Health cohort of patients with primary hyperaldosteronism: an infrequent genetic cause of Conn's syndrome. Endocr Relat Cancer 19:255–260

Chapter 5
From Genetic Abnormalities to Pathophysiological Mechanisms

Maria-Christina Zennaro and Sheerazed Boulkroun

Abstract Maintenance of an appropriate zona glomerulosa cell membrane potential is crucial for the regulation of aldosterone biosynthesis. Cell membrane depolarization is one of the main triggers for the chain of intracellular events that ultimately leads to increased aldosterone biosynthesis. Potassium channels play a key role in the maintenance of the membrane resting potential of zona glomerulosa cells. Among the different K^+ channels, the TASK (TWIK-related acid-sensitive potassium) channels are highly expressed in the adrenal cortex. Their role in the regulation of aldosterone biosynthesis has been highlighted by the analysis of different mouse models of TASK channel invalidation. Recently, mutations in different genes coding for proteins involved in the regulation of the zona glomerulosa cell membrane potential and ionic homeostasis have been identified in tumoral (somatic) DNA from sporadic aldosterone-producing adenoma and in germline DNA from patients with familial hyperaldosteronism. Although little is known about their specific function in the adrenal gland, in this chapter we describe their structure and function and discuss, based on the knowledge in other tissues and published work, the role of these proteins in normal aldosterone production and in the pathogenesis of primary aldosteronism (PA).

Keywords Aldosterone-producing adenoma • Potassium channel • ATPase • KCNJ5 • ATP1A1 • ATP2B3 • Somatic mutation • Membrane potential • Calcium signaling

M.-C. Zennaro (✉) • S. Boulkroun
INSERM, UMRS_970, Paris Cardiovascular Research Center, Paris, France

University Paris Descartes, Sorbonne Paris Cité, Paris, France

Assistance Publique-Hôpitaux de Paris, Hôpital Européen Georges Pompidou, Service de Génétique, Paris, France
e-mail: maria-christina.zennaro@inserm.fr

P. Hellman (ed.), *Primary Aldosteronism: Molecular Genetics, Endocrinology, and Translational Medicine*, DOI 10.1007/978-1-4939-0509-6_5,

Calcium Signaling and the Regulation of Aldosterone Biosynthesis

The human adrenal cortex is constituted by three distinct morphological zones with specific functional properties [3] (Fig. 5.1, left panel): the zona glomerulosa (ZG), which is located immediately underneath the capsule, produces mineralocorticoids

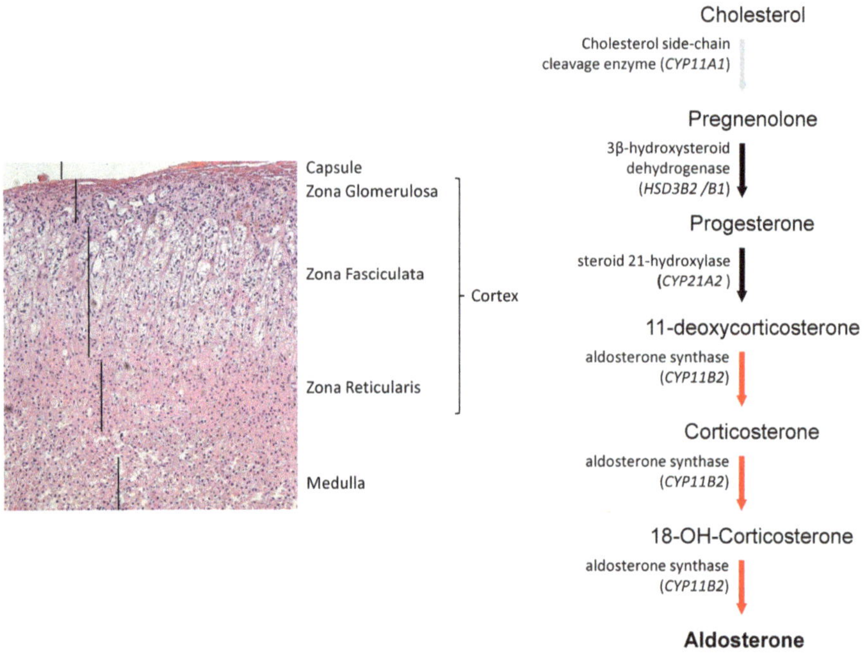

Fig. 5.1 *Histological structure of the adrenal cortex and aldosterone biosynthesis pathway.* (*Left panel*) The adrenal gland is composed of two distinct anatomical structures of different origin and function: the cortex and the medulla. The cortex, located in the periphery, produces adrenal steroid hormones, while the medulla is responsible for catecholamine biosynthesis. The cortex is divided into three different morphological and functional zones: the zona glomerulosa, located underneath the capsule, produces mineralocorticoids (aldosterone), and the zona fasciculata produces glucocorticoids, whereas biosynthesis of sexual steroids takes place in the inner zona reticularis. (*Right panel*) Aldosterone is synthesized from cholesterol through a series of sequential enzymatic reactions involving cytochrome P450 enzymes (*right panel*). Conversion of cholesterol into pregnenolone is catalyzed by the cholesterol side-chain cleavage enzyme (*CYP11A1*) in the mitochondria. Pregnenolone is released into the cytosol and converted to progesterone by 3β-hydroxysteroid dehydrogenase (*HSD3B1/B2*). The 21-hydroxylation of progesterone by the steroid 21-hydroxylase (*CYP21A2*) produces 11-deoxycorticosterone (DOC). The aldosterone synthase (*CYP11B2*) catalyzes the last three reactions allowing conversion of DOC into aldosterone: the 11β-hydroxylation of DOC to form corticosterone, the 18-hydroxylation to yield 18-hydroxycorticosterone (18-OH-B), and finally the 18-methyloxidation to form aldosterone. *Grey arrows* represent reactions taking place in the mitochondria and *black arrows* reactions taking place in the endoplasmic reticulum of all three zones of the adrenal cortex. *Red arrows* indicate reactions taking place in mitochondria of zona glomerulosa only. It has to be noted that conversion of DOC to corticosterone also takes place in the zona fasciculata where it is catalyzed by the activity of 11β-hydroxylase (not shown)

involved in the regulation of sodium and potassium homeostasis and blood pressure. The zona fasciculata (ZF), the thickest zone of the cortex, produces glucocorticoid hormones that play important roles in stress response and energy homeostasis, while biosynthesis of sexual steroids takes place in the inner zona reticularis. Aldosterone and cortisol are synthesized from cholesterol by a series of specific enzymatic reactions [16] with the final steps catalyzed by the isozymes aldosterone synthase (encoded by *CYP11B2*) and 11β-hydroxylase (encoded by *CYP11B1*), respectively. These enzymes are highly homologous, and their genes are located in tandem on chromosome 8q21-q22. 11β-hydroxylase catalyzes the 11β-hydroxylation of 11-deoxycortisol to cortisol and of 11-deoxycorticosterone (DOC) to corticosterone. Aldosterone synthase catalyzes the 11β-hydroxylation of DOC to corticosterone, 18-hydroxylation of corticosterone to 18-hydroxycorticosterone (18-OHB), and 18-oxidation of 18-OHB to aldosterone (Fig. 5.1, right panel). Acute aldosterone production is controlled by rapid signaling events that increase cholesterol influx into the mitochondria, where cholesterol is converted into pregnenolone, the first step of aldosterone biosynthesis. Chronic and sustained regulation of aldosterone production involves the increased expression of *CYP11B2* [27].

Aldosterone biosynthesis is tightly regulated in an exquisite endocrine regulatory loop to maintain electrolyte and fluid homeostasis by the kidney. The principal regulators are the renin–angiotensin system and extracellular potassium (K^+) concentration. While the renin–angiotensin system is the main effector responsible for increasing aldosterone production in conditions of volume and salt depletion, K^+ exerts greater amplitude of regulatory control over a wide range of concentrations with maximal hormone production that is attained between 8 and 10 mmol/L [55, 58]. It was shown very early that alterations in K^+ concentrations can change the steroid output of zona glomerulosa cells even after maximal stimulation by other secretagogues [58]. Furthermore, angiotensin II (AngII) and K^+ synergize to regulate aldosterone production: in cases where one of the two agonists is below a certain threshold, stimulation of aldosterone biosynthesis by the other is impaired. On the other hand, only small changes of either AngII or K^+ are required to elicit robust stimulation of aldosterone production when the other agonist is present at modest to high concentration [66]. Remarkably, it has been demonstrated that plasma K^+ is also a central component of an AngII-independent mechanism regulating aldosterone production in conditions of sodium depletion [46].

The key molecular pathway involved in aldosterone production is calcium (Ca^{2+}) signaling [55]. Increased intracellular calcium levels affect aldosterone biosynthesis in many ways: by increasing the activity of cholesterol ester hydrolase, with subsequent release of deesterified cholesterol from its cytoplasmic stores; by increasing cholesterol delivery to the outer mitochondrial membrane; by promoting the transfer of cholesterol to the inner mitochondrial membrane through increased expression of the steroid acute regulatory (StAR) protein; by increasing the formation of cofactors necessary for the p450 cytochrome enzymes involved in aldosterone biosynthesis; and by stimulating the transcription of *CYP11B2* (reviewed in [55]). This last step involves activation of the Ca^{2+} signaling pathway, with binding of Ca^{2+} to calmodulin, and activation of Ca^{2+}/calmodulin-dependent protein kinases, which regulate by phosphorylation the activity of several transcriptional activators that regulate expression of *CYP11B2*, in particular the nuclear receptor subfamily four group A (NR4A) members 1 and 2 (NURR77 or NGF1B and NURR1), the cyclic AMP-dependent transcription factor ATF-1, and the cyclic AMP-responsive element-binding protein (CREB) [6].

AngII signals through the AngII type 1 receptor (AT1R) to stimulate inositol trisphosphate-dependent Ca^{2+} release from the endoplasmic reticulum. In addition, stimulation by AngII or K^+ results in depolarization of the zona glomerulosa cell membrane and opening of voltage-dependent Ca^{2+} channels, a major mechanism controlling intracellular Ca^{2+} concentration. Indeed, Ca^{2+} transport through the plasma membrane is regulated by the ionic concentration gradient and the membrane potential, which depends on the distribution of diffusible ions and their selective conductance across the membrane. The concentration gradient of major cations between the intracellular and extracellular space, which is required for the establishment of the membrane potential, is generated among others by the activity of the Na^+, K^+-ATPase, which transports two K^+ ions into and three sodium ions out of the cell, and by Ca^{2+} pumps. In the adrenal zona glomerulosa the main ionic conductance is that of K^+ due to the expression of different types of K^+ channels. As a consequence, the cell membrane potential closely follows the equilibrium potential of K^+ over a large range of extracellular K^+ concentrations [5]. Elevation of extracellular K^+ concentration, decrease of intracellular K^+ concentration, inhibition of the Na^+, K^+-ATPase, or closure of TASK potassium channels all lead to cell membrane depolarization, allowing opening of voltage-dependent Ca^{2+} channels. AngII inhibits Na^+, K^+-ATPase activity in rat adrenal glomerulosa cells, which might represent an additional mechanism contributing to its stimulation of aldosterone production [26].

Potassium Channels and the Regulation of Aldosterone Biosynthesis

Patch-clamp studies have revealed inwardly rectifying, outwardly (delayed) rectifying, Ca^{2+}-activated as well as background potassium currents in glomerulosa cells. Among the different K^+ channels, the TASK (TWIK-related acid-sensitive potassium) channels are highly expressed in the adrenal cortex. TASK channels are responsible for the background (or leak) potassium current and exert a significant role in the generation of the strongly negative resting membrane potential (>80 mV) in glomerulosa cells. Their role in the regulation of aldosterone biosynthesis has been highlighted by the analysis of different mouse models of TASK channel invalidation displaying different phenotypes of aldosterone excess [18, 24, 29, 47]. Genetic invalidation of the TASK1 channel in mice leads to ectopic expression of *CYP11B2* in zona fasciculata due to adrenocortical cell depolarization [29]. Female homozygous TASK1 knockout mice present low-renin, glucocorticoid-remediable hyperaldosteronism; until puberty, male TASK1 knockout mice display the same phenotype but normalize subsequently in terms of adrenal zonation and aldosterone secretion. Indeed, androgen-dependent expression of TASK3 in adult male mice, and possibly other mechanisms, compensates for the loss of TASK1 function [29]. When both TASK1 and TASK3 channels are deleted, mice present a phenotype reminiscent of patients with idiopathic primary hyperaldosteronism (IHA) [18]. No abnormal adrenal cortex zonation is observed, but profound ZG membrane depolarization leads to elevated plasma aldosterone levels and low circulating renin, with aldosterone production not suppressed by a high-salt diet. In contrast to the previous models, mice lacking TASK3 channels display a mild hyperaldosteronism that is associated with low renin levels and an increased aldosterone-to-renin ratio. These animals show partially autonomous aldosterone production, which is not suppressed by high-sodium or low-potassium diets [47], suggesting that constitutive depolarization of zona glomerulosa cells in these animals leads to partially autonomous aldosterone production, which is counterbalanced by decreased activity of the renin–angiotensin system. Altogether, these models suggest that TASK channels serve a dual function, with TASK1 controlling the functional zonation in terms of *CYP11B2* expression, while TASK3 is responsible for the control of zona glomerulosa cell membrane potential [47]. Although these models suggest that abnormalities in TASK1 and/or TASK3 channels may be involved in the pathogenesis of PA in humans, no causative mutations of these genes have been identified so far [15] (Zennaro et al. unpublished results).

G Protein-Activated Inward Rectifier Potassium Channels, ATPases, and Primary Aldosteronism

Until recently, TASK channels were presumed to be the principal actors in the maintenance of zona glomerulosa membrane potential and regulation of aldosterone biosynthesis. A major advance in our understanding of the pathogenesis of PA has come from the identification of a few recurrent sporadic and germline mutations in the *KCNJ5* gene coding for the G protein-activated inward rectifier potassium channel 4 (GIRK4) in aldosterone-producing adenoma (APA) and familial hyperaldosteronism type III [14, 15, 40, 52] (see Fig. 5.2). All mutations identified so far are located near or within the selectivity filter of GIRK4, which contains the consensus GYG motif for potassium selectivity (see below). Expression of mutated channels in different cell lines demonstrated that these gain-of-function mutations affect the ion selectivity of the channel, with increased Na^+ conductance leading to chronic membrane depolarization [15, 40, 52]. It has been shown that these changes are responsible for increased Ca^{2+} influx into the cell through activation of voltage-gated Ca^{2+} channels leading to increased Ca^{2+}/calmodulin signaling and constitutive secretion of aldosterone [45]. Inherited *KNCJ5* mutations also lead to increased cell proliferation in familial hyperaldosteronism type III, where subjects show massive bilateral adrenal hyperplasia requiring bilateral adrenalectomy to control blood pressure [23]. However, overexpression of mutated GIRK4 channels in human embryonic kidney cells [52] or adrenal H295R cells [45] results in Na^+-dependent cell death or decreased proliferation, most likely due to lethal intracellular Na^+

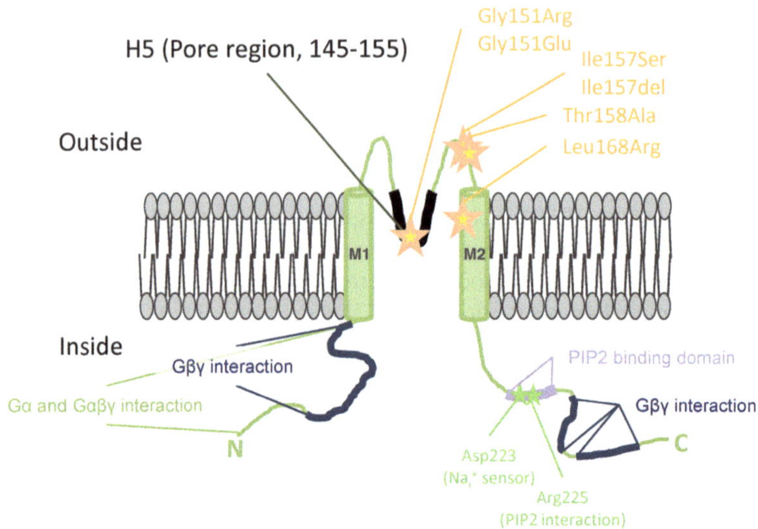

Fig. 5.2 *Schematic representation of the GIRK4 subunit.* GIRK4 subunits of GIRK channels present two transmembrane domains (M1 and M2), a putative pore region (H5, indicated in *black*) and intracellular N- and C-termini. Regions involved in Gβγ interaction are indicated in *blue*, those involved in interaction with Gα and Gαβγ are indicated in *green*, the PIP2-binding domain is indicated in *purple*, and amino acids involved in Na_i^+ sensing and in PIP2 interaction are identified by *green stars*. GIRK4 mutations identified in sporadic and familial forms of primary aldosteronism are indicated by *yellow stars*

accumulation in these systems. The fact that somatic GIRK4 mutations lead to increased cell proliferation in APA therefore awaits formal demonstration in experimental systems.

Several studies have shown that somatic *KCNJ5* mutations are present in ~40 % of APA from Western countries [1, 4, 9, 39] and as high as 65 % of patients from Japan [57]. *KCNJ5* mutations are associated with female gender, younger age, and a more severe phenotype of the disease in terms of preoperative aldosterone levels and hypokalemia. They are however not consistently associated with tumor size, blood pressure levels, and postoperative outcome after surgery [9]. While germline *KCNJ5* mutations are involved in the pathogenesis of bilateral adrenal hyperplasia in familial forms of the disease, similar mutations have not been identified in patients with IHA, which together with APA represents the other most frequent form of sporadic PA [9].

More recently, whole-exome sequencing performed in 9 APA has identified recurrent somatic mutations in *ATP1A1*, coding for the α1 subunit of the Na^+, K^+-ATPase, and *ATP2B3*, coding for the plasma membrane calcium-transporting ATPase 3 (PMCA3) [7] (Fig. 5.3). These mutations are present in ~7 % of tumors in a large European multicenter study including 308 APA samples. Mutations were more frequent in males and were associated with higher preoperative aldosterone levels and significantly lower serum potassium concentrations [7].

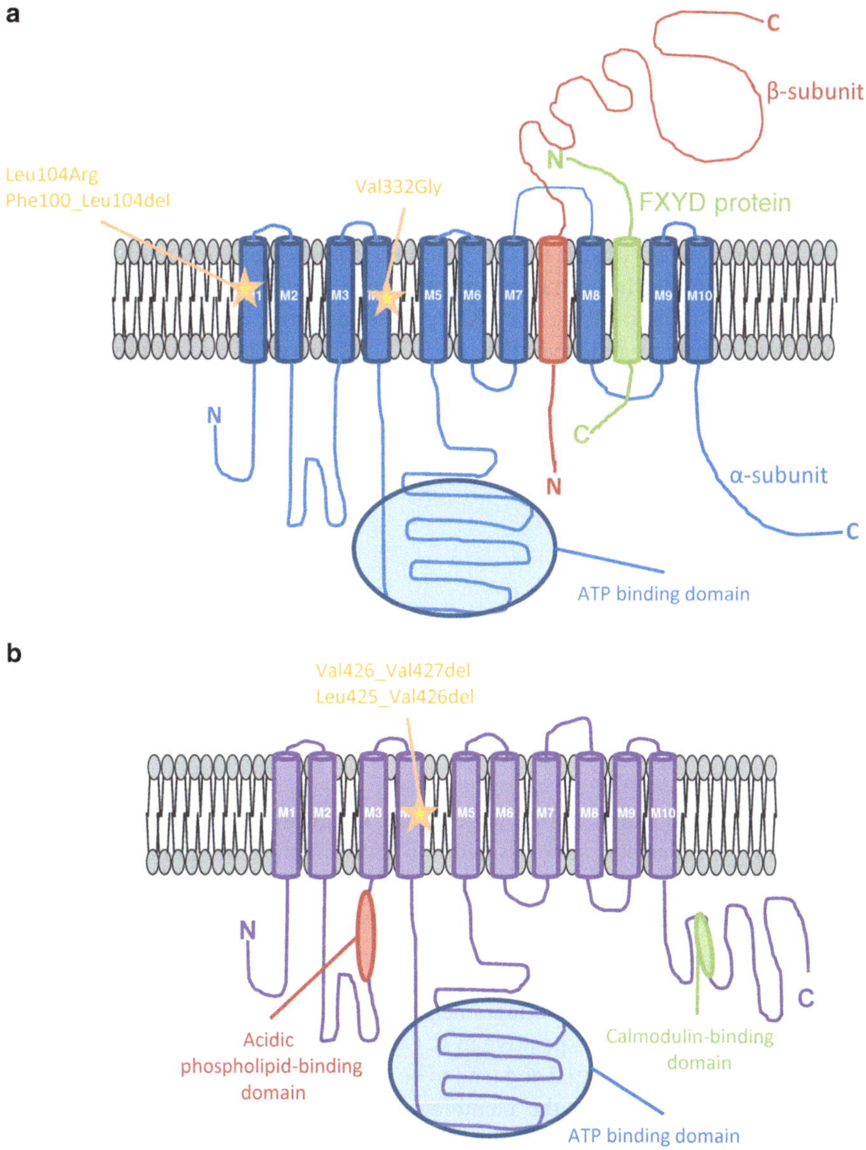

Fig. 5.3 *Schematic representation of Na⁺, K⁺-ATPase and plasma membrane calcium transporting ATPase 3 (PMCA3).* The Na^+, K^+-ATPase and PMCA3 belong to the P-type ATPase family. (**a**) The Na^+, K^+-ATPase is composed of two subunits, α and β. The α subunit presents ten transmembrane domains (M1–M10), and the N- and C-termini are intracellular. The ATP-binding region, located in the second intracellular loop of the α subunit, is encased in a *blue circle*. The β subunit has a single membrane crossing with a cytoplasmic N-terminus and is located close to the M7/M10 transmembrane domain. FXYD proteins possess one transmembrane domain with an extracellular N-terminus; they are not integral part of the Na^+, K^+-ATPase but modulate the pump activity. Mutations identified in primary aldosteronism are indicated by *yellow stars*. (**b**) Similar to the Na^+, K^+-ATPase, the PMCA pump possesses ten transmembrane domains (M1–M10) and the ATP-binding region is located in the second intracellular loop (*blue circle*). The acidic phospholipid-binding domain, located in the first intracellular loop, and the calmodulin-binding domain, located in the C-terminal tail, are indicated in *red* and in *green*, respectively. Mutations identified in primary aldosteronism are indicated by *yellow stars*

Mutations in the α1 subunit of the Na^+, K^+-ATPase affect amino acids in the transmembrane α-helix M1 or the juxtaposed α-helix M4, which are involved in potassium ion binding and gating [19]. The small deletions found in PMCA3 involve the homologous region of the M4 transmembrane helix, where according to the known structure of a homologous rabbit sarcoplasmic reticulum-type Ca^{2+}-ATPase, a glutamate is crucial for Ca^{2+} binding. Both ATPases are highly expressed in the adrenal cortex. In vitro experiments in cell models have shown that mutations in the α1 subunit of the Na^+, K^+-ATPase lead to a complete loss of pump activity and a strongly reduced affinity for K^+. Furthermore, electrophysiological studies performed on primary adrenal adenoma cells demonstrated an inappropriate depolarization of cells expressing mutated *ATP1A1* genes. Although mutations in PMCA3 have not been investigated experimentally, deletions are predicted to cause a major distortion of the Ca^{2+}-binding site, therefore affecting intracellular Ca^{2+} clearance [7].

G Protein-Activated Inward Rectifier Potassium Channels

Structure and Function of G Protein-Activated Inward Rectifier Potassium Channels

GIRK channels are members of a large family of inwardly rectifying K^+ channels (Kir1–Kir7). Kir channels are classified into seven families but can be categorized into four functional groups: (1) the classical Kir channels (Kir2.x); (2) the G protein-gated Kir channels (Kir3.x, now referred to us as GIRKx); (3) the ATP-sensitive K^+ channels (Kir6.x); and (4) the K^+-transport channels (Kir1.x, Kir4.x, Kir5.x, and Kir7.x). "Inward rectifiers" are a class of K^+ channels that can conduct much larger inward currents at membrane voltages negative to the K^+ equilibrium potential than outward currents at voltages positive to it. Consequently Kir channels operate near the resting membrane potential and tend to be silenced when voltage-dependent Na^+ or Ca^{2+} channels depolarize the membrane [36]. In the adrenal gland, however, under physiological conditions, Kir channel opening will lead to a K^+ outflow rather than potassium inflow (see below).

GIRK channels comprise four members (GIRK1, GIRK2, GIRK3, and GIRK4) showing 36 % sequence identity. GIRK1 was first cloned from a rat heart cDNA library, based on sequence similarity with cloned inwardly rectifying K^+ channels, ROMK1 (Kir1.1) and IRK1 [35]. The encoded protein presented similar structure to ROMK and IRK1 with two transmembrane regions (M1 and M2), a putative pore region (H5), and intracellular N- and C-termini. Although in *Xenopus* oocytes GIRK1 displays many of the properties of the G protein-coupled muscarinic K^+ channel (I_{KACh}) from the heart [35], in mammalian cell lines expression of GIRK1 alone does not produce a functional K^+ channel [34]. The effects observed in *Xenopus* oocytes were, in fact, due to GIRK1 heteromeric assembly with Kir3.5/XIR, a homolog of GIRK4 [28]. GIRK1 generally forms heteromultimers with other GIRK subunits to form functional K^+ channels. In heart, GIRK1 and GIRK4 physically associate to form the I_{KACh} channel. The quaternary structure of this channel was determined by different approaches. Corey *et al.* showed that GIRK proteins form tetramers and that native I_{KACh} is most likely a tetramer composed of two GIRK1 and two GIRK4 subunits. Surprisingly, both of the possible arrangements of subunits, GIRK1–GIRK4–GIRK1–GIRK4 or $(GIRK1)_2$–$(GIRK4)_2$, around the pore may be viable [17].

Comparison of the solved structures of the cytoplasmic domains of GIRK1, GIRK2, and IRK1 (Kir2.1) highlighted a conserved secondary structure for inwardly rectifying K^+ channels, consisting of 14 β-strands and 2 α-helices. Two-thirds of the amino acid sequence of GIRK channels is represented by large hydrophilic N- and C-terminal domains, which form a large "cytoplasmic pore" structure. Electrophysiological studies revealed the importance of this cytoplasmic pore. First, it extends the effective length of the pore. The cytoplasmic pore contains some of the acidic residues essential for the voltage-dependent high-affinity block of the channel by Mg^{2+} and polyamines from the intracellular side. This binding, which physically blocks the channel, underlies the voltage gating and the inward rectification of the channel. The mechanism of inward rectification also involves the M2 helix, with GIRK4 possessing a crucial Asn and GIRK1 an Asp in this position as polyamine-binding site. This gives rise to large inward currents at hyperpolarized potentials and small outward currents at more positive potentials. In contrast to voltage-gated K-channels, GIRKs lack an intrinsic voltage sensor segment. Second, the cytoplasmic pore is the structural component through which gating of GIRK channels can be modulated by regulatory proteins, ATP, Na^+, or pH. Resolution of the crystal structure of a protein formed by the N- and C-termini of GIRK1 showed that a single subunit forms a globular, mainly β sheet protein with a prominent α helix, which can assemble as a tetramer of identical subunits to form a pore [43]. The cytoplasmic pore increases the length of the ion pathway and is wide enough to allow K^+ to remain hydrated; it constitutes more a long tunnel than a wide vestibule. Phosphatidylinositol 4,5-bisphosphate (PIP2)-binding domains have also been localized to the N- and C-termini by mutagenesis studies. Indeed, gating of GIRKs is dependent on the membrane content of PIP2, with PIP2 enhancing GIRK currents and PIP2 depletion reducing GIRK currents.

Each subunit of the tetrameric channel is made up of two transmembrane domains flanking a highly conserved pore-forming helix. In terms of ion selectivity, GIRK channel subunits all present the same signature sequence: TXG(Y/F)G. In the "weaver" mouse, mutation of the Gly156 to serine in the selectivity filter of the GIRK2 channel results in the loss of K^+ selectivity [41]. However, residues outside the selectivity filter of GIRK channels have also been found to contribute to K^+ selectivity. Residues involved in the selectivity filter of channels formed by GIRK1/GIRK4 subunits have been identified by homologies with the Kir2.1 channel. Mutation of the Thr141 in the pore loop and Ser165 in M2 of Kir2.1 has been shown to alter both cesium (Cs^+) block and rubidium (Rb^+) permeation and mutations in the same position in GIRK4, Thr148, or Ala172 have the same effect, whereas similar mutations in GIRK1 at position Ala142 or Ser166 did not affect the channel characteristics [37]. Molecular modelling suggested that residues Glu145 and Arg155 in GIRK4 and residues Glu139 and Arg149 in GIRK1 form a salt bridge behind the selectivity filter and probably act to maintain the structure rigid. Disruption of the salt bridge renders the selectivity filter floppy and has dramatic effects on permeation, inward rectification, and agonist activation, similar to those observed when residues involved in the selectivity filter are mutated.

Regulation of GIRK Channels by G Proteins

The intracellular domains of GIRK channels, which also include the cytoplasmic pore region, are crucial for modulation of channel activity by many regulators and for establishing the voltage dependence of inward rectification [67]. In these domains, the sequence identity increases to ≥80 %. GIRKs are coupled to many different G protein-coupled receptors (GPCRs), like the muscarinic M_2, δ-opioid, dopamine D4, and somatostatin receptors. GIRKs are effectors of Gβγ signaling. Gβγ has roles in channel trafficking and assembly in addition to cell signaling. Gβγ binds to the intracellular N- and C-terminal domains and induces a configuration change that is transduced to the lower M2 region which is rotated. While there exist 2–3 separate Gβγ-binding segments on each GIRK, with the channel tetramer having 8–12 putative Gβγ-binding sites, cross-linking experiments have established that each channel subunit binds to one Gβγ, with a total of four Gβγ per channel tetramer [67]. Mutations within the Gβγ-binding segment of the C-terminal region of GIRKs eliminate agonist-induced receptor activation of the channel but preserve Gβγ-dependent basal activities, indicating that some binding sites are required for early interactions between Gβγ and GIRKs during channel biosynthesis and channel assembly, while other sites may be required to mediate channel activation at the cell surface. The cytoplasmic region of GIRKs is critically involved in channel gating. Gβγ specificity is dependent upon the specific Gα subunit with which they are associated; Gα (Gαi subunit, but not Gαs or Gαq) plays a central role in determining receptor-coupling specificity to GIRKs. Interestingly, in native tissue, only Gαi-coupled receptors activate GIRKs [49]; as all heterotrimers release Gβγ, it is hypothesized that this specificity may derive from spatial restriction of heterotrimers composed of Gαs or Gαq in the membrane lipid bilayer, preventing interaction with GIRKs [53].

GIRKs are also regulated by regulators of G protein signaling (RGS) proteins. RGS have mostly negative modulatory roles on GPCR-mediated signal transduction [61]. They act as GTPase-activating proteins (GAPs), thus terminating the activation cycle of Gα by promoting its intrinsic GTPase activity. On GIRK channels, RGS proteins accelerate both the activation and the deactivation kinetics of the channel [51]. The impact on deactivation is explained by their GAP activity, which terminates Gα activation by promoting GTP hydrolysis, increasing GαGDP which sequesters Gβγ into an inactive complex. The mechanisms of GIRK activation by

RGS are less well understood. It has been described that RGS4 can form a stable complex with the $GABA_B$ receptor, Gαo and GIRK, indicating that they may act as accessory proteins forming part of a larger signaling complex [67].

Regulation by PIP2 and Sodium

GIRKs are regulated by plasma membrane PIP2; receptor-mediated hydrolysis of PIP2 via Gαq leads to K-current desensitization of GIRK1/4 complexes through the activation of phospholipase C (PLC) [33]. This occurs also after activation of signaling pathways not involving heterotrimeric G proteins, like the epidermal growth factor receptor, which directly couples to PLCγ. The extent of agonist-induced desensitization depends upon the strength of the GIRK–PIP2 interaction. The mechanistic basis for K^+-current inhibition by PIP2 hydrolysis is a direct interaction between PIP2 and GIRKs [33]. The interaction between PIP2 and GIRKs is weak, and at the low PIP2 concentrations of the plasma membrane PIP2 does not normally gate GIRK channels. PIP2 produced via hydrolysis of ATP causes prolonged unitary channel openings, which sensitize the channel to gating molecules like Gβγ or sodium [56]. Gβγ subunits require PIP2 to stimulate and maintain the activity of GIRKs. Gating molecules vice versa stabilize channel interactions with PIP2, suggesting that gating proceeds by modulating channel PIP2 interactions. GIRKs seem therefore to be regulated by the balance of two pathways: one activating pathway, via GPCRs coupled to Gαi and gating by Gβγ interacting directly with the channel to stabilize its interaction with PIP2 leading to channel opening: one inhibitory pathway, via PLC-dependent hydrolysis of PIP2, therefore limiting channel activity [33].

Intracellular Na^+ (Na_i^+) can activate GIRK channels which contain GIRK2 or GIRK4 subunits independently of G protein activation. This mechanism involves two processes: (1) a modification of the functional state of the channel which depends on ATP hydrolysis and (2) a subsequent gating of the ATP-modified channel by Na^+ [56]. This mechanism of K_{ACh} channel activation was shown to be operative during Na_i^+ accumulation, produced for instance by blocking the Na^+, K^+-ATPase, and is likely to be involved in the "direct" electrophysiological effects of cardiac glycosides, such as digitalis, drugs widely used in heart failure or for improvement of the inotropic state of the heart [56]. Studies aimed at identifying regions of GIRK channels that mediate their activation by Na^+ have converged to a region located in the C-terminus close to the plasma membrane. In GIRK4, this region was found to include residues 214–252. Aspartate at position 223 in GIRK4, located in the CD loop between the βC- and βD-strands, is considered to be the Na_i^+ sensor. At the equivalent position, GIRK1 possesses an asparagine (Asn217) probably explaining its sodium insensitivity.

Intracellular Na^+ also strengthens the interaction between GIRKs and PIP2, increasing and accelerating GIRK activation by PIP2 [30]. Na_i^+ can activate channels containing GIRK4 by modifying the three-dimensional structure of the loop to increase the channel's sensitivity to PIP2. In GIRK4, a highly conserved arginine (Arg225) in the loop that contains the crucial Asp223 has been shown to be crucial in the sensitivity of the channel to PIP2. Asp223 inhibits electrostatic interactions between PIP2 and Arg225, while Na^+ binding attenuates this inhibition, allowing the arginine residue to enhance the channel's sensitivity to PIP2. Na^+ plays the role of a switch that breaks the hydrogen bonding between the aspartate and the arginine. Na^+ sensitivity of GIRK channels involves also the backbone carbonyls of two more residues and a water molecule. The existence of a specific Na^+-binding motif, DXRXXH, especially in GIRK channels, was proposed [50].

Recently, the structural basis for GIRK channel regulation by G proteins, PIP2, and sodium has been elucidated by establishment of the crystal structure of the GIRK2 channel [60]. These studies show that GIRK channels contain two functional gates, an inner helix gate (formed by the inner helices of the transmembrane domain) and a G loop gate (formed by the G loop at the apex of the C-terminal domain), that are regulated by a combination of cytoplasmic and membrane stimuli. The Na^+-binding site is located between the βC-βD and βE-βG loops and is dependent on a negatively charged Asp residue. PIP2 binds at the interface between the transmembrane and cytoplasmic domains and is coordinated by several positively charged residues.

GIRK as Part of Larger Signaling Complexes

GIRKs are part of large macromolecular signaling complexes, which are organized in transient interactions to stable signalosomes, depending on the need for either signal amplification with no need for specificity or rather rapid and highly specific signaling events [67]. Many proteins have been shown to associate in those complexes, for example GIRK1/4 with β2-adrenergic receptors, or D2 and D4 receptors, which remain intact throughout the signaling process. Receptor–Gβγ interactions initially occur in the endoplasmic reticulum, after which they are trafficked to the cell membrane. These early complexes may also contain GIRKs and RGS proteins. Other proteins associated with GIRKs are GPCR-kinases (GRKs), protein kinases (PK)A and PKC, and protein phosphatases (PP)I and PP2A. Tyrosine phosphorylation has been shown to inhibit GIRK activity. Channel inactivation has been linked to activation of Gαq-coupled receptors and could involve PKC-mediated phosphorylation of the channel or PLC-mediated PIP2 depletion. It is most likely that GIRK inhibition is initially mediated by PIP2 depletion and that subsequently increased DAG can lead to PKC stimulation, which inactivates the channel through phosphorylation and reduced interaction with PIP2. Gβγ subunits stabilize interactions with PIP2 and lead to persistent channel activation. Activation of PLC hydrolyzes PIP2 and limits Gβγ-stimulated activity, indicating that PIP2 itself is a receptor-regulated second messenger, downregulation of which accounts for GIRK desensitization [33].

The Na^+, K^+-ATPase and PMCA

The Na^+, K^+-ATPase or Sodium Pump

ATPases are classified into five types and nine subtypes. The Na^+, K^+-ATPase is a member of the P-type ATPase family whose members are characterized by the presence of a specific motif DKTGTLT. The Na^+, K^+-ATPase is composed of two subunits, α and β. Four isoforms of the α subunits have been identified, α1–α4. They are composed of about 1,000 amino acids, with 10 transmembrane segments (M1–M10); the N- and C-termini have been shown to be intracellular [31]. The β subunit is a type II membrane protein, and three isoforms have been identified, β1–β3. β subunits are composed of about 370 amino acids and have a single membrane crossing with a cytoplasmic N-terminus. Crystallographic data predict that the β subunit is located close to the M7/M10 transmembrane domain of the α subunit. Both α and β subunits are needed to form a functional ATPase (Fig. 5.3a). Although β subunits facilitate the correct membrane integration acting as a chaperone protein, they are also involved in the mechanism of active transport. Depending on the association of α subunits with different β subunits affinity for potassium can be modified [32].

The reaction mechanism of the Na^+, K^+-ATPase involves different conformational changes: the first conformation (E_1) presents high affinity for both Na^+ and ATP (0.2 μM), whereas the second one (E_2) has only low affinity for ATP (150 mM). Binding of ATP to E_1 permits the binding of three intracellular Na^+ and leads to E_1 phosphorylation (E_1P). The bound Na^+ ions are occluded, and a new conformational change occurs allowing Na^+ to be released at the extracellular surface (E_2P). The E_2P conformation is sensitive to aqueous hydrolysis and binds two K^+ at the outer surface, inducing enzyme dephosphorylation (E_2) and K^+ occluding. The binding of ATP to the low-affinity site of the enzyme allows release of the two K^+ ions at the intracellular side. The enzyme returns to the conformation (E_1) with high affinity for Na^+, and ATP and is available for a new cycle.

Remarkably the catalytic activity of the enzyme and the ionic transport are performed by two separate regions. Different approaches (chemical labeling, site-directed mutagenesis) demonstrated that all the residues involved in nucleotide binding are located in the second extracellular loop between the M4 and M5 transmembrane domain (which are the domains carrying the recurrent somatic mutations found in APA, see above). Proteolysis experiments revealed that the cation transport domain is formed by transmembrane segments of the protein. In particular, the glutamate at position 779 in the M5 transmembrane domain is a key residue in the ability of the enzyme to occlude ions, while residues involved in cation coordination are located in M4, M5, and M6 transmembrane domains. Indeed several negatively charged amino acids are present in these domains and are not compensated by positive charges strongly suggesting that transported cations are involved not only in charge neutralization but also in enzyme stability.

Due to its role, the Na+, K+-ATPase is ubiquitously expressed. In the adrenal cortex, the α1 subunit is predominantly expressed in zona glomerulosa and, to a less extent, in zona fasciculata [31, 59].

Regulation of the Na^+, K^+-ATPase

The activity of the Na^+, K^+-ATPase is regulated by several factors, including FXYD proteins, ouabain and other cardiotonic steroids, and hormones. The FXYD protein family is composed of seven members (FXYD1–FXYD7). They possess one transmembrane domain with an extracellular N-terminus and are characterized by the presence of an extracellular FXYD motif, two conserved glycine residues located in the transmembrane domain, and one intracellular serine residue. The FXYD proteins are not an integral part of the Na^+, K^+-ATPase but modulate the pump activity by changing the apparent affinity for Na^+, K^+ or ATP. Their expression is tissue specific allowing adaptation of Na^+, K^+-ATPase activity to the tissue [22].

Cardiotonic steroids (comprising especially digoxin and ouabain), named due to their positive effect on heart performance, play an important role in the control of blood pressure but also in the control of many cellular functions (proliferation, differentiation) due to the activation of specific cellular pathways; modification of endogenous levels of cardiotonic steroids could be involved in chronic renal and heart failure, hypertension, and cancer. They constitute also an important class of Na^+, K^+-ATPase inhibitors. Indeed, the Na^+, K^+-ATPase not only acts as a Na^+ and K^+ transporter but also as a receptor for this class of molecules. The Na^+, K^+-ATPase interacts with cytoskeleton proteins (ankyrins and adducins) or membrane proteins (caveolins); this kind of interactions can play a role in targeting and stabilizing the pump into specialized membrane signaling microdomains. The α2 and α3 subunits are located in specific plasma membrane microdomains adjacent to the endoplasmic reticulum and in close proximity to the Na^+/Ca^{2+} exchanger, thus forming a functional structure named PLasmERosome [8]. Binding of ouabain induces an increase in Ca^{2+} signaling. The α1 subunits reside in caveolae where they interact with Src kinase, phosphoinositide 3-kinase, ankyrin, and inositol triphosphate receptor, forming a functional structure called signalosome [48]. Binding of ouabain can result in the activation of the MAPK and PI3K pathway and in the generation of specific second messengers [mitochondrial reactive oxygen species (ROS), PLC, and Ca^{2+}] [54].

Short- and long-term regulation of the Na^+, K^+-ATPase also involves a variety of hormones. The short-term effects implicate either (1) a direct effect on the kinetic behavior of the enzyme or (2) a translocation to the membrane of preexisting pumps; long-term effects involve de novo pump synthesis. Among others, aldosterone has been shown to increase the expression of the α subunit of the Na^+, K^+-ATPase in the distal tubule of the kidney [20]. The mineralocorticoid receptor is strongly expressed in the zona glomerulosa of the adrenal cortex [10]. Whether aldosterone-mediated activation of the Na^+, K^+-ATPase may represent a short autocrine regulatory loop restricting aldosterone production in the adrenal zona glomerulosa awaits further investigation.

The Plasma Membrane Calcium-Transporting ATPase

The plasma membrane calcium-transporting ATPase (PMCA) pumps allow extruding Ca^{2+} from the cell and are key regulators of cellular Ca^{2+} homeostasis. The family comprises four members (PMCA1–PCMA4) composed of about 1,200 amino acids, with 10 transmembrane segments (M1–M10) (Fig. 5.3b). Similarly to the Na^+, K^+-ATPase, the PMCA belongs to the P-type ATPase family. The Ca^{2+} ATPase reaction cycle involves two conformational states E_1 and E_2. In the E_1 state, intracellular Ca^{2+} binds to the pump with a high affinity, whereas in the E_2 conformational state, the affinity of the pump for Ca^{2+} decreases, leading to its release at the extracellular side. The PMCA pumps have only one Ca^{2+}-binding site instead of two described in the Sarco(Endo)plasmic reticulum Ca^{2+}-ATPase (SERCA). In addition to the ATP-binding site located in the second intracellular loop, the first intracellular loop contains a domain (~40 amino acids) which binds activating acidic phospholipids, and the intracellular C-tail contains a calmodulin-binding site. In the absence of calmodulin, the C-tail interacts also with two specific sites located in the first intracellular loop, leading to an auto-inhibitory conformation [21]; calmodulin binding removes the C-terminal tail from the inhibitory sites, restoring the pump activity. While PCMA1 and PCMA4 are ubiquitously expressed, PMCA2 and PMCA3 are expressed in a very limited number of tissues, essentially in the nervous system. PMCA2 is also expressed in the mammary gland and PMCA3 in the adrenal cortex [11].

In addition to the activating effect of calmodulin reported above, PMCA pumps can be activated by other mechanisms, such as (1) binding of acidic phospholipids in the first intracellular loop, which reduce the Ca^{2+} Km of the pump; (2) its dimerization through the calmodulin-binding domain; and (3) phosphorylation of the calmodulin-binding domain, by protein kinase C, which prevents the interaction of the auto-inhibitory calmodulin-binding domain with the first intracellular loop. Finally, calpain can irreversibly activate the pump by cleavage of the C-terminal part which contains the auto-inhibitory calmodulin-binding domain [12].

How Do GIRK4 Channels and ATPases Regulate Physiological Aldosterone Production?

As described above, the activity of the Na^+, K^+-ATPase and of different Ca^{2+} pumps is essential for the establishment of the membrane potential of zona glomerulosa cells and for maintaining intracellular calcium homeostasis. The finding that GIRK4 and ATPase mutations were responsible for sporadic and familial hyperaldosteronism opens the question as to whether GIRK channels, Na^+, K^+-ATPase, and PMCA3 also play an important role in the physiology of zona glomerulosa cells and aldosterone production. GIRK4, Na^+, K^+-ATPase, and PMCA3 are highly expressed in the adrenal cortex and in APA (Fig. 5.4). GIRK4 is particularly expressed in the zona

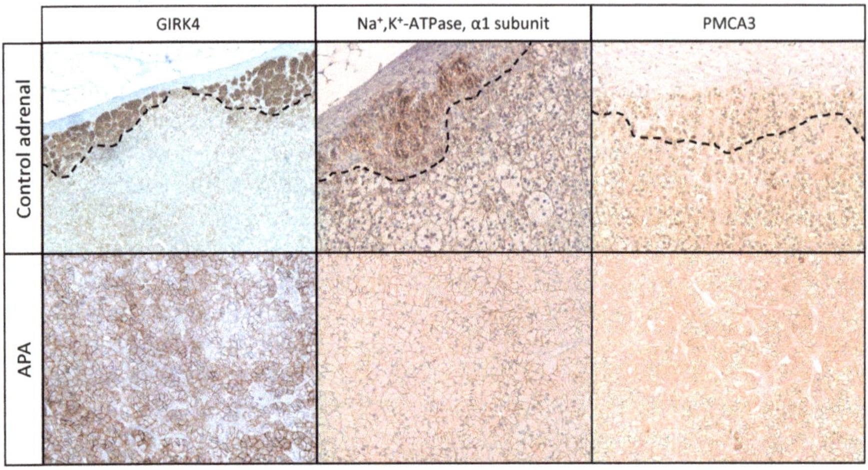

Fig. 5.4 *Immunolocalization of GIRK4, Na^+, K^+-ATPase α1, and PMCA3 in control adrenal cortex and APA*. In control adrenal, GIRK4 and the α1 subunit of the Na^+, K^+-ATPase are strongly expressed in zona glomerulosa and to a less extent in zona fasciculata, while PMCA3 is expressed in the entire cortex. GIRK4, Na^+, K^+-ATPase α1, and PMCA3 are all expressed in APA. The *dotted line* delineates the zona glomerulosa underneath the capsule in control adrenal. Magnification ×200

glomerulosa, although its heteromerization partner has not been formally identified so far in this tissue. As GIRK channels act as inward rectifiers at membrane voltages negative to the K^+ equilibrium potential, in the zona glomerulosa, where the membrane potential is usually slightly more depolarized than the K^+ equilibrium potential, GIRK channels conduct outward potassium currents [15]. GIRK channels may therefore contribute to maintaining the hyperpolarized state of the zona glomerulosa cell membrane, providing a GPCR-coupled effector regulated by the balance of different pathways. Activating pathways would involve different GPCRs expressed in the zona glomerulosa coupled to Gαi and gating by Gβγ, or increased Na_i^+, leading to channel opening: inhibitory pathways may act via PLC-dependent hydrolysis of PIP2, therefore limiting channel activity.

AngII was found to inhibit each type of the hitherto described K^+ channels, in particular TASK channels. Maneuvers applied to activate PLC, Gq, and PKC, or to increase the concentration of cytoplasmic Ca^2 and IP3, led to the conclusion that the action of AngII on K^+ channels is mediated by the breakdown of PIP2 in the plasma membrane [55]. In a model of adrenocortical cells, it has been shown that activation of GIRK4 inhibits AngII-stimulated changes in membrane voltage and aldosterone secretion; similarly, GIRK4 overexpression leads to a decrease in membrane voltage, decreased intracellular Ca^{2+} and aldosterone production, and reduced mRNA expression of *StAR*, *CYP11A1*, *HSD3B2*, *CYP21A2*, *CYP17A1*, *CYP11B1*, and *CYP11B2*, coding for the major steroidogenic enzymes involved in aldosterone biosynthesis [44] (Fig. 5.1). The mechanistic basis for this effect has been attributed to AngII-dependent downregulation of *KCNJ5* mRNA expression and GIRK4 protein levels, involving Ca^{2+} signaling [44]. It has been therefore suggested that GIRK4 containing channels in the zona glomerulosa continuously transfer K^+ from inside to out of the cells to regulate membrane voltage, an action that is inhibited by AngII [44]. In addition to regulating GIRK4 channel expression, an additional mechanism whereby AngII could negatively regulate GIRK4 channel function is Gαq-mediated PLC-dependent PIP2 hydrolysis. Conversely, the inhibitory effect of AngII on Na^+, K^+-ATPase activity which leads to cell membrane depolarization [26] may have an opposite effect on GIRK activity, as increase in Na_i^+ can activate GIRK channels [30]. These may serve as negative feedback mechanism during intense stimulation with AngII, similarly to the effect of increased intracellular Ca^{2+} leading to pump activation [64]. Indeed, under conditions where extracellular K^+ stimulates aldosterone secretion, i.e., 4–10 mM, it also stimulates the Na^+, K^+-ATPase by direct binding to the pump as well as through increased intracellular Ca^{2+} [64]. In rat glomerulosa cells, the predominant form of Na^+, K^+-ATPase is the α-isoenzyme [55]. Inhibition of the Na^+, K^+-ATPase by ouabain has been shown to rapidly increase the release of aldosterone from rat glomerulosa cells, an effect involving calcium influx through voltage-gated calcium channels [65]. Furthermore, prolonged infusion of ouabain in rats results in raised plasma concentrations of aldosterone and corticosterone, without effect on plasma renin activity, that is associated with marked hypertrophy of the zona glomerulosa, indicating that prolonged treatment with ouabain selectively stimulates the growth and steroidogenic capacity of adrenal zona glomerulosa cells [42]. AngII reduces the activity of the Na^+, K^+-ATPase through the AT1R [26], an effect that possibly involves the activation of a tyrosine phosphatase [63]. Inhibition of Na^+, K^+-ATPase contributes to membrane depolarization and generation of a calcium signal, finally leading to increased aldosterone production.

The adrenal cortex is a complex tissue, where cords of steroidogenic cells are in close contact with endothelial cells from blood vessels, chromaffin cells from the adrenal medulla, immune cells (mast cells, lymphocytes, macrophages), and nerve terminations. All those different cellular components constitute the basis for a paracrine and autocrine control of aldosterone production, involving catecholamines and neurotransmitters (adrenalin, noradrenalin, dopamine, and serotonin), cytokines (TGFβ, interleukins), vasoactive peptides (endothelin, nitric oxide), and growth factors (IGF, EGF). Among them, different molecules involve signaling via GPCRs coupled to different effector mechanisms. Whereas the role of these factors in regulating aldosterone production under physiological circumstances is still debated, a few of them might involve coupling to GIRK channels to exert their effects. The neurotransmitter dopamine is a well-known inhibitor of aldosterone biosynthesis [55]. In bovine adrenal glands as well as in humans, administration of the dopaminergic antagonist metoclopramide causes a rise in plasma aldosterone levels [13, 38]. Both D2 and D4 dopamine receptors are expressed in the adrenal gland [62]. A large amount of data indicates that dopamine inhibits aldosterone production via the D2 receptor coupled to Gαi signaling [62]; animals inactivated for the D2 dopamine receptor show twofold increased aldosterone levels [2]. This regulation may involve Gαi-mediated decrease in PKA signaling but also a Gβγ-dependent stimulatory effect on GIRK4 channel function. Indeed, a potentiation of GIRK channel activity by dopamine via the D2 receptor is a characteristic feature of GIRK1/GIRK4 heterotetramers [34]. A second factor possibly implicating GIRK channels to regulate aldosterone production is vasopressin. Vasopressin is a Ca^{2+}-mobilizing agonist binding to the V1 receptor in glomerulosa cells. In glomerulosa cell-enriched primary cultures, vasopressin increased aldosterone secretion and was found to be as potent as AngII in stimulating aldosterone secretion, phosphoinositide turnover, and Ca^{2+} mobilization [25]. Similarly to AngII, the action of vasopressin on V1 involves Gαq-PLC-mediated PIP2 hydrolysis, with increased calcium signaling resulting from mobilization of Ca^{2+} from intracellular IP3-dependent stores [55]. In addition, it has been shown that vasopressin increases intracellular Ca^{2+} concentrations via increased Ca^{2+} influx. This latter mechanism may involve inhibition of GIRK activity via PLC-mediated PIP2 hydrolysis (see above).

Conclusion

Different recurrent somatic mutations of *KCNJ5*, *ATP1A1*, and *ATP2B3* have been identified in APA as well as germline mutations of *KCNJ5* in familial hyperaldosteronism type III. These mutations affect the zona glomerulosa cell membrane potential and ionic homeostasis, leading to increased calcium signaling which promotes increased aldosterone biosynthesis and possible cell proliferation. Gene expression studies in a large series of APA did not identify distinctive molecular features of APA carrying mutations compared with non-mutated tumors [9]. This suggests that eventually the remaining 50 % of APA without identified mutations harbor genomic changes (structural changes, gene expression changes) that converge to altered ionic homeostasis as a central pathogenic mechanism of primary aldosteronism.

References

1. Akerstrom T, Crona J, Delgado Verdugo A, Starker LF, Cupisti K, Willenberg HS, Knoefel WT, Saeger W, Feller A, Ip J, Soon P, Anlauf M, Alesina PF, Schmid KW, Decaussin M, Levillain P, Wangberg B, Peix JL, Robinson B, Zedenius J, Backdahl M, Caramuta S, Iwen KA, Botling J, Stalberg P, Kraimps JL, Dralle H, Hellman P, Sidhu S, Westin G, Lehnert H, Walz MK, Akerstrom G, Carling T, Choi M, Lifton RP, Bjorklund P (2012) Comprehensive Re-Sequencing of Adrenal Aldosterone Producing Lesions Reveal Three Somatic Mutations near the KCNJ5 Potassium Channel Selectivity Filter. PLoS One 7(7):e41926
2. Armando I, Wang X, Villar VA, Jones JE, Asico LD, Escano C, Jose PA (2007) Reactive oxygen species-dependent hypertension in dopamine D2 receptor-deficient mice. Hypertension 49(3):672–678
3. Arnold J (1866) Ein Beitrag zur feineren Struktur und dem Chemismus des Nebennieren. Virchows Arch Patholog Anatomie Physiol Klin Med 35:64–107
4. Azizan EA, Murthy M, Stowasser M, Gordon R, Kowalski B, Xu S, Brown MJ, O'Shaughnessy KM (2012) Somatic Mutations Affecting the Selectivity Filter of KCNJ5 Are Frequent in 2 Large Unselected Collections of Adrenal Aldosteronomas. Hypertension 59(3):587–591
5. Bandulik S, Penton D, Barhanin J, Warth R (2010) TASK1 and TASK3 potassium channels: determinants of aldosterone secretion and adrenocortical zonation. Horm Metab Res 42(6):450–457

6. Bassett MH, White PC, Rainey WE (2004) The regulation of aldosterone synthase expression. Mol Cell Endocrinol 217(1–2):67–74
7. Beuschlein F, Boulkroun S, Osswald A, Wieland T, Nielsen HN, Lichtenauer UD, Penton D, Schack VR, Amar L, Fischer E, Walther A, Tauber P, Schwarzmayr T, Diener S, Graf E, Allolio B, Samson-Couterie B, Benecke A, Quinkler M, Fallo F, Plouin PF, Mantero F, Meitinger T, Mulatero P, Jeunemaitre X, Warth R, Vilsen B, Zennaro MC, Strom TM, Reincke M (2013) Somatic mutations in ATP1A1 and ATP2B3 lead to aldosterone-producing adenomas and secondary hypertension. Nat Genet 45(4):440–444
8. Blaustein MP, Juhaszova M, Golovina VA (1998) The cellular mechanism of action of cardiotonic steroids: a new hypothesis. Clin Exp Hypertens 20(5–6):691–703
9. Boulkroun S, Beuschlein F, Rossi GP, Golib-Dzib JF, Fischer E, Amar L, Mulatero P, Samson-Couterie B, Hahner S, Quinkler M, Fallo F, Letizia C, Allolio B, Ceolotto G, Cicala MV, Lang K, Lefebvre H, Lenzini L, Maniero C, Monticone S, Perrocheau M, Pilon C, Plouin PF, Rayes N, Seccia TM, Veglio F, Williams TA, Zinnamosca L, Mantero F, Benecke A, Jeunemaitre X, Reincke M, Zennaro MC (2012) Prevalence, Clinical, and Molecular Correlates of KCNJ5 Mutations in Primary Aldosteronism. Hypertension 59(3):592–598
10. Boulkroun S, Samson-Couterie B, Dzib JF, Lefebvre H, Louiset E, Amar L, Plouin PF, Lalli E, Jeunemaitre X, Benecke A, Meatchi T, Zennaro MC (2010) Adrenal cortex remodeling and functional zona glomerulosa hyperplasia in primary aldosteronism. Hypertension 56(5):885–892
11. Brini M, Cali T, Ottolini D, Carafoli E (2013) The plasma membrane calcium pump in health and disease. FEBS J 280(21):5385–5397
12. Carafoli E, Brini M (2000) Calcium pumps: structural basis for and mechanism of calcium transmembrane transport. Curr Opin Chem Biol 4(2):152–161
13. Carey RM, Thorner MO, Ortt EM (1980) Dopaminergic inhibition of metoclopramide-induced aldosterone secretion in man. Dissociation of responses to dopamine and bromocriptine. J Clin Invest 66(1):10–18
14. Charmandari E, Sertedaki A, Kino T, Merakou C, Hoffman DA, Hatch MM, Hurt DE, Lin L, Xekouki P, Stratakis CA, Chrousos GP (2012) A Novel Point Mutation in the KCNJ5 Gene Causing Primary Hyperaldosteronism and Early-Onset Autosomal Dominant Hypertension. J Clin Endocrinol Metab 97(8):E1532–E1539
15. Choi M, Scholl UI, Yue P, Bjorklund P, Zhao B, Nelson-Williams C, Ji W, Cho Y, Patel A, Men CJ, Lolis E, Wisgerhof MV, Geller DS, Mane S, Hellman P, Westin G, Akerstrom G, Wang W, Carling T, Lifton RP (2011) K+ channel mutations in adrenal aldosterone-producing adenomas and hereditary hypertension. Science 331(6018):768–772
16. Connell JM, Davies E (2005) The new biology of aldosterone. J Endocrinol 186(1):1–20
17. Corey S, Clapham DE (1998) Identification of native atrial G-protein-regulated inwardly rectifying K+ (GIRK4) channel homomultimers. J Biol Chem 273(42):27499–27504
18. Davies LA, Hu C, Guagliardo NA, Sen N, Chen X, Talley EM, Carey RM, Bayliss DA, Barrett PQ (2008) TASK channel deletion in mice causes primary hyperaldosteronism. Proc Natl Acad Sci U S A 105(6):2203–2208
19. Einholm AP, Andersen JP, Vilsen B (2007) Importance of Leu99 in transmembrane segment M1 of the Na+, K+-ATPase in the binding and occlusion of K+. J Biol Chem 282(33): 23854–23866
20. Escoubet B, Coureau C, Bonvalet JP, Farman N (1997) Noncoordinate regulation of epithelial Na channel and Na pump subunit mRNAs in kidney and colon by aldosterone. Am J Physiol 272(5 Pt 1):C1482–C1491
21. Falchetto R, Vorherr T, Carafoli E (1992) The calmodulin-binding site of the plasma membrane Ca2+ pump interacts with the transduction domain of the enzyme. Protein Sci 1(12): 1613–1621
22. Geering K (2008) Functional roles of Na, K-ATPase subunits. Curr Opin Nephrol Hypertens 17(5):526–532
23. Geller DS, Zhang J, Wisgerhof MV, Shackleton C, Kashgarian M, Lifton RP (2008) A novel form of human Mendelian hypertension featuring nonglucocorticoid-remediable aldosteronism. J Clin Endocrinol Metab 93(8):3117–3123

24. Guagliardo NA, Yao J, Hu C, Schertz EM, Tyson DA, Carey RM, Bayliss DA, Barrett PQ (2012) TASK-3 channel deletion in mice recapitulates low-renin essential hypertension. Hypertension 59(5):999–1005
25. Guillon G, Trueba M, Joubert D, Grazzini E, Chouinard L, Cote M, Payet MD, Manzoni O, Barberis C, Robert M et al (1995) Vasopressin stimulates steroid secretion in human adrenal glands: comparison with angiotensin-II effect. Endocrinology 136(3):1285–1295
26. Hajnoczky G, Csordas G, Hunyady L, Kalapos MP, Balla T, Enyedi P, Spat A (1992) Angiotensin-II inhibits Na+/K+ pump in rat adrenal glomerulosa cells: possible contribution to stimulation of aldosterone production. Endocrinology 130(3):1637–1644
27. Hattangady NG, Olala LO, Bollag WB, Rainey WE (2012) Acute and chronic regulation of aldosterone production. Mol Cell Endocrinol 350(2):151–162
28. Hedin KE, Lim NF, Clapham DE (1996) Cloning of a Xenopus laevis inwardly rectifying K+ channel subunit that permits GIRK1 expression of IKACh currents in oocytes. Neuron 16(2):423–429
29. Heitzmann D, Derand R, Jungbauer S, Bandulik S, Sterner C, Schweda F, El Wakil A, Lalli E, Guy N, Mengual R, Reichold M, Tegtmeier I, Bendahhou S, Gomez-Sanchez CE, Aller MI, Wisden W, Weber A, Lesage F, Warth R, Barhanin J (2008) Invalidation of TASK1 potassium channels disrupts adrenal gland zonation and mineralocorticoid homeostasis. Embo J 27(1): 179–187
30. Hibino H, Inanobe A, Furutani K, Murakami S, Findlay I, Kurachi Y (2010) Inwardly rectifying potassium channels: their structure, function, and physiological roles. Physiological reviews 90(1):291–366
31. Jorgensen PL, Hakansson KO, Karlish SJ (2003) Structure and mechanism of Na, K-ATPase: functional sites and their interactions. Annu Rev Physiol 65:817–849
32. Kaplan JH (2002) Biochemistry of Na, K-ATPase. Annu Rev Biochem 71:511–535
33. Kobrinsky E, Mirshahi T, Zhang H, Jin T, Logothetis D (2000) Receptor-mediated hydrolysis of plasma membrane messenger PIP2 leads to K+-current desensitization. Nat Cell Biol 2(8):507–514
34. Krapivinsky G, Gordon EA, Wickman K, Velimirovic B, Krapivinsky L, Clapham DE (1995) The G-protein-gated atrial K+ channel IKACh is a heteromultimer of two inwardly rectifying K(+)-channel proteins. Nature 374(6518):135–141
35. Kubo Y, Baldwin TJ, Jan YN, Jan LY (1993) Primary structure and functional expression of a mouse inward rectifier potassium channel. Nature 362(6416):127–133
36. Lu Z (2004) Mechanism of rectification in inward-rectifier K+ channels. Annu Rev Physiol 66:103–129. doi:10.1146/annurev.physiol.66.032102.150822
37. Makary SM, Claydon TW, Dibb KM, Boyett MR (2006) Base of pore loop is important for rectification, activation, permeation, and block of Kir3.1/Kir3.4. Biophys J 90(11):4018–4034
38. McKenna TJ, Island DP, Nicholson WE, Liddle GW (1979) Dopamine inhibits angiotensin-stimulated aldosterone biosynthesis in bovine adrenal cells. J Clin Invest 64(1):287–291
39. Monticone S, Hattangady NG, Nishimoto K, Mantero F, Rubin B, Cicala MV, Pezzani R, Auchus RJ, Ghayee HK, Shibata H, Kurihara I, Williams TA, Giri JG, Bollag RJ, Edwards MA, Isales CM, Rainey WE (2012) Effect of KCNJ5 Mutations on Gene Expression in Aldosterone-Producing Adenomas and Adrenocortical Cells. J Clin Endocrinol Metab 97(8):E1567–E1572
40. Mulatero P, Tauber P, Zennaro MC, Monticone S, Lang K, Beuschlein F, Fischer E, Tizzani D, Pallauf A, Viola A, Amar L, Williams TA, Strom TM, Graf E, Bandulik S, Penton D, Plouin PF, Warth R, Allolio B, Jeunemaitre X, Veglio F, Reincke M (2012) KCNJ5 mutations in European families with nonglucocorticoid remediable familial hyperaldosteronism. Hypertension 59(2):235–240
41. Navarro B, Kennedy ME, Velimirovic B, Bhat D, Peterson AS, Clapham DE (1996) Nonselective and G betagamma-insensitive weaver K+ channels. Science 272(5270):1950–1953
42. Neri G, De Toni R, Tortorella C, Rebuffat P, Bova S, Cargnelli G, Petrelli L, Spinazzi R, Nussdorfer GG (2006) Ouabain chronic infusion enhances the growth and steroidogenic capacity of rat adrenal zona glomerulosa: the possible involvement of the endothelin system. Int J Mol Med 18(2):315–319

43. Nishida M, MacKinnon R (2002) Structural basis of inward rectification: cytoplasmic pore of the G protein-gated inward rectifier GIRK1 at 1.8 A resolution. Cell 111(7):957–965
44. Oki K, Plonczynski M, Lam M, Gomez-Sanchez E, Gomez-Sanchez C (2012) The potassium channel, Kir3.4 participates in angiotensin II-stimulated aldosterone production by a human adrenocortical cell line. Endocrinology 153(9):4328–4335
45. Oki K, Plonczynski MW, Luis Lam M, Gomez-Sanchez EP, Gomez-Sanchez CE (2012) Potassium Channel Mutant KCNJ5 T158A Expression in HAC-15 Cells Increases Aldosterone Synthesis. Endocrinology 153(4):1774–1782
46. Okubo S, Niimura F, Nishimura H, Takemoto F, Fogo A, Matsusaka T, Ichikawa I (1997) Angiotensin-independent mechanism for aldosterone synthesis during chronic extracellular fluid volume depletion. J Clin Invest 99(5):855–860
47. Penton D, Bandulik S, Schweda F, Haubs S, Tauber P, Reichold M, Cong LD, El Wakil A, Budde T, Lesage F, Lalli E, Zennaro MC, Warth R, Barhanin J (2012) Task3 potassium channel gene invalidation causes low renin and salt-sensitive arterial hypertension. Endocrinology 153(10):4740–4748
48. Pierre SV, Xie Z (2006) The Na, K-ATPase receptor complex: its organization and membership. Cell Biochem Biophys 46(3):303–316
49. Robillard L, Ethier N, Lachance M, Hebert TE (2000) Gbetagamma subunit combinations differentially modulate receptor and effector coupling in vivo. Cell Signal 12(9–10):673–682
50. Rosenhouse-Dantsker A, Sui JL, Zhao Q, Rusinova R, Rodriguez-Menchaca AA, Zhang Z, Logothetis DE (2008) A sodium-mediated structural switch that controls the sensitivity of Kir channels to PtdIns(4,5)P(2). Nat Chem Biol 4(10):624–631
51. Saitoh O, Kubo Y, Miyatani Y, Asano T, Nakata H (1997) RGS8 accelerates G-protein-mediated modulation of K+ currents. Nature 390(6659):525–529
52. Scholl UI, Nelson-Williams C, Yue P, Grekin R, Wyatt RJ, Dillon MJ, Couch R, Hammer LK, Harley FL, Farhi A, Wang WH, Lifton RP (2012) Hypertension with or without adrenal hyperplasia due to different inherited mutations in the potassium channel KCNJ5. Proc Natl Acad Sci U S A 109(7):2533–2538
53. Schwarzer S, Nobles M, Tinker A (2010) Do caveolae have a role in the fidelity and dynamics of receptor activation of G-protein-gated inwardly rectifying potassium channels? J Biol Chem 285(36):27817–27826
54. Silva E, Soares-da-Silva P (2012) New insights into the regulation of Na+, K+-ATPase by ouabain. Int Rev Cell Mol Biol 294:99–132
55. Spat A, Hunyady L (2004) Control of aldosterone secretion: a model for convergence in cellular signaling pathways. Physiol Rev 84(2):489–539
56. Sui JL, Chan KW, Logothetis DE (1996) Na+activation of the muscarinic K+ channel by a G-protein-independent mechanism. J Gen Physiol 108(5):381–391
57. Taguchi R, Yamada M, Nakajima Y, Satoh T, Hashimoto K, Shibusawa N, Ozawa A, Okada S, Rokutanda N, Takata D, Koibuchi Y, Horiguchi J, Oyama T, Takeyoshi I, Mori M (2012) Expression and Mutations of KCNJ5 mRNA in Japanese Patients with Aldosterone-Producing Adenomas. J Clin Endocrinol Metab 97(4):1311–1319
58. Tait JF, Tait SA (1976) The effect of changes in potassium concentration on the maximal steroidogenic response of purified zona glomerulosa cells to angiotensin II. J Steroid Biochem 7(9):687–690
59. Wang HY, O'Doherty GA (2012) Modulators of Na/K-ATPase: a patent review. Expert Opin Ther Pat 22(6):587–605
60. Whorton MR, MacKinnon R (2011) Crystal structure of the mammalian GIRK2 K+ channel and gating regulation by G proteins, PIP2, and sodium. Cell 147(1):199–208
61. Willars GB (2006) Mammalian RGS proteins: multifunctional regulators of cellular signalling. Semin Cell Dev Biol 17(3):363–376
62. Wu KD, Chen YM, Chu TS, Chueh SC, Wu MH, Bor-Shen H (2001) Expression and localization of human dopamine D2 and D4 receptor mRNA in the adrenal gland, aldosterone-producing adenoma, and pheochromocytoma. J Clin Endocrinol Metab 86(9):4460–4467
63. Yingst D, Davis J, Schiebinger R (2000) Inhibitors of tyrosine phosphatases block angiotensin II inhibition of Na(+) pump. Eur J Pharmacol 406(1):49–52

64. Yingst D, Davis J, Schiebinger R (2001) Effects of extracellular calcium and potassium on the sodium pump of rat adrenal glomerulosa cells. Am J Physiol Cell Physiol 280(1):25
65. Yingst DR, Davis J, Krenz S, Schiebinger RJ (1999) Insights into the mechanism by which inhibition of Na, K-ATPase stimulates aldosterone production. Metabolism 48(9):1167–1171
66. Young DB, Smith MJ Jr, Jackson TE, Scott RE (1984) Multiplicative interaction between angiotensin II and K concentration in stimulation of aldosterone. Am J Physiol 247(3 Pt 1): E328–E335
67. Zylbergold P, Ramakrishnan N, Hebert T (2010) The role of G proteins in assembly and function of Kir3 inwardly rectifying potassium channels. Channels (Austin) 4(5):411–421

Chapter 6
Familial Hyperaldosteronism Type I

Paolo Mulatero, Silvia Monticone, Franco Veglio, and Tracy Ann Williams

Abstract Primary aldosteronism comprises sporadic and genetic forms. Three forms of familial hyperaldosteronism have been described so far. In this chapter we discuss the genetic basis, clinical phenotypes, and diagnosis and therapy of familial hyperaldosteronism type I. This condition is caused by the presence of the chimeric CYP11B1/CYP11B2 gene and displays unique characteristics such as the normalization of blood pressure and aldosterone levels after dexamethasone administration, the hyperproduction of the hybrid steroids 18-hydroxycortisol and 18-oxocortisol, and an increased rate of cerebrovascular events.

Keywords Glucocorticoid-remediable aldosteronism • Familial hyperaldosteronism • Primary aldosteronism • Aldosterone

Abbreviations

ACTH	Adrenocorticotropic hormone
APA	Aldosterone-producing adenoma
B	Corticosterone
BAH	Bilateral adrenal hyperplasia
CYP11B1	11β-Hydroxylase
CYP11B2	Aldosterone synthase
CYP17	17α-Hydroxylase
CYP21	21-Hydroxylase
DOC	Deoxycorticosterone

P. Mulatero, M.D. (✉) • S. Monticone • F. Veglio • T.A. Williams, Ph.D
Division of Internal Medicine and Hypertension, Department of Medical Sciences, University of Torino, Medicina Interna 4, Via Genova 3, Torino 10126, Italy
e-mail: paolo.mulatero@unito.it

P. Hellman (ed.), *Primary Aldosteronism: Molecular Genetics, Endocrinology, and Translational Medicine*, DOI 10.1007/978-1-4939-0509-6_6,

DST	Dexamethasone-suppression test
FH-I	Familial hyperaldosteronism type I
GRA	Glucocorticoid-remediable aldosteronism
MRA	Mineralocorticoid receptor antagonist
18OHB	18-Hydroxycorticosterone
18OHF	18-Hydroxycortisol
18oxoF	18-Oxocortisol
PA	Primary aldosteronism
PCR	Polymerase chain reaction
PRA	Plasma renin activity
SNP	Single-nucleotide polymorphism
UAH	Unilateral adrenal hyperplasia

Introduction

Primary aldosteronism (PA) was first described by Conn in 1955, when a condition of severe hypertension and hypokalemia in a 34-year-old woman was relieved after the removal of a 40 mm adrenocortical adenoma [1]. PA is now considered the most common secondary form of hypertension [2]. In addition, it has become also clear that aldosterone is responsible for cardiovascular inflammation and fibrosis [3] and that PA patients undergo cardiovascular events significantly more often than essential hypertensives [4]. PA subtype diagnosis is fundamental to address patients to the most appropriate therapy, surgical for aldosterone-producing adenoma (APA) and unilateral adrenal hyperplasia (UAH) and medical with mineralocorticoid receptor antagonists (MRA) for bilateral adrenal hyperplasia (BAH) patients. Together with sporadic PA, familial forms have also been described [5–7]. Early detection of these conditions is of paramount importance to allow targeted therapy, thereby preventing the damage associated with long-life inappropriate aldosterone production. In this chapter we describe the genetic cause, clinical and biochemical phenotypes, and diagnosis and therapy of familial hyperaldosteronism type I.

Historical Description

Familial hyperaldosteronism type I (FH-I) has also been defined in the past as dexamethasone-suppressible hyperaldosteronism and subsequently as glucocorticoid-remediable aldosteronism (GRA). FH-I was first described by Sutherland et al. [5] in a father and son (41 and 16 years old, respectively), both affected by hypertension and hypokalemic alkalosis. Interestingly, of the 11 uncles and aunties of the father 3 died of cerebrovascular events, 2 in their 40s, and 1 in his 60s. The father was hypertensive since he was 19 years old and the boy since he was 13. Electrocardiogram revealed left ventricular hypertrophy. Plasma renin activity (PRA) was undetectable in both subjects, both under normal and low-sodium diet. In the father, urinary aldosterone levels were markedly elevated and therefore he underwent left adrenalectomy; after surgery aldosterone levels were reduced by half but were still elevated. Adrenal exploration was undertaken because Conn's syndrome was suspected; no adenomas were found, and the left adrenal was removed because of its greater size compared to the contralateral. The adrenal showed multiple nodules of 1–4 mm composed of *zona fasciculata* cells [5]. The son also displayed high urinary aldosterone levels. Surprisingly, when dexamethasone 2 mg/day was given to patients, a normalization of blood pressure, plasma potassium levels, and PRA and a sustained inhibition of aldosterone secretion were observed.

A few months later, New and Peterson reported the case of a 12-year-old boy with hypertension and hypokalemic alkalosis, who was hypertensive since he was 2 years old and with a long history of polyuria, polydipsia, enuresis, and severe headache [8]. The patient displayed low PRA and high aldosterone levels. Again, dexamethasone determined a reduction of blood pressure and suppression of aldosterone to undetectable levels. Consistently, intravenous ACTH infusion determined an increase in blood pressure and aldosterone levels.

Subsequently, Miura et al. [9] reported a similar case in a 17 years old Japanese boy. Interestingly, the patient underwent complete removal of the left adrenal and half of the right adrenal without showing improvement of hypertension and hypokalemia; histology revealed in this case diffuse hyperplasia of the *zona fasciculata–reticularis* without nodules.

These three reports shed light on a new form of PA completely different from APA and with a familial basis.

Clinical Diagnosis

Between 1966 and 1992, diagnosis of FH-I was exclusively made on a clinical basis. In most cases, a positive diagnosis was made when a complete suppression of aldosterone levels was achieved during a dexamethasone-suppression test (DST) (Liddle JCEM 1960). The test is usually performed over 2–4 days when dexamethasone 0.5 mg is administered every 6 h [10, 11]. Consistently, ACTH infusion was shown to determine increased blood pressure and hypokalemia [12] and a greater increase in the plasma aldosterone and 18-hydroxycorticosterone (18OHB) compared to low-renin essential hypertensives, PA patients, and normal subjects [13]. Furthermore, aldosterone levels show a circadian rhythm similar to cortisol and are unresponsive to posture [14], in agreement with a dependency from ACTH and not from angiotensin II stimulation; however, normal angiotensin II response is restored during chronic dexamethasone therapy [15]. Interestingly, chronic ACTH administration determines a persistent increase in aldosterone production in contrast with normal subjects, where ACTH induces a transient increase in aldosterone secretion followed by return to normal levels in 1–2 days [12, 16]. Another distinct feature of FH-I is the abnormal production of the 17-hydroxylated analogs of 18OHB and aldosterone, 18-hydroxycortisol (18OHF) and 18-oxocortisol (18oxoF), also called "hybrid steroids" [16, 17]. Before the discovery of the genetic cause of FH-I, the increased production of 18OHF and 18oxoF in this disease suggested the possibility that FH-I could be caused by a disorder of the adrenal transitional zone in cells expressing both the 17-hydroxylase and the P-450-corticosterone methyl oxidase complex necessary for the 18-hydroxylation and 18-oxidation of corticosterone [16].

Genetic Cause of FH-I

The genetic cause of FH-I was demonstrated in 1992 to be due to a chimeric CYP11B1/CYP11B2 gene [18, 19]. This hybrid gene results from an unequal crossing over between CYP11B1 and CYP11B2 genes during meiosis, thereby forming a fusion gene comprising sequences from CYP11B1 at the 5′ end (including ACTH regulatory sequences) and sequences from CYP11B2 at the 3′ end, enough to confer aldosterone synthase activity to the chimeric enzyme [20] (Fig. 6.1).

CYP11B2 encodes aldosterone synthase, a mitochondrial cytochrome P450 enzyme that synthesizes aldosterone from deoxycorticosterone (DOC). Aldosterone synthase catalyzes three reactions: 11β-hydroxylation of DOC to corticosterone (B),

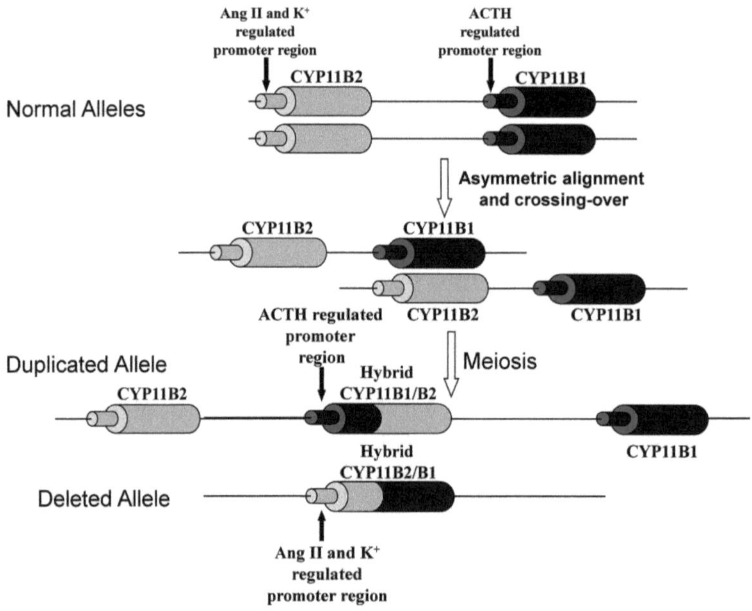

Fig. 6.1 The asymmetric alignment and crossing over between CYP11B1 (in *black*) and CYP11B2 (in *grey*) genes produce a hybrid CYP11B1/CYP11B2 gene with the promoter region of CYP11B1 (regulated by ACTH) and a portion of CYP11B2 sufficient to confer aldosterone synthase activity to the encoded hybrid enzyme. In the deleted allele, CYP11B2 is at the 5′ end and CYP11B1 at the 3′ end (see text)

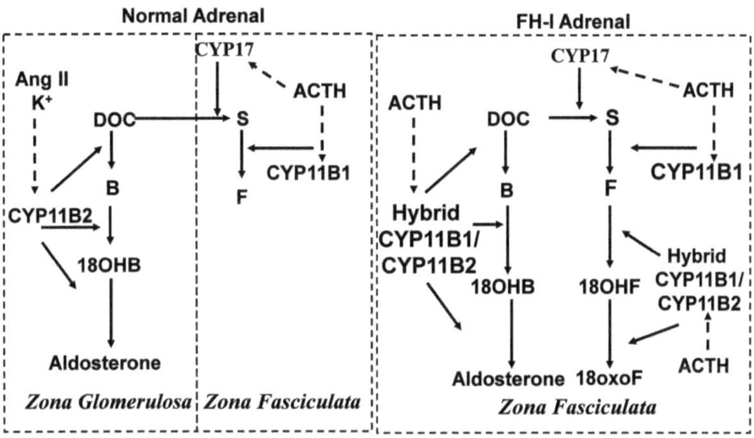

Fig. 6.2 In the normal zonation of the adrenal cortex, in the zona glomerulosa CYP11B2, under the control of angiotensin II and potassium, converts DOC to B, 18OHB, and aldosterone, whereas CYP11B1, under the control of ACTH, converts S to F. When biochemical zonation is disturbed by the simultaneous expression of the hybrid CYP11B1/CYP11B2 enzyme and CYP17, the hybrid enzyme, under the control of ACTH, is able to convert DOC to aldosterone and F to 18OHF and 18oxoF

18-hydroxylation of B to 18OHB, and, finally, 18-oxidation of 18OHB to aldosterone [21, 22]. CYP11B2 is located in chromosomal region 8q24.3, at a distance of 40 kb from CYP11B1, that encodes 11β-hydroxylase [23, 24]. This enzyme synthesizes cortisol from the precursor 11-deoxycortisol (Fig. 6.2). Different expression patterns ensure differential steroid production and zonation in the adrenal cortex: CYP11B1 is expressed throughout the entire cortex and is mainly regulated by ACTH, CYP11B2 is exclusively expressed in the *zona glomerulosa* and is regulated by angiotensin II and potassium levels, and CYP17 (17α-hydroxylase that converts 11-deoxycortisol to cortisol) is selectively expressed in the *zona fasciculata* (Fig. 6.2). Therefore aldosterone is exclusively produced in the *zona glomerulosa* and cortisol in the *zona fasciculata–reticularis*. The simultaneous presence of the hybrid enzyme and of CYP17 determines the abnormal production of the hybrid steroids [25] (Fig. 6.2).

The recombination between the two genes allows the diagnosis of FH-I by Southern blot analysis in which a new band, specific for the hybrid gene, appears with BamHI and EcoR1 restriction enzyme digestion [18, 20, 26]. The asymmetrical recombination between the two genes is made possible by the high degree of homology between the two genes (95 % in the coding regions, 90 % in the introns, and 93 % identity of the amino acid sequence) [25]. The hybrid enzyme is expressed in the *zona fasciculata* of the adrenal cortex and produces aldosterone, 18OHF, and 18oxoF under the regulatory control of ACTH [26, 27]. To date, chimeric genes responsible for FH-I have always been shown to have the point of recombination between intron 2 and exon 4 [28] (Fig. 6.3). Subsequently, it was shown that only two residues are

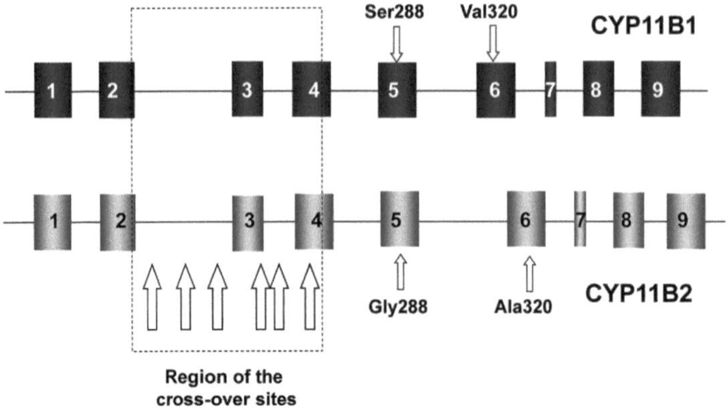

Fig. 6.3 Schematic description of CYP11B1 and CYP11B2 gene structures, displaying a high degree of homology (95 % of identity in coding sequences) except for a small insertion in intron 5 of CYP11B2. The region in which the crossing over occurs is indicated as is the location of nucleotides encoding residues 288 and 320 which are fundamental for the 18-hydroxylase and 18-oxidase activities of CYP11B2, respectively

indispensable for aldosterone synthase activity: Gly288 and Ala320 [29] (Fig. 6.3). Glycine 288 is responsible for the 18-hydroxylase activity and alanine 320 for 18-oxidase activity; consistent with these observations, the substitution of Ser288 and Val320 in CYP11B1 with the corresponding residues in CYP11B2 confers 18-hydroxylase and 18-oxidase activities so that the new enzyme can synthesize aldosterone from DOC. Similarly the substitution of Gly288 in CYP11B2 with a serine disrupts aldosterone synthase activities [26, 29]. Theoretically, FH-I could also be determined by a gene conversion between CYP11B1 and CYP11B2 genes rather than by the asymmetrical crossing over [26, 30]. Gene conversion is a non-reciprocal recombination involving the transfer of genetic information from one allele or homologous gene to another that is a frequent cause of 21-hydroxylase deficiency due to a recombination between CYP21 and CYP21P (homologous pseudogene carrying deleterious mutations) [31]. However, despite intensive investigations, this type of recombination has never been demonstrated in PA and FH-I patients [26]. Since aldosterone secretion is frequently regulated by ACTH rather than by angiotensin II in APA, the presence of the chimeric gene, or mutations in residues 288 and 320 of CYP11B1 converting it into an aldosterone-producing enzyme, was investigated in the DNA extracted from APA: none of the APA patients displayed the chimeric gene or mutations in exons 5 and 6 of CYP11B1 [32, 33].

Interestingly, the deleted allele carrying the hybrid CYP11B2/CYP11B1 gene complementary to that responsible for FH-I has been shown to be responsible for a clinical phenotype of congenital adrenal hyperplasia associated with 11β-hydroxylase deficiency [34].

Diagnosis, Prevalence, and Phenotypes

FH-I diagnosis became even easier after 1995 [35] with the introduction of the long-polymerase chain reaction (PCR) strategy for the amplification of the hybrid gene [10, 26, 35]. This rapid and efficient method substituted the DST and the hybrid steroid measurement for FH-I diagnosis; it should be emphasized that DST could result in a relatively high rate of falsely positive diagnoses of FH-I [10, 36]. Furthermore, the increase in hybrid steroid production is not pathognomonic of FH-I, because these steroids can also be produced in variable amounts in patients with APA [37, 38] and in some FH-III families [7]. Therefore, the clinical tests have been progressively abandoned and FH-I diagnosis is currently performed by long-PCR amplification of the hybrid CYP11B1/CYP11B2 gene.

Current guidelines of the Endocrine Society [39] suggest to test for FH-I in all patients with the onset of PA earlier than 20 years of age and in those who have a family history of PA or of strokes at young age (<40 years). However, due to the benefit of an early diagnosis and the requirement of a specific therapy, some authors, including our group, prefer to systematically test all PA patients [40, 41]. The prevalence of FH-I has been found to be inferior to 1 % of all PA patients [42, 43]. Random screening of hypertensive patients has proven to be unsuccessful [26, 36, 44–46]. However, screening in targeted patients (hypertensive individuals with a history of resistant hypertension, with a family history of intracranial hemorrhage or resistant hypertension and or a history of hypokalemia) resulted in the detection of new FH-I cases [47].

Another subgroup of patients in which FH-I (and in general genetic forms of PA) should be considered is hypertensive children: it has been recently shown that among untreated hypertensive children (4–16 years old), the prevalence of FH-I was 3.1 % [48].

The possibility of performing FH-I diagnosis with an easy and relatively inexpensive test enabled clinicians to recognize many FH-I patients with mild clinical phenotypes [49] and even asymptomatic normotensive individuals [36].

The clinical phenotypes of FH-I families cover the whole spectrum of hypertension severity, from resistant hypokalemic hypertension to normokalemic mild hypertension and to asymptomatic normotension. The possible reason for such a wide variation in the severity of hypertension has been extensively investigated: the role of sodium intake has been ruled out by many authors [50, 51] as well as the possibility of a different gene expression dependent on the site of the crossing over [20]. The role of aldosterone and 18OHF and 18oxoF levels (as an index of the hybrid enzyme activity) has been shown by some authors [38, 51] but not by others [28]. Also the protective role of urinary kallikrein has been shown in some families [28] but not in others [38]. Finally, some authors have reported higher blood pressure in males [51] and in patients inheriting the hybrid gene from their mothers who also had higher aldosterone levels [52]. This last observation was interpreted as being the result of chronic exposure in utero to elevated aldosterone levels that could determine increased aldosterone responsiveness later in life.

It should be noted that the extreme phenotypic variability applies not only in comparisons between families but also between members of the same pedigree [28, 38, 51–53]. Interestingly, in some cases, patients with florid biochemical hyperaldosteronism showed normal blood pressure levels, but also subjects carrying the hybrid gene displayed normal aldosterone and unsuppressed renin [53]. The most probable explanation for the clinical variability is the effect of genetic variations at genes encoding proteins involved in sodium handling or in modulating the mineralocorticoid response: for example SNPs on the bradykinin B2 receptor and in the alpha-adducin gene have been shown to affect blood pressure levels in patients with sporadic PA [54].

As in sporadic PA, most FH-I patients are normokalemic [50], and therefore, genetic screening should not be restricted to the hypokalemic patient.

Generally, patients with FH-I display normal adrenals at CT scanning. However, in the few cases that have been adrenalectomized, a diffuse hyperplasia of the zona fasciculata, with or without nodules, has been observed [5, 9]. In one French family comprising seven affected individuals, two also had adrenal adenomas and two others had micronodular adrenal hyperplasia [27]. The reason for the hyperplasia/adrenal nodules in those subjects is still unknown.

Patients with FH-I display a high risk of cerebrovascular complications, around 20 % of the patients and 50 % of the families [55]. The most frequent event is cerebral hemorrhage (70 % of cases) due to ruptured intracranial aneurysms, which is often fatal (60 % mortality). The mean age of the event is 32 years [55]. It has been hypothesized that hypertension and/or the excess of aldosterone during early phases of the cerebrovascular development could favor the formation of aneurysms [55]. FH-I women display increased prevalence of pregnancy-aggravated hypertension but not of preeclampsia [56]. Interestingly, FH-I subjects display evidence of abnormal left ventricular structure and function already in the normotensive stage of the disease [57], consistent with the hypothesis that increased aldosterone levels are associated with target organ damage at least in part independent of the effects on blood pressure levels. This raises the question whether FH-I subjects should be treated with dexamethasone and/or MR antagonists even if blood pressure is still normal.

Therapy

FH-I treatment is based primarily on glucocorticoid administration in order to inhibit the ACTH-stimulated aldosterone production [39]. Dexamethasone and prednisone are the most used steroids for their long half-lives and should be taken at bed time to suppress the morning ACTH peak. In adult patients, doses of dexamethasone of 0.125–0.25 mg/day (or prednisone 2.5–5 mg/day) are usually sufficient to control hyperaldosteronism and hypokalemia (if present). The minimum dose necessary to control blood pressure should be suggested in order to avoid cushingoid side effects [39, 58]. MR antagonists such as spironolactone and eplerenone can be associated to glucocorticoids to obtain blood pressure control.

The use of eplerenone may be preferred in FH-I children to avoid potential growth retardation and antiandrogenic effects associated with glucocorticoids and spironolactone, respectively [39, 59]. In all FH-I patients sodium intake should be restricted even in the normotensive phase.

Conclusions

Familial hyperaldosteronism type I is a rare but often severe and potentially fatal form of genetic hyperaldosteronism that should be carefully excluded in at least some subgroups of patients, such as subjects with the onset of PA earlier than 20 years of age and in those who have a family history of PA or of strokes at a young age, who have been shown to have an increased risk of suffering from this disease. Recent studies have shown that FH-I may be relatively frequent in hypertensive children, and therefore, this category of patients should also be tested. The existence of specific therapy for FH-I and the high risk of cerebrovascular complications may suggest that all PA patients should be tested to offer them and their affected relatives the appropriate treatment.

References

1. Conn JW (1955) Primary aldosteronism. J Lab Clin Med 45:661–664
2. Mulatero P, Stowasser M, Loh KC, Fardella CE, Gordon RD, Mosso L, Gomez-Sanchez CE, Veglio F, Young WF Jr (2004) Increased diagnosis of primary aldosteronism, including surgically correctable forms, in centers from five continents. J Clin Endocrinol Metab 89:1045–1050
3. Mulatero P, Milan A, Williams TA, Veglio F (2006) Mineralocorticoid receptor blockade in the protection of target organ damage. Cardiovasc Hematol Agents Med Chem 4:75–91
4. Milliez P, Girerd X, Plouin PF, Blacher J, Safar ME, Mourad JJ (2005) Evidence for an increased rate of cardiovascular events in patients with primary aldosteronism. J Am Coll Cardiol 45:1243–1248
5. Sutherland DJ, Ruse JL, Laidlaw JC (1966) Hypertension, increased aldosterone secretion and low plasma renin activity relieved by dexamethasone. Can Med Assoc J 95:1109–1119
6. Gordon RD, Stowasser M, Tunny TJ, Klemm SA, Finn WL, Krek AL (1991) Clinical and pathological diversity of primary aldosteronism, including a new familial variety. Clin Exp Pharmacol Physiol 18:283–286
7. Geller DS, Zhang J, Wisgerhof MV, Shackleton C, Kashgarian M, Lifton RP (2008) A novel form of human Mendelian hypertension featuring nonglucocorticoid-remediable aldosteronism. J Clin Endocrinol Metab 93:3117–3123
8. New MI, Peterson RE (1967) A new form of congenital adrenal hyperplasia. J Clin Endocrinol Metab 27:300–305
9. Miura K, Yoshinaga K, Goto K, Katsushima I, Maebashi M, Demura H, Iino M, Demura R, Torikai T (1968) A case of glucocorticoid-responsive hyperaldosteronism. J Clin Endocrinol Metab 28:1807–1815
10. Mulatero P, Veglio F, Pilon C, Rabbia F, Zocchi C, Limone P, Boscaro M, Sonino N, Fallo F (1998) Diagnosis of glucocorticoid-remediable aldosteronism in primary aldosteronism: aldosterone response to dexamethasone and long polymerase chain reaction for chimeric gene. J Clin Endocrinol Metab 83:2573–2575

11. Litchfield WR, New MI, Coolidge C, Lifton RP, Dluhy RG (1997) Evaluation of the dexamethasone suppression test for the diagnosis of glucocorticoid-remediable aldosteronism. J Clin Endocrinol Metab 82:3570–3573
12. New MI, Peterson RE, Saenger P, Levine LS (1976) Evidence for an unidentified ACTH-induced steroid hormone causing hypertension. J Clin Endocrinol Metab 43:1283–1293
13. Ganguly A, Weinberger MH, Guthrie GP, Fineberg NS (1984) Adrenal steroid responses to ACTH in glucocorticoid-suppressible aldosteronism. Hypertension 6:563–567
14. Ganguly A, Grim CE, Weinberger MH (1981) Anomalous postural aldosterone response in glucocorticoid-suppressible hyperaldosteronism. N Engl J Med 305:991–993
15. Connell JM, Kenyon CJ, Corrie JE, Fraser R, Watt R, Lever AF (1986) Dexamethasone-suppressible hyperaldosteronism. Adrenal transition cell hyperplasia? Hypertension 8:669–676
16. Gomez-Sanchez CE, Gill JR Jr, Ganguly A, Gordon RD (1988) Glucocorticoid-suppressible aldosteronism: a disorder of the adrenal transitional zone. J Clin Endocrinol Metab 67: 444–448
17. Ulick S, Chan CK, Gill JR Jr, Gutkin M, Letcher L, Mantero F, New MI (1990) Defective fasciculata zone function as the mechanism of glucocorticoid-remediable aldosteronism. J Clin Endocrinol Metab 71:1151–1157
18. Lifton RP, Dluhy RG, Powers M, Rich GM, Cook S, Ulick S, Lalouel JM (1992) A chimaeric 11 beta-hydroxylase/aldosterone synthase gene causes glucocorticoid-remediable aldosteronism and human hypertension. Nature 355:262–265
19. Lifton RP, Dluhy RG, Powers M, Rich GM, Gutkin M, Fallo F, Gill JR Jr, Feld L, Ganguly A, Laidlaw JC, Murnaghan DJ, Kaufman C, Stockigt JR, Ulick S, Lalouel J-M (1992) Hereditary hypertension caused by chimaeric gene duplications and ectopic expression of aldosterone synthase. Nat Genet 2:66–74
20. Pascoe L, Curnow KM, Slutsker L, Connell JM, Speiser PW, New MI, White PC (1992) Glucocorticoid-suppressible hyperaldosteronism results from hybrid genes created by unequal crossovers between CYP11B1 and CYP11B2. Proc Natl Acad Sci U S A 89:8327–8331
21. Curnow KM, Tusie-Luna MT, Pascoe L, Natarajan R, Gu JL, Nadler JL, White PC (1991) The product of the CYP11B2 gene is required for aldosterone biosynthesis in the human adrenal cortex. Mol Endocrinol 5:1513–1522
22. Kawamoto T, Mitsuuchi Y, Toda K, Yokoyama Y, Miyahara K, Miura S, Ohnishi T, Ichikawa Y, Nakao K, Imura H et al (1992) Role of steroid 11 beta-hydroxylase and steroid 18-hydroxylase in the biosynthesis of glucocorticoids and mineralocorticoids in humans. Proc Natl Acad Sci U S A 89:1458–1462
23. Taymans SE, Pack S, Pak E, Torpy DJ, Zhuang Z, Stratakis CA (1998) Human CYP11B2 (aldosterone synthase) maps to chromosome 8q24.3. J Clin Endocrinol Metab 83:1033–1036
24. Brand E, Chatelain N, Mulatero P, Féry I, Curnow K, Jeunemaitre X, Corvol P, Pascoe L, Soubrier F (1998) Structural analysis and evaluation of the aldosterone synthase gene in hypertension. Hypertension 32:198–204
25. Pascoe L, Curnow KM (1995) Genetic recombination as a cause of inherited disorders of aldosterone and cortisol biosynthesis and a contributor to genetic variation in blood pressure. Steroids 60:22–27
26. Mulatero P, Curnow KM, Aupetit-Faisant B, Foekling M, Gomez-Sanchez C, Veglio F, Jeunemaitre X, Corvol P, Pascoe L (1998) Recombinant CYP11B genes encode enzymes that can catalyze conversion of 11-deoxycortisol to cortisol, 18-hydroxycortisol, and 18-oxocortisol. J Clin Endocrinol Metab 83:3996–4001
27. Pascoe L, Jeunemaitre X, Lebrethon MC, Curnow KM, Gomez-Sanchez CE, Gasc JM, Saez JM, Corvol P (1995) Glucocorticoid-suppressible hyperaldosteronism and adrenal tumors occurring in a single French pedigree. J Clin Invest 96:2236–2246
28. Dluhy RG, Lifton RP (1995) Glucocorticoid-remediable aldosteronism (GRA): diagnosis, variability of phenotype and regulation of potassium homeostasis. Steroids 60:48–51
29. Curnow KM, Mulatero P, Emeric-Blanchouin N, Aupetit-Faisant B, Corvol P, Pascoe L (1997) The amino acid substitutions Ser288Gly and Val320Ala convert the cortisol producing enzyme, CYP11B1, into an aldosterone producing enzyme. Nat Struct Biol 4:32–35

30. Mulatero P, Morello F, Veglio F (2004) Genetics of primary aldosteronism. J Hypertens 22: 663–670
31. Tusié-Luna MT, White PC (1995) Gene conversions and unequal crossovers between CYP21 (steroid 21-hydroxylase gene) and CYP21P involve different mechanisms. Proc Natl Acad Sci U S A 92:10796–10800
32. Carroll J, Dluhy R, Fallo F, Pistorello M, Bradwin G, Gomez-Sanchez CE, Mortensen R (1996) Aldosterone-producing adenomas do not contain glucocorticoid-remediable aldosteronism chimeric gene duplications. J Clin Endocrinol Metab 81:4310–4312
33. Pilon C, Mulatero P, Barzon L, Veglio F, Garrone C, Boscaro M, Sonino N, Fallo F (1999) Mutations in CYP11B1 gene converting 11beta-hydroxylase into an aldosterone-producing enzyme are not present in aldosterone-producing adenomas. J Clin Endocrinol Metab 84:4228–4231
34. Portrat S, Mulatero P, Curnow KM, Chaussain JL, Morel Y, Pascoe L (2001) Deletion hybrid genes, due to unequal crossing over between CYP11B1 (11beta-hydroxylase) and CYP11B2 (aldosterone synthase) cause steroid 11beta-hydroxylase deficiency and congenital adrenal hyperplasia. J Clin Endocrinol Metab 86:3197–3201
35. Jonsson JR, Klemm SA, Tunny TJ, Stowasser M, Gordon RD (1995) A new genetic test for familial hyperaldosteronism type I aids in the detection of curable hypertension. Biochem Biophys Res Commun 207:565–571
36. Fardella CE, Mosso L, Gómez-Sánchez C, Cortés P, Soto J, Gómez L, Pinto M, Huete A, Oestreicher E, Foradori A, Montero J (2000) Primary hyperaldosteronism in essential hypertensives: prevalence, biochemical profile, and molecular biology. J Clin Endocrinol Metab 85:1863–1867
37. Morra di Cella S, Veglio F, Mulatero P, Christensen V, Aycock K, Zhu Z, Gomez-Sanchez EP, Gomez-Sanchez CE (2002) A time-resolved fluoroimmunoassay for 18-oxocortisol and 18-hydroxycortisol. Development of a monoclonal antibody to 18-oxocortisol. J Steroid Biochem Mol Biol 82:83–88
38. Mulatero P, di Cella SM, Monticone S, Schiavone D, Manzo M, Mengozzi G, Rabbia F, Terzolo M, Gomez-Sanchez EP, Gomez-Sanchez CE, Veglio F (2012) 18-hydroxycorticosterone, 18-hydroxycortisol, and 18-oxocortisol in the diagnosis of primary aldosteronism and its subtypes. J Clin Endocrinol Metab 97:881–889
39. Funder JW, Carey RM, Fardella C, Gomez-Sanchez CE, Mantero F, Stowasser M, Young WF Jr, Montori VM (2008) Endocrine Society. Case detection, diagnosis, and treatment of patients with primary aldosteronism: an endocrine society clinical practice guideline. J Clin Endocrinol Metab 93:3266–3281
40. Stowasser M, Gordon RD (2004) Primary aldosteronism—careful investigation is essential and rewarding. Mol Cell Endocrinol 217:33–39
41. Mulatero P, Bertello C, Verhovez A, Rossato D, Giraudo G, Mengozzi G, Limerutti G, Avenatti E, Tizzani D, Veglio F (2009) Differential diagnosis of primary aldosteronism subtypes. Curr Hypertens Rep 11:217–223
42. Stowasser M, Pimenta E, Gordon RD (2011) Familial or genetic primary aldosteronism and Gordon syndrome. Endocrinol Metab Clin North Am 40:343–368
43. Mulatero P, Tizzani D, Viola A, Bertello C, Monticone S, Mengozzi G, Schiavone D, Williams TA, Einaudi S, La Grotta A, Rabbia F, Veglio F (2011) Prevalence and characteristics of familial hyperaldosteronism: the PATOGEN study (Primary Aldosteronism in TOrino-GENetic forms). Hypertension 58:797–803
44. Pizzolo F, Trabetti E, Guarini P, Mulatero P, Ciacciarelli A, Blengio GS, Corrocher R, Olivieri O (2005) Glucocorticoid remediable aldosteronism (GRA) screening in hypertensive patients from a primary care setting. J Hum Hypertens 19:325–327
45. Strauch B, Zelinka T, Hampf M, Bernhardt R, Widimsky J Jr (2003) Prevalence of primary hyperaldosteronism in moderate to severe hypertension in the Central Europe region. J Hum Hypertens 17:349–352
46. Stowasser M, Gordon RD, Gunasekera TG, Cowley DC, Ward G, Archibald C, Smithers BM (2003) High rate of detection of primary aldosteronism, including surgically treatable forms, after 'non-selective' screening of hypertensive patients. J Hypertens 21:2149–2157

47. Gates LJ, Benjamin N, Haites NE, MacConnachie AA, McLay JS (2001) Is random screening of value in detecting glucocorticoid-remediable aldosteronism within a hypertensive population? J Hum Hypertens 15:173–176
48. Aglony M, Martínez-Aguayo A, Carvajal CA, Campino C, García H, Bancalari R, Bolte L, Avalos C, Loureiro C, Trejo P, Brinkmann K, Giadrosich V, Mericq V, Rocha A, Avila A, Perez V, Inostroza A, Fardella CE (2011) Frequency of familial hyperaldosteronism type 1 in a hypertensive pediatric population: clinical and biochemical presentation. Hypertension 57: 1117–1121
49. Mulatero P, di Cella SM, Williams TA, Milan A, Mengozzi G, Chiandussi L, Gomez-Sanchez CE, Veglio F (2002) Glucocorticoid remediable aldosteronism: low morbidity and mortality in a four-generation Italian pedigree. J Clin Endocrinol Metab 87:3187–3191
50. Rich GM, Ulick S, Cook S, Wang JZ, Lifton RP, Dluhy RG (1992) Glucocorticoid-remediable aldosteronism in a large kindred: clinical spectrum and diagnosis using a characteristic biochemical phenotype. Ann Intern Med 116:813–820
51. Stowasser M, Bachmann AW, Huggard PR, Rossetti TR, Gordon RD (2000) Severity of hypertension in familial hyperaldosteronism type I: relationship to gender and degree of biochemical disturbance. J Clin Endocrinol Metab 85:2160–2166
52. Jamieson A, Slutsker L, Inglis GC, Fraser R, White PC, Connell JM (1995) Glucocorticoid-suppressible hyperaldosteronism: effects of crossover site and parental origin of chimaeric gene on phenotypic expression. Clin Sci 88:563–570
53. Fallo F, Pilon C, Williams TA, Sonino N, Morra Di Cella S, Veglio F, De Iasio R, Montanari P, Mulatero P (2004) Coexistence of different phenotypes in a family with glucocorticoid-remediable aldosteronism. J Hum Hypertens 18:47–51
54. Mulatero P, Williams TA, Milan A, Paglieri C, Rabbia F, Fallo F, Veglio F (2002) Blood pressure in patients with primary aldosteronism is influenced by bradykinin B(2) receptor and alpha-adducin gene polymorphisms. J Clin Endocrinol Metab 87:3337–3343
55. Litchfield WR, Anderson BF, Weiss RJ, Lifton RP, Dluhy RG (1998) Intracranial aneurysm and hemorrhagic stroke in glucocorticoid-remediable aldosteronism. Hypertension 31:445–450
56. Wyckoff JA, Seely EW, Hurwitz S, Anderson BF, Lifton RP, Dluhy RG (2000) Glucocorticoid-remediable aldosteronism and pregnancy. Hypertension 35:668–672
57. Stowasser M, Sharman J, Leano R, Gordon RD, Ward G, Cowley D, Marwick TH (2005) Evidence for abnormal left ventricular structure and function in normotensive individuals with familial hyperaldosteronism type I. J Clin Endocrinol Metab 90:5070–5076
58. Stowasser M, Bachmann AW, Huggard PR, Rossetti TR, Gordon RD (2000) Treatment of familial hyperaldosteronism type I: only partial suppression of adrenocorticotropin required to correct hypertension. J Clin Endocrinol Metab 85:3313–3318
59. Dluhy RG, Anderson B, Harlin B, Ingelfinger J, Lifton R (2001) Glucocorticoid-remediable aldosteronism is associated with severe hypertension in early childhood. J Pediatr 138: 715–720

Chapter 7
Familial Hyperaldosteronism Type II

Michael Stowasser and Richard Douglas Gordon

Abstract As originally defined, the term familial hyperaldosteronism type II (FH-II) refers to the occurrence in families of at least two members with primary aldosteronism (PA) that is not glucocorticoid suppressible and not associated with the hybrid *CYP11B1/2* gene mutation responsible for familial hyperaldosteronism type I (FH-I, glucocorticoid-remediable aldosteronism). FH-II appears to be much more common than FH-I and is probably genetically heterogeneous. As in apparently non-familial PA, PA in the majority of patients with FH-II is due to either unilateral aldosterone-producing adenoma or bilateral adrenal hyperplasia which may be diffuse or nodular and responds favorably to unilateral adrenalectomy (for unilateral forms) or specific medical treatment antagonizing aldosterone action. So far, the only gene found to be mutated in the germ line of affected members of families with PA (after exclusion of FH-I by genetic testing for the hybrid gene) is *KCNJ5*, encoding a potassium channel, but this appears to be a rare cause of familial PA. The search for other underlying genetic mutations is ongoing.

Keywords Primary aldosteronism • Familial • Familial hyperaldosteronism type II • Genetics • Prevalence • Phenotype • Definition • Clinical features

M. Stowasser, M.B.B.S., F.R.A.C.P., Ph.D. (✉)
Endocrine Hypertension Research Centre, University of Queensland
School of Medicine, Princess Alexandra Hospital, Ipswich Road,
Woolloongabba, Brisbane, QLD 4102, Australia
e-mail: m.stowasser@uq.edu.au

R.D. Gordon, M.B.B.S., M.D., Ph.D., F.R.A.C.P., F.R.C.P.
Endocrine Hypertension Research Centre, University of Queensland
School of Medicine, Greenslopes Hospital, Brisbane, QLD 4120, Australia

P. Hellman (ed.), *Primary Aldosteronism: Molecular Genetics, Endocrinology, and Translational Medicine*, DOI 10.1007/978-1-4939-0509-6_7,

Introduction and Definition

Twenty-five years after Sutherland and co-workers [31] first described the familial occurrence of glucocorticoid-suppressible primary aldosteronism (PA) (see Chap. 4), a second familial variety of PA, in which aldosterone is not glucocorticoid suppressible, was described by the Greenslopes Hospital Hypertension Unit (GHHU) in Brisbane, Australia, in 1991 [15]. Additional families were subsequently also reported from other countries [11, 19]. This condition was labelled familial hyperaldosteronism type II (FH-II) [29] in order to distinguish it from the glucocorticoid-suppressible form (familial hyperaldosteronism type I, FH-I). The GHHU and its sister unit at Princess Alexandra Hospital (also in Brisbane) are now following 45 Australian families (110 patients) with FH-II [14, 27, 28]. In each family, PA was confirmed by fludrocortisone suppression testing (FST), and FH-I was excluded by demonstrating the absence of the *CYP11B1/B2* hybrid gene mutation by genetic testing and/or failure of dexamethasone to suppress aldosterone.

In 2008, Geller and co-workers described an American family with an affected father and two daughters with PA which, like FH-II, was not glucocorticoid suppressible and not associated with the hybrid gene mutation but, unlike FH-II, was characterized by severe, childhood-onset hypertension, 18-hydroxy- and 18-oxo-cortisol levels which were markedly elevated (to a much greater degree than in FH-I) and resected adrenals showing marked, diffuse hyperplasia of zona fasciculata (ZF), with the combined adrenal weight in one daughter reaching 81 g (normal <12 g) [12]. The description of this family led Mulatero to coin the term "familial hyperaldosteronism type III" (FH-III) [21]. As is discussed in Chap. 6, the affected members of this family were later found by Choi et al. [6] to carry a germline mutation in *KCNJ5*, which encodes a potassium channel. Since that report, several other families with PA and germline *KCNJ5* mutations have been reported, some of them demonstrating much milder phenotypes which resembled those of families with FH-II (see below and Chap. 6). This overlap has raised an issue in terms of the definitions of these two familial forms of PA. Given that Mulatero's use of the term "FH-III" was based on the description of a new form of clinical presentation, it could be argued that the term be reserved for families which show similar early-onset non-glucocorticoid-suppressible severe PA with markedly enlarged adrenals. This, however, creates uncertainty in how to label patients with milder PA and *KCNJ5* mutations. Another approach, which is possibly preferable, is to define FH-III genetically (that is, familial PA due to inherited germline mutations of *KCNJ5*) with FH-II remaining a diagnosis of exclusion (that is, all forms of familial PA for which the underlying genetic mutation remains unknown) (Table 7.1). Defined in this way, the phenotype of FH-III becomes quite variable, ranging from mild to very severe PA and with adrenal morphology ranging from apparently normal (on radiological imaging) to grossly hyperplastic.

The nomenclature for familial forms of hypertension is evolving and may change, as each approach has strengths and weaknesses. For example, retaining FH-II as a diagnosis of exclusion and using the term FH-III for families with germline *KCNJ5* mutations imply that as new causative mutations are discovered, an ever-increasing

Table 7.1 Clinicopathological features of familial hyperaldosteronism type I, II, and III

	FH-I	FH-II	FH-III
Genetic basis	Hybrid *CYP11B1/CYP11B2* mutation	Unknown	Missense (so far) point mutations in *KCNJ5*
Pattern of transmission	Autosomal dominant	Variable—autosomal dominant in some families; possibly autosomal recessive in others	Autosomal dominant
Prevalence	<1 % of PA	At least 6 % of PA	≪1 % of PA
Age of onset of HT	Childhood–early adulthood	Adulthood	Childhood (less than 18 years)
Severity of HT	Variable—from normotensive to severely hypertensive	Variable—from normotensive to severely hypertensive	Variable—from mildly to severely hypertensive
Prevalence of hypokalemia	20–25 %	20–25 %	>90 %
Glucocorticoid suppressibility	Yes	No	No
Hybrid steroids (18-oxo-cortisol and 18-hydroxy-cortisol)	Elevated	Elevated in patients with angiotensin-unresponsive APA; normal otherwise	Markedly elevated in one family; normal to mildly elevated in another
Adrenal morphology	Usually normal; occasional nodules	Variable—most commonly either unilateral nodule or diffuse or nodular bilateral hyperplasia	Normal to marked, diffuse hyperplasia
Treatment	Low doses of glucocorticoids; alternatively aldosterone antagonist agents	Unilateral adrenalectomy (for unilateral forms); aldosterone antagonist agents	Bilateral adrenalectomy (for severe forms with marked adrenal hyperplasia); aldosterone antagonist agents

FH familial hyperaldosteronism, *PA* primary aldosteronism, *HT* hypertension, *CT* computed tomography list of numerical FH designations (for example, FH-IV, FH-V) will emerge. Some investigators will find this confusing and possibly unacceptable. Indeed, this has not been the practice for other genetically heterogeneous conditions such as Liddle syndrome (caused by activating mutations in the genes coding either the gamma or the beta subunits of the sodium epithelial channel) and familial hyperkalemic hypertension (also known as Gordon syndrome, so far known to be caused by mutations in *WNK1* or *WNK4*, encoding two of the with no lysine [K] family of kinases which regulate the sodium/potassium co-transporter, and in *CUL3* or *KLCH3*, thought to encode proteins involved in ubiquitination of WNK1 and WNK4 kinases). The optimal approach to the classification of familial forms of PA is an issue worthy of further discussion.

Clinical Features

Patients with FH-II have demonstrated substantial diversity in phenotypic expression [27, 28]. Among the 110 patients identified so far by our Brisbane group, ages at presentation ranged from 14 to 78 years; 56 (51 %) were female, and 27 (25 %) were hypokalemic. Thirty-one (28 %) have undergone unilateral adrenalectomy. Of these, 27 had unilateral PA confirmed by preoperative adrenal venous sampling (AVS) and/or postoperative cure of hypertension and biochemical PA, 1 "almost" lateralized on AVS but with incomplete contralateral suppression, and 3 had bilateral PA but were unable to tolerate aldosterone antagonist treatment in the doses required to control hypertension. Two (2 %) other patients have undergone bilateral adrenalectomy, one for bilateral giant macronodular hyperplasia causing autonomous adrenal aldosterone and cortisol production and the other in another institution for severe, medically unresponsive, hypokalemic PA associated with bilateral macronodular hyperplasia. The remaining 77 (70 %) patients, in whom hypertension has been treated medically with agents that block aldosterone action, comprise 56 with bilateral PA confirmed by AVS, 1 with unilateral PA who opted for medical treatment, and 20 in whom AVS either has not yet been performed ($n = 12$) or gave inconclusive results ($n = 8$).

In this series of families with FH-II, mode of transmission of phenotype has followed a dominant pattern in 18 families but remains uncertain in the other 27. Interestingly, several families have included affected members with differing forms of PA. For example, in one family, a 37-year-old female underwent removal in 1987 of a 2.2 cm right aldosterone-producing adenoma (APA) with cure of hypertension and hypokalemia. Preoperatively, here plasma aldosterone levels failed to rise in response to either the assumption of upright posture or an intravenous infusion of angiotensin II (AII), consistent with the AII-unresponsive variety of APA. In 1990, her hypertensive, normokalemic father was found, at age 63 years, to have PA due to a 0.5 cm right AII-responsive APA, the removal of which led to marked improvement in hypertension control. Ten years later, her 46-year-old hypertensive, normokalemic sister was diagnosed as having PA due to bilateral adrenal hyperplasia (BAH) and was commenced on spironolactone treatment. In a second family, hypokalemia was cured and hypertension markedly improved in a 78-year-old woman following removal of a 6 mm left AII-responsive APA in 1993 [14]. In the following year, her 46-year-old hypertensive, normokalemic daughter was diagnosed as having PA due to a 14 mm left AII-unresponsive APA, the removal of which led to cure of hypertension. While the mother's tumor was almost entirely composed of zona glomerulosa (ZG)-like cells and hybrid cells (cells having morphological characteristics of both ZG and ZF), the daughter's tumor was composed predominantly of ZF-like cells [14]. This is consistent with our previously reported observations in patients with apparently non-familial PA that AII-responsive APAs usually demonstrate a predominance (at least 80 %) of non-ZF-like cells, while AII-unresponsive APAs tend to be composed mainly (at least 50 %) of ZF-like cells [34].

Prevalence

Because clinical, biochemical, and morphological characteristics of patients with FH-II do not differ significantly from those with apparently non-familial PA [13, 27, 28], it is possible that mutations underlying FH-II may be relatively common among the broader PA population.

In the Brisbane experience, FH-II appears to be at least seven times more common than FH-I. From 1992 to 2004, 912 patients were diagnosed as having PA after screening all newly referred hypertensives by aldosterone/renin ratio (ARR) testing and confirming the diagnosis by FST, and all underwent either dexamethasone suppression testing or genetic testing for the hybrid gene mutation responsible for FH-I. Of these 912 patients, 29 (3.2 %) represented new families with FH-II (their affected relatives being subsequently identified) and only 4 (0.4 %) were from new families with FH-I.

Mulatero and colleagues [23] assessed prevalence rates for familial PA among 300 patients consecutively diagnosed in their institution (after excluding those referred with a form of familial PA in mind). Hybrid gene testing yielded only two (0.7 %) with FH-I. Of the remaining 298, 199 had relatives available for, and consenting to, biochemical screening by ARR testing and, where positive, definitive confirmation or exclusion of PA by intravenous saline infusion testing. Twelve had at least one affected relative, giving a prevalence of FH-II of at least 6 % (almost ten times that of FH-I) in that study. The prevalence may have been higher given that another 54 families remained of "uncertain" affectation status, either because not all hypertensive members underwent ARR testing or because tested family members were considered to have "uncertain" status [23].

Why Look for Mutations Causing FH-II?

Unlike in FH-I, the genetic defect/s underlying FH-II has/have not yet been elucidated. Identification of such defects would further the understanding of the pathogenesis of FH-II, as has occurred in the case of FH-I since elucidation of the hybrid gene defect [18], and has important implications for patient management. As in apparently non-familial PA, detection of FH-II currently involves biochemical screening by ARR testing and confirmation of PA by FST. As has already been observed in FH-I, elucidation of mutations causing FH-II should lead to the development of new genetic screening tests which greatly simplify diagnosis, being absolutely specific for a particular mutation, clearly much more sensitive and specific than biochemical testing. This would permit earlier and more frequent detection of those affected, provided that identification of the responsible mutations had been achieved.

Candidate Gene Studies in FH-II

The search for genetic abnormalities causing FH-II has involved both candidate gene and genome-wide search approaches. We have excluded the hybrid gene mutation responsible for FH-I in all of our patients with FH-II [27, 28]. Sequencing studies performed within Yutaka Shizuta's laboratory in Kochi, Japan, on peripheral blood DNA from one of our Australian patients with FH-II did not reveal mutations in the coding region of *CYP11B2* (personal communication, Yutaka Shizuta, Department of Medical Chemistry, Kochi Medical School, Japan, 1992).

It is possible in vitro to introduce point mutations into *CYP11B1* which confer aldosterone synthase activity to its gene product [8]. Fallo's group, however, found no evidence of such mutations in peripheral blood DNA from Italian patients with FH-II [11] or from ten Australian patients (four families) with FH-II from the GHHU/PAHHU series [unpublished observations]. This group also excluded both the −344T and the intron conversion alleles of *CYP11B2* (which have been implicated in PA) in all four of their patients with FH-II [11].

Single-strand conformation polymorphism analysis of the *p53* tumor-suppressor gene revealed no evidence of germline mutations in 14 patients with FH-II or somatic mutations in tumor DNA from the 7 of these who underwent removal of an aldosterone-producing tumor [2].

Linkage Analysis Studies in FH-II

Linkage studies performed in collaboration with Stratakis et al. (NIH, Bethesda, MD, USA) involving one large, informative family from the GHHU series revealed no evidence of cosegregation of phenotype with polymorphisms within the *CYP11B2*, *AT1*, or *MEN1* loci [32, 33]. A genome-wide search in this family, however, demonstrated linkage between FH-II and a locus at chromosome 7p22 with a maximum paired logarithm of odds (LOD) score of 3.26 [17]. Subsequent work involving a second Australian family and a South American family identified by Dr. Maria New (New York Presbyterian Hospital) increased the multipoint LOD score for the locus to 4.61 [25]. Recombination events in our largest Australian family of eight affected individuals narrowed the locus by 1.8 Mbp, allowing the exclusion of almost half the candidate genes in the original locus [25]. Linkage to 7p22 has also been verified in two Italian FH-II families identified by Dr. Paolo Mulatero (University of Torino). The combined multipoint LOD score for the five families that are informative for the 7p22 locus (two Australian, one South American, and two Italian) would appear to have put the LOD score beyond reasonable doubt at 5.22 [30].

Although Fallo and co-workers were unable to demonstrate LOH at the 7p22 locus in APAs removed from patients with FH-II [10], this would not exclude causative mutations unable to be detected by the LOH approach.

Sequencing at Chromosome 7p22 and Beyond in FH-II

There are approximately 50 genes residing within the linked 7p22 locus. Initial sequencing efforts were directed towards the more likely candidates among these genes including *PRKAR1B* [9], *RBaK* [16, 26], *PMS2* and *GNA12* [16], and *ZNF12*, *RPA3*, and *GLCCI* (unpublished data). All were relevant as they are involved either in cell cycle control or steroid action, and adrenal cortical hyperplasia and neoplasia and abnormal steroid regulation are characteristic features of FH-II. In each case, gDNA from two affected and two unaffected subjects from our largest 7p22-linked FH-II family was used to sequence the gene followed by further genotyping of interesting single-nucleotide polymorphisms (SNPs) in additional affected and unaffected members from FH-II families as well as unrelated normotensive controls. However, no mutations likely to be causative for FH-II were identified by this approach [9, 16, 26].

Later efforts involved intensive examination of this region using next-generation sequencing methodology, which generates sequencing data much more quickly than traditional PCR and direct sequencing approaches. This also permitted a wider search to include whole-genome linkage analysis and whole-exomic sequencing to identify candidate SNPs both within 7p22 and elsewhere. Of the high-priority targets thus identified, however, the great majority were excluded after Sanger sequencing because of incomplete segregation with phenotype [4], and the search for causative mutations in FH-II remains intensive and ongoing.

Genetic Heterogeneity in FH-II

FH-II, and PA in general, is likely to be genetically heterogeneous. For example, for two Australian families with FH-II, linkage at the 7p22 region was excluded [25]. This genetic heterogeneity is not surprising given the high degree of clinical and biochemical phenotypic diversity observed in FH-II and other forms of PA. Genetic heterogeneity has been reported in other inherited forms of hypertension such as Liddle syndrome [35] and Gordon syndrome [3, 7, 20].

Relevance of *KCNJ5* Mutations to Families Designated as Having FH-II

Choi and colleagues [6] recently reported somatic mutations (G151R and L168R) in *KCNJ5*, encoding an inwardly rectifying potassium channel, in 8 of 22 APAs removed from Swedish patients with apparently non-familial PA. As mentioned in the opening section of this chapter, these authors also identified a third *KCNJ5* mutation (T158A) in the germ line of an American family with a familial form of PA reported in 2008 [12] associated with very severe, early-onset PA and sufficiently different clinically (and in the case of FH-I, genetically) from FH-I and -II to be labelled "FH-III" by Mulatero [21]. The authors proposed that the *KCNJ5* mutations, by causing increased channel Na^+ permeability (extracellular concentrations of which are much higher than K^+), predispose to chronic adrenocortical cell membrane depolarization and consequently to influx of Ca^{2+} which, in turn, leads to upregulation of enzymes involved in aldosterone synthesis and cell proliferation [6].

Subsequently, Mulatero et al. [22] reported somatic *KCNJ5* mutations (one each of the three mutations reported by Choi et al.) in 3 of 11 APAs removed from patients with FH-II. They also described a novel germline mutation (G151E) in both affected members (mother and daughter) of 1 of 21 families with FH-II studied. Both had early-onset hypertension and moderately severe biochemical PA, but, unlike the family studied by Geller et al. [12], the adrenals appeared normal on computed tomography (CT) and hybrid steroid levels were only slightly elevated. The novel mutation again demonstrated loss of K^+/Na^+ selectivity when expressed in HEK cells [22]. Hence, a family previously designated as having FH-II was found to carry a germline mutation in the gene mutated in FH-III.

Scholl et al. described two more families (six subjects) with germline G151E mutations associated with early-onset but mild PA controllable with spironolactone and not associated with abnormal adrenal morphology on CT [24]. However, two other pedigrees (four subjects) with germline G151R mutations had a much more severe phenotype with very-early-onset and severe PA that was poorly responsive to spironolactone and, in three of these patients, eventually required bilateral adrenalectomy (performed before the age of 5 years in each case) to achieve control. The removed adrenals demonstrated hyperplasia of both ZF and ZG in two, while the youngest (18 months) operated subject's adrenals were histologically normal. Surprisingly, G151E-mutated channels showed markedly higher (more abnormal) sodium conductance and conferred greater lethality to transfected HEK 293T cells than G151R-mutated channels. This increased lethality may explain the lack of adrenal hyperplasia occurring clinically in patients bearing germline G151E (versus G151R) mutations [24].

Another novel germline *KCNJ5* mutation (I157S) was detected in a mother and daughter with severe early-onset PA and bilateral massive adrenal hyperplasia [5]. When expressed in HEK cells, this mutation again resulted in loss of channel ion selectivity and less negative cell membrane potentials.

In collaboration with Kevin O'Shaughnessy and Morris Brown in Cambridge, UK, we reported somatic *KCNJ5* mutations in 30 (41 %) of 73 APAs (10 of 27 from Australia and 20 of 46 from the UK) from patients with apparently non-familial PA [1]. We have not, however, identified germline *KCNJ5* mutations among any of our patients with FH-II (32 families so far studied) ([1] and unpublished observations), but testing of all the remaining available families (with particular focus on those with more pronounced bilaterally abnormal adrenal morphology) is ongoing. It is likely that further reports of germline *KCNJ5* mutations in families previously designated as having FH-II will appear. Whether they should then be labelled as having FH-III, or an entirely new labelling system devised, is a matter worthy of debate.

Conclusions

The study of familial forms of PA has led to a much greater understanding of the genetic mechanisms underlying regulation of aldosterone synthesis and adrenal growth and the molecular basis of PA itself. FH-II is the most common variety and will almost certainly prove to be genetically heterogeneous. Although the genetics of FH-II remains to be elucidated, the emergence of new technologies that have streamlined the analysis of large regions of DNA has greatly enhanced the likelihood of success and, as has recently occurred with the discovery of germline *KCNJ5* mutations, promises to deliver further insights into the causation/s of this phenotypically diverse condition.

References

1. Azizan EA, Murthy M, Stowasser M, Gordon R, Kowalski B, Xu S, Brown MJ, O'Shaughnessy KM (2012) Somatic mutations affecting the selectivity filter of KCNJ5 are frequent in 2 large unselected collections of adrenal aldosteronomas. Hypertension 59(3):587–591
2. Ballantine DM, Klemm SA, Tunny TJ, Stowasser M, Gordon RD (1996) PCR-SSCP analysis of the p53 gene in tumours of the adrenal gland. Clin Exp Pharmacol Physiol 23(6–7):582–583
3. Boyden LM, Choi M, Choate KA, Nelson-Williams CJ, Farhi A, Toka HR, Tikhonova IR, Bjornson R, Mane SM, Colussi G, Lebel M, Gordon RD, Semmekrot BA, Poujol A, Valimaki MJ, De FME, Sanjad SA, Gutkin M, Karet FE, Tucci JR, Stockigt JR, Keppler-Noreuil KM, Porter CC, Anand SK, Whiteford ML, Davis ID, Dewar SB, Bettinelli A, Fadrowski JJ, Belsha CW, Hunley TE, Nelson RD, Trachtman H, Cole TR, Pinsk M, Bockenhauer D, Shenoy M, Vaidyanathan P, Foreman JW, Rasoulpour M, Thameem F, Al-Shahrouri HZ, Radhakrishnan J, Gharavi AG, Goilav B, Lifton RP (2012) Mutations in kelch-like 3 and cullin 3 cause hypertension and electrolyte abnormalities. Nature 482(7383):98–102
4. Carss KJ, Stowasser M, Gordon RD, O'Shaughnessy KM (2011) Further study of chromosome 7p22 to identify the molecular basis of familial hyperaldosteronism type II. J Hum Hypertens 25(9):560–564

5. Charmandari E, Sertedaki A, Kino T, Merakou C, Hoffman DA, Hatch MM, Hurt DE, Lin L, Xekouki P, Stratakis CA, Chrousos GP (2012) A novel point mutation in the KCNJ5 gene causing primary hyperaldosteronism and early-onset autosomal dominant hypertension. J Clin Endocrinol Metab 97(8):E1532–E1539
6. Choi M, Scholl UI, Yue P, Bjorklund P, Zhao B, Nelson-Williams C, Ji W, Cho Y, Patel A, Men CJ, Lolis E, Wisgerhof MV, Geller DS, Mane S, Hellman P, Westin G, Akerstrom G, Wang W, Carling T, Lifton RP (2011) K+ channel mutations in adrenal aldosterone-producing adenomas and hereditary hypertension. Science 331(6018):768–772
7. Cope G, Golbang A, O'Shaughnessy KM (2005) WNK kinases and the control of blood pressure. Pharmacol Ther 106(2):221–231
8. Curnow KM, Mulatero P, Emeric-Blanchouin N, Aupetit-Faisant B, Corvol P, Pascoe L (1997) The amino acid substitutions Ser288Gly and Val320Ala convert the cortisol producing enzyme, CYP11B1, into an aldosterone producing enzyme. Nat Struct Biol 4(1):32–35
9. Elphinstone MS, Gordon RD, So A, Jeske YW, Stratakis CA, Stowasser M (2004) Genomic structure of the human gene for protein kinase A regulatory subunit R1-beta (PRKAR1B) on 7p22: no evidence for mutations in familial hyperaldosteronism type II in a large affected kindred. Clin Endocrinol (Oxf) 61(6):716–723
10. Fallo F, Pilon C, Barzon L, Pistorello M, Sonino N, Veglio F, Mulatero P (2004) Retention of heterozygosity at chromosome 7p22 and 11q13 in aldosterone-producing tumours of patients with familial hyperaldosteronism not remediable by glucocorticoids. J Hum Hypertens 18(11):829–830
11. Fallo F, Veglio F, Mulatero P, Sonino N, Pilon C, Barzon L, Trimarchi F, Boscaro M, Benvenga S (2000) Genetic studies in familial aldosteronism not suppressible by dexamethasone. J Endocr Genet 1:159–164
12. Geller DS, Zhang J, Wisgerhof MV, Shackleton C, Kashgarian M, Lifton RP (2008) A novel form of human Mendelian hypertension featuring nonglucocorticoid-remediable aldosteronism. J Clin Endocrinol Metab 93(8):3117–3123
13. Gordon RD, Klemm SA, Tunny TJ, Stowasser M (1992) Primary aldosteronism: hypertension with a genetic basis. Lancet 340(8812):159–161
14. Gordon RD, Stowasser M (1998) Familial forms broaden horizons in primary aldosteronism. Trends Endocrinol Metab 9:220–227
15. Gordon RD, Stowasser M, Tunny TJ, Klemm SA, Finn WL, Krek AL (1991) Clinical and pathological diversity of primary aldosteronism, including a new familial variety. Clin Exp Pharmacol Physiol 18(5):283–286
16. Jeske YW, So A, Kelemen L, Sukor N, Willys C, Bulmer B, Gordon RD, Duffy D, Stowasser M (2008) Examination of chromosome 7p22 candidate genes RBaK, PMS2 and GNA12 in familial hyperaldosteronism type II. Clin Exp Pharmacol Physiol 35(4):380–385
17. Lafferty AR, Torpy DJ, Stowasser M, Taymans SE, Lin JP, Huggard P, Gordon RD, Stratakis CA (2000) A novel genetic locus for low renin hypertension: familial hyperaldosteronism type II maps to chromosome 7 (7p22). J Med Genet 37(11):831–835
18. Lifton RP, Dluhy RG, Powers M, Rich GM, Cook S, Ulick S, Lalouel JM (1992) A chimaeric 11 beta-hydroxylase/aldosterone synthase gene causes glucocorticoid-remediable aldosteronism and human hypertension. Nature 355(6357):262–265
19. London N, Swales J, Hollinrake K, Bell P, Heagerty A (1992) Familial Conn's syndrome. Postgrad Med J 68(806):976–977
20. Louis-Dit-Picard H, Barc J, Trujillano D, Miserey-Lenkei S, Bouatia-Naji N, Pylypenko O, Beaurain G, Bonnefond A, Sand O, Simian C, Vidal-Petiot E, Soukaseum C, Mandet C, Broux F, Chabre O, Delahousse M, Esnault V, Fiquet B, Houillier P, Bagnis CI, Koenig J, Konrad M, Landais P, Mourani C, Niaudet P, Probst V, Thauvin C, Unwin RJ, Soroka SD, Ehret G, Ossowski S, Caulfield M, Bruneval P, Estivill X, Froguel P, Hadchouel J, Schott JJ, Jeunemaitre X (2012) KLHL3 mutations cause familial hyperkalemic hypertension by impairing ion transport in the distal nephron. Nat Genet 44(4):456–460, S451-453
21. Mulatero P (2008) A new form of hereditary primary aldosteronism: familial hyperaldosteronism type III. J Clin Endocrinol Metab 93(8):2972–2974

22. Mulatero P, Tauber P, Zennaro MC, Monticone S, Lang K, Beuschlein F, Fischer E, Tizzani D, Pallauf A, Viola A, Amar L, Williams TA, Strom TM, Graf E, Bandulik S, Penton D, Plouin PF, Warth R, Allolio B, Jeunemaitre X, Veglio F, Reincke M (2012) KCNJ5 mutations in European families with nonglucocorticoid remediable familial hyperaldosteronism. Hypertension 59(2):235–240
23. Mulatero P, Tizzani D, Viola A, Bertello C, Monticone S, Mengozzi G, Schiavone D, Williams TA, Einaudi S, La GA, Rabbia F, Veglio F (2011) Prevalence and characteristics of familial hyperaldosteronism: the PATOGEN Study (Primary Aldosteronism in TOrino-GENetic forms). Hypertension 58(5):797–803
24. Scholl UI, Nelson-Williams C, Yue P, Grekin R, Wyatt RJ, Dillon MJ, Couch R, Hammer LK, Harley FL, Farhi A, Wang WH, Lifton RP (2012) Hypertension with or without adrenal hyperplasia due to different inherited mutations in the potassium channel KCNJ5. Proc Natl Acad Sci U S A 109(7):2533–2538
25. So A, Duffy DL, Gordon RD, Jeske YW, Lin-Su K, New MI, Stowasser M (2005) Familial hyperaldosteronism type II is linked to the chromosome 7p22 region but also shows predicted heterogeneity. J Hypertens 23(8):1477–1484
26. So A, Jeske YW, Gordon RD, Duffy D, Kelemen L, Stowasser M (2006) No evidence for coding region mutations in the retinoblastoma-associated Kruppel-associated box protein gene (RBaK) causing familial hyperaldosteronism type II. Clin Endocrinol (Oxf) 65(6):829–831
27. Stowasser M, Gordon RD (2001) Familial hyperaldosteronism. J Steroid Biochem Mol Biol 78(3):215–229
28. Stowasser M, Gordon RD (2003) Primary aldosteronism: from genesis to genetics. Trends Endocrinol Metab 14(7):310–317
29. Stowasser M, Gordon RD, Tunny TJ, Klemm SA, Finn WL, Krek AL (1992) Familial hyperaldosteronism type II: five families with a new variety of primary aldosteronism. Clin Exp Pharmacol Physiol 19(5):319–322
30. Sukor N, Mulatero P, Gordon RD, So A, Duffy D, Bertello C, Kelemen L, Jeske Y, Veglio F, Stowasser M (2008) Further evidence for linkage of familial hyperaldosteronism type II at chromosome 7p22 in Italian as well as Australian and South American families. J Hypertens 26(8):1577–1582
31. Sutherland DJ, Ruse JL, Laidlaw JC (1966) Hypertension, increased aldosterone secretion and low plasma renin activity relieved by dexamethasone. Can Med Assoc J 95(22):1109–1119
32. Torpy DJ, Gordon RD, Lin JP, Huggard PR, Taymans SE, Stowasser M, Chrousos GP, Stratakis CA (1998) Familial hyperaldosteronism type II: description of a large kindred and exclusion of the aldosterone synthase (CYP11B2) gene. J Clin Endocrinol Metab 83(9):3214–3218
33. Torpy DJ, Stratakis CA, Gordon RD (1998) Linkage analysis of familial hyperaldosteronism type II–absence of linkage to the gene encoding the angiotensin II receptor type 1. J Clin Endocrinol Metab 83(3):1046
34. Tunny TJ, Gordon RD, Klemm SA, Cohn D (1991) Histological and biochemical distinctiveness of atypical aldosterone-producing adenomas responsive to upright posture and angiotensin. Clin Endocrinol (Oxf) 34(5):363–369
35. Warnock DG (2001) Liddle syndrome: genetics and mechanisms of Na+ channel defects. Am J Med Sci 322(6):302–307

Chapter 8
Familial Hyperaldosteronism Type III

Tracy Ann Williams, Silvia Monticone, Franco Veglio, and Paolo Mulatero

Abstract Primary aldosteronism is a frequent form of endocrine hypertension comprising both sporadic and familial forms. Three forms of familial hyperaldosteronism have been described to date. In this chapter we discuss the clinical phenotypes and the genetic basis of familial hyperaldosteronism type III. This condition is caused by a mutation in the KCNJ5 gene, encoding the potassium channel GIRK4 (also called Kir 3.4), that alters the selectivity filter of the ion channel. In the presence of these mutations, aldosterone secretion is increased leading to a particularly severe form of hyperaldosteronism with early-onset hypertension that is usually resistant to pharmacological treatment and requires bilateral adrenalectomy.

Keywords Familial hyperaldosteronism • Primary aldosteronism • Aldosterone • Hybrid steroids • Adrenal hyperplasia

Abbreviations

ACTH	Adrenocorticotropic hormone
ADX	Adrenalectomy
APA	Aldosterone-producing adenoma
CYP11B1	11β-Hydroxylase
CYP11B2	Aldosterone synthase
DBP	Diastolic blood pressure

T.A. Williams, Ph.D. (✉) • S. Monticone • F. Veglio • P. Mulatero, M.D.
Division of Internal Medicine and Hypertension, Department of Medical Sciences, University of Torino, Medicina Interna 4, Via Genova 3, Torino 10126, Italy
e-mail: tracyann.williams@unito.it

P. Hellman (ed.), *Primary Aldosteronism: Molecular Genetics, Endocrinology, and Translational Medicine*, DOI 10.1007/978-1-4939-0509-6_8,

FH-III	Familial hyperaldosteronism type III
PA	Primary aldosteronism
PRA	Plasma renin activity
SBP	Systolic blood pressure

Introduction

After the first description by Jerome Conn [1], primary aldosteronism (PA) was considered a frequent form of secondary hypertension. However, this hypothesis was subsequently challenged by most clinical researchers [2], until the use of the aldosterone/plasma renin activity (PRA) ratio (ARR) as a screening test in most hypertensive patients [3]. The widespread use of the ARR led to the recognition of PA as the most frequent and potentially curable form of endocrine hypertension. This stimulated further research studies that demonstrated a pivotal role of aldosterone excess in cardiac, vascular and renal damage [4] resulting in an increased rate of cardiovascular events in PA patients compared to essential hypertensives [5].

The subtype diagnosis of PA is of paramount importance both for sporadic forms, to address patients to the appropriate therapy, and for familial forms, to perform an early diagnosis of affected relatives.

Familial forms comprise familial hyperaldosteronism type I (FH-I) also known as glucocorticoid-remediable aldosteronism, determined by the presence of a chimeric enzyme that results from the recombination of CYP11B1 and CYP11B2 genes [6]; familial hyperaldosteronism type II (FH-II) for which the causative gene has not been identified but has been shown in some cases to be linked to chromosomal region 7p22 [7]; and familial hyperaldosteronism type III (FH-III) that is discussed in this chapter.

Historical Description

In 2008 Geller et al. described a family with a peculiar clinical and hormonal phenotype associated with PA [8] that was defined as FH-III [9]. The index case was the father, whose particular condition was firstly described in 1959 [10] at the age of 9 years when he had been suffering from headache since he was 3 years old and had severe polyuria, polydipsia, and enuresis, and developed generalised myalgia. Blood pressure readings at 5 years ranged between 160 and 200/115–140 with a highest recorded value of 300/190. A chest X-ray and electrocardiogram showed left ventricular hypertrophy [10]. Plasma potassium levels were between 2.1 and 3.0 mEq/L; 3-day average urinary aldosterone levels were 67 μg/day (normal values 4–8) and 17-ketosteroids were slightly above the normal level. Corticotropin administration determined a twofold increase of urinary aldosterone levels together with a reported marked increase in 17-ketosteroid and 17-hydroxysteroid excretion. The boy was diagnosed with PA and underwent adrenal exploration: both adrenal glands were enlarged, and the patient underwent bilateral adrenalectomy [10]. The adrenals displayed an increased size and nodular hyperplasia with the *zona fasciculata* occupying most of the gland. After surgery, polyuria decreased from 6.5 to 1.2 L/day, blood pressure fell to 110/65, and potassium increased to normal levels [10]. Twenty-six years later the two daughters of the patient displayed severe childhood hypertension (at 7 and 4 years of age) [8]. Biochemical and hormonal evaluations showed marked hypokalaemia (K^+ <2 mEq/L in both sisters) and very high levels of serum aldosterone (137.4 and 185.1 ng/dL; normal values 3–39.5) with suppressed PRA. Surprisingly, during a 3-week dexamethasone administration, aldosterone levels paradoxically increased whereas blood pressure levels were unchanged [8]. The two girls were lost to follow-up for 8 years after which they were seen again for markedly resistant hypertension and hypokalaemia despite multidrug regimens including spironolactone and amiloride and robust potassium supplementation. Hormone measurements showed suppressed ACTH and markedly increased aldosterone and its precursors deoxycorticosterone and 18-hydroxycorticosterone. Cortisol levels were within the normal range. Similar results were obtained with urinary steroid measurements. Finally, 18-hydroxycortisol and 18-oxocortisol were particularly elevated, and even greater than the levels reported for FH-I [11]. The dexamethasone suppression test was repeated with similar results to those obtained 8 years previously, but unexpectedly, cortisol levels were not suppressed during the test, suggesting a global alteration of the regulation of aldosterone and cortisol in the adrenal cortex [8]. Both girls underwent bilateral adrenalectomy: adrenals were markedly enlarged and at histology demonstrated a diffuse hyperplasia of the *zona fasciculata* without evidence of nodularity.

Genetic Cause of FH-III

The genetic cause of FH-III is due to the presence of a germline mutation in the *KCNJ5* gene located on chromosome 11q24 [12, 13]. *KCNJ5* encodes the G-protein-activated inward rectifier K^+ channel 4 (GIRK4, also known as Kir3.4) that is implicated in the regulation of heart rate [14] and in the pathogenesis of atrial fibrillation [15]. A heterozygous Gly387Arg loss-of-function KCNJ5 mutation is present in all affected members of a family with long QT syndrome, an inherited cardiac disorder predisposing affected individuals to sudden death from cardiac arrhythmias [16]. In the adrenal gland, GIRK4 is localised to the zona glomerulosa and to the outer part of the zona fasciculata [12, 17, 18]. Mutations in KCNJ5 that cause FH-III are located around the highly conserved GlyTyrGly motif in the K^+ selectivity filter in the pore domain of the channel. These mutations interfere with ion selectivity and result in an increase in Na^+ entry and membrane depolarisation [12, 19–21]. In the zona glomerulosa cells of the adrenal gland, membrane depolarisation leads to the opening of voltage-gated calcium channels and an increase in intracellular Ca^{2+} [13].

The first described KCNJ5 mutation responsible for FH-III was Thr158Ala [12] which has also been described as a somatic mutation in aldosterone-producing adenomas [19]. Expression of the KCNJ5 Thr158Ala mutation in a human adrenal cortical cell line (HAC15) resulted in Na^+ and Ca^+ influx and an increase in *CYP11B2* (the gene encoding aldosterone synthase) expression and a marked increase in aldosterone secretion that could be inhibited using the calcium channel blocker nifedipine [22].

A total of seven families with FH-III caused by KCNJ5 mutations have now been described (Table 8.1). These mutations comprise Thr158Ala in three members of a single family [8, 12]; Gly151Glu in seven members of three families [19, 20]; Gly151Arg in four members of two families [20]; and Ile157Ser in two members of one family [21]. The Gly151Glu genotype is correlated with a notably milder phenotype compared with patients harbouring the other mutations [20]. As with the other described KCNJ5 FH-III mutations, Gly151Glu results in Na^+ influx and membrane depolarisation [19]; however, the Na^+ conductance of cells expressing this mutation was surprisingly much greater than those expressing Gly151Arg [20]. The Gly151Glu mutation resulted in a Na^+-dependent cell lethality, and it is this increased cell death that may account for the reduced adrenocortical hyperplasia and the milder phenotype observed in patients carrying this form of mutated KCNJ5 [20].

Patients carrying the Thr158Ala KCNJ5 FH-III mutation exhibit a massive overproduction of hybrid steroids, a paradoxical increase in aldosterone levels in response to dexamethasone administration and decreased androgen production [8]. The family with three patients carrying the Thr158Ala mutation comprises the boy first described in 1959 [10] who later fathered the two sisters with FH-III [8]. This family exhibited severe primary aldosteronism and hypertension that was resistant to a multi-drug therapy and required bilateral adrenalectomy [8]. In contrast, FH-III patients with the Gly151Glu KCNJ5 mutation were treated with medical therapy that included mineralocorticoid receptor antagonists and amiloride, which successfully controlled both the blood pressure and hypokalaemia [19, 20]. The adrenals appeared normal on CT scanning with no evidence of hyperplasia [19, 20]. Hybrid steroids were produced at lower levels compared to Thr158Ala and were within the range of hybrid steroids produced by patients with sporadic primary aldosteronism. In addition, blood pressure and aldosterone levels were not increased upon dexamethasone administration. The FH-III Ile157Ser and Gly151Arg KCNJ5 mutations cause a clinical profile more reminiscent of Thr158Ala, rather than Gly151Glu, with patients displaying severe aldosteronism and early-onset hypertension, uncontrolled with medical therapy, and massive bilateral adrenal hyperplasia, thus requiring bilateral adrenalectomy [20, 21].

Table 8.1 Clinical and biochemical parameters of FH-III families

Families (references)	Sex (M/F)	Age at diagnosis of hypertension (years, range)	Serum potassium (mEq/L, range)	Serum aldosterone (ng/dL)	SBP/DBP (mmHg)	CT scanning	Therapy
Thr158Ala [8, 10]	1/2	4–7	1.8–2.1	137–185	190–300/140–190	Marked bilateral hyperplasia	Bilateral ADX
Gly151Glu [19, 25]	0/2	2–18	2.8–2.9	41.2–113	130–190/80–115	Normal adrenals	Medical
Gly151Glu [20, 26, 27]	2/2	0.2–12	2.6–4.4	91–297	135–160/85–120	Normal adrenals	Medical/ADX
Gly151Glu [20]	2/0	1–4	n.a. (low)	n.a. (high)	n.a. (high)	n.a.	Medical/Bil.ADX
Gly151Arg [20]	0/3	1	1.4–3.2	88	120–175/70–90	Marked bilateral hyperplasia	Bilateral ADX
Gly151Arg [20]	0/1	4	1.7	23	125/80	n.a.	n.a.
Ile157Ser [21]	0/2	2–7	2.7	118	150–170/100	Marked bilateral hyperplasia	Bilateral ADX

M/F male/female, *SBP* systolic blood pressure, *DBP* diastolic blood pressure, *ADX* adrenalectomy, *n.a.* not available

Diagnosis, Prevalence and Phenotypes

The diagnosis of FH-III was at first based on the particular clinical features of the first described family [8, 9, 23]. However, it soon became clear that these features were specific to this family and not of FH-III in general [19]. For this reason the only consistent way to diagnose FH-III is by KCNJ5 DNA sequencing and the identification of mutations that alter the selectivity filter of the ion channel.

Prevalence of FH-III has not been investigated systematically in large populations. In our centre we found a single family [19] among 12 with familial hyperaldosteronism (8.3 %) that were identified in the PATOGEN (Primary Aldosteronism in TOrino-GENetic forms) study [24]. On the basis of these results, FH-III accounts for less than 1 % of PA patients.

Clinical phenotypes have been shown to vary between families and according to the causative mutation. We describe here the most important clinical features of the published pedigrees.

Thr158Ala [8, 10, 12]—This was the mutation causing the first described case of FH-III [10], and only one family has been described to date with this mutation. The clinical and biochemical phenotypes associated with this mutation are described in the previous paragraphs (Table 8.1).

Gly151Glu [19, 20, 25–27]—Three families with this mutation have been described. The Italian family is of particular interest since the index case became hypertensive when she was 18 which is the oldest age of diagnosis of hypertension in all FH-III cases published so far [19] (Table 8.1). Interestingly, she had a history of polyuria in the first decade of life that subsequently disappeared which suggests that aldosterone overproduction and hypokalaemia were already present. After PA diagnosis, blood pressure levels were normalized with a three-drug treatment including low-dose spironolactone (25 mg). The daughter was referred at 2 years of age to the hospital for polyuria and polydipsia, and she was severely hypertensive and hypokalaemic. Aldosterone levels were particularly high (>100 ng/dL) and not modified after dexamethasone administration [25]. The same test was performed to the mother with similar results (cortisol displayed normal suppression in contrast with the family described by Geller) [8]. Blood pressure and hypokalaemia were controlled with canrenone and amiloride [25]. She also displayed hypercalciuria and nephrocalcinosis, and the latter was also present in the mother. Both patients had normal appearance of the adrenal glands at CT scanning and displayed levels of 18-hydroxycortisol and 18-oxocortisol in the range of sporadic PA patients [28] or slightly higher but much lower than the levels measured in FH-I patients and in the family described by Geller [8].

In the American family K1486 reported by Scholl [20] the first patient was described in 1955 [26] (Table 8.1). He was a 13-year-old boy with polyuria and nicturia since early childhood, with hypertension (up to 200/150) and severe hypokalaemia (1.8–2.2 mEq/L). PA diagnosis was made, and the patient underwent removal of the right and four-fifths of the left adrenal gland. After surgery the patient became normotensive except when he underwent a high-sodium diet [26].

His daughter was found hypertensive at the age of 2 years: even in this case polyuria and polydipsia were present. Potassium levels were 3.5 mEq/L, PRA was suppressed and aldosterone was elevated. During dexamethasone administration, cortisol levels were suppressed and aldosterone unchanged [26]. Blood pressure levels were normalized with spironolactone therapy. In adulthood she had two children with PA, hypertension and hypokalaemia before the age of 2 years: in both cases spironolactone normalized blood pressure and potassium levels [20].

The last family described with G151E mutations (K124) [20] had two affected members: the son was hypertensive and hypokalaemic since 4 years of age and was effectively treated with spironolactone. The father underwent bilateral adrenalectomy at 6 years of age for PA that was diagnosed at the age of 1 because spironolactone was not yet available (Table 8.1).

Gly151Arg [20]—Two families with this mutation have been described. In the first family, the mother and the two daughters all had hypertension and hypokalaemia before 2 years of age. Spironolactone and unilateral adrenalectomy were uneffective, and only bilateral adrenalectomy successfully normalized blood pressure and potassium levels. Adrenal glands were markedly enlarged with hyperplasia of the *zona glomerulosa* and of the *zona fasciculata* [20].

In the last patient (K 409) [20] G151R was probably a de novo mutation since both parents were normotensive. She had hypokalaemic hypertension since the age of 4 years when PA was diagnosed. She was lost at follow-up [20].

Ile157Ser [21]—The family described with this mutation comprises two affected members, a mother and daughter. The daughter was hypertensive and hypokalaemic since 2 years of age when severe PA was diagnosed [21]. Dexamethasone suppression testing was negative; she was treated with spironolactone until the age of 15 when she underwent removal of the entire left and half of the right adrenal because of resistant hypertension despite multiple-drug treatment including spironolactone. The adrenals were markedly enlarged with diffuse adrenocortical hyperplasia. Despite normalisation of the hypertension and hypokalaemia by the surgical intervention, the remaining right adrenal subsequently became hyperplastic and the patient again developed resistant hypertension: she was awaiting further removal of the right adrenal gland at the time of her description [21]. The mother was hypertensive and hypokalaemic for PA since 7 years of age and underwent bilateral adrenalectomy for massive bilateral adrenal hyperplasia at 13 years [21].

In summary, with the exception of an Italian woman, all FH-III patients suffered from severe hypertension and hypokalaemia in early childhood (before the age of 7) which was in most cases associated with polyuria and polydipsia. This last feature is probably determined by a hypokalaemic tubulopathy with a urinary concentrating defect associated with reduced expression of aquaporin-2 [29]. It should be noted that only the family described by Geller [8] displayed aldosterone hypersecretion associated with deregulated cortisol production and a paradoxical increase in aldosterone secretion during dexamethasone administration: therefore, this feature should no longer be considered as characteristics of FH-III. Bilateral adrenal hyperplasia has been shown in all families except in those carrying the Gly151Glu mutation that causes an increase in cell death [20]. Finally, hypokalaemia was marked in most patients, again with the exception of some patients carrying the Gly151Glu mutation. Finally, aldosterone levels were particularly increased and much higher than those reported for FH-I and FH-II patients [24].

Therapy

With the exception of families with the Gly151Glu mutation, in which hypertension and hypokalaemia were reported to be controlled by mineralocorticoid receptor antagonists and amiloride, in all other patients bilateral adrenalectomy was requested.

Conclusions

FH-III is a rare and particularly aggressive form of genetic hyperaldosteronism, associated in most cases with severe hypertension and hypokalaemia requiring bilateral adrenalectomy. This condition is determined by mutations in the KCNJ5 gene encoding the potassium channel GIRK4.

References

1. Conn JW (1955) Primary aldosteronism. J Lab Clin Med 45:661–664
2. Ganguly A (1998) Primary aldosteronism. N Engl J Med 339:1828–1834
3. Mulatero P, Stowasser M, Loh KC, Fardella CE, Gordon RD, Mosso L, Gomez-Sanchez CE, Veglio F, Young WF Jr (2004) Increased diagnosis of primary aldosteronism, including surgically correctable forms, in centers from five continents. J Clin Endocrinol Metab 89:1045–1050
4. Mulatero P, Milan A, Williams TA, Veglio F (2006) Mineralocorticoid receptor blockade in the protection of target organ damage. Cardiovasc Hematol Agents Med Chem 4:75–91
5. Milliez P, Girerd X, Plouin PF, Blacher J, Safar ME, Mourad JJ (2005) Evidence for an increased rate of cardiovascular events in patients with primary aldosteronism. J Am Coll Cardiol 45:1243–1248
6. Lifton RP, Dluhy RG, Powers M, Rich GM, Cook S, Ulick S, Lalouel JM (1992) A chimaeric 11 beta-hydroxylase/aldosterone synthase gene causes glucocorticoid-remediable aldosteronism and human hypertension. Nature 355:262–265
7. Sukor N, Mulatero P, Gordon RD, So A, Duffy D, Bertello C, Kelemen L, Jeske Y, Veglio F, Stowasser M (2008) Further evidence for linkage of familial hyperaldosteronism type II at chromosome 7p22 in Italian as well as Australian and South American families. J Hypertens 26:1577–1582
8. Geller DS, Zhang J, Wisgerhof MV, Shackleton C, Kashgarian M, Lifton RP (2008) A novel form of human Mendelian hypertension featuring nonglucocorticoid-remediable aldosteronism. J Clin Endocrinol Metab 93:3117–3123
9. Mulatero P (2008) A new form of hereditary primary aldosteronism: familial hyperaldosteronism type III. J Clin Endocrinol Metab 93:2972–2974
10. Therien B, Mellinger RC, Caldwell JR, Howard PJ (1959) Primary aldosteronism due to adrenal hyperplasia; occurrence in a boy aged 10 years. AMA J Dis Child 98:90–99

11. Rich GM, Ulick S, Cook S, Wang JZ, Lifton RP, Dluhy RG (1992) Glucocorticoid-remediable aldosteronism in a large kindred: clinical spectrum and diagnosis using a characteristic biochemical phenotype. Ann Intern Med 116:813–820
12. Choi M, Scholl UI, Yue P, Björklund P, Zhao B, Nelson-Williams C, Ji W, Cho Y, Patel A, Men CJ, Lolis E, Wisgerhof MV, Geller DS, Mane S, Hellman P, Westin G, Åkerström G, Wang W, Carling T, Lifton RP (2011) K+ channel mutations in adrenal aldosterone-producing adenomas and hereditary hypertension. Science 331:768–772
13. Mulatero P, Monticone S, Rainey WE, Veglio F, Williams TA (2013) Role of KCNJ5 in familial and sporadic primary aldosteronism. Nat Rev Endocrinol 9(2):104–112. doi:10.1038/nrendo.2012.230
14. Wickman K, Nemec J, Gendler SJ, Clapham DE (1998) Abnormal heart rate regulation in GIRK4 knockout mice. Neuron 20:103–114
15. Kovoor P, Wickman K, Maguire CT, Pu W, Gehrmann J, Berul CI, Clapham DE (2001) Evaluation of the role of I(KACh) in atrial fibrillation using a mouse knockout model. J Am Coll Cardiol 37:2136–2143
16. Yang Y, Yang Y, Liang B, Liu J, Li J, Grunnet M, Olesen SP, Rasmussen HB, Ellinor PT, Gao L, Lin X, Li L, Wang L, Xiao J, Liu Y, Liu Y, Zhang S, Liang D, Peng L, Jespersen T, Chen YH (2010) Identification of a Kir3.4 mutation in congenital long QT syndrome. Am J Hum Genet 86:872–880
17. Monticone S, Hattangady NG, Nishimoto K, Mantero F, Rubin B, Cicala MV, Pezzani R, Auchus RJ, Ghayee HK, Shibata H, Kurihara I, Williams TA, Giri JG, Bollag RJ, Edwards MA, Isales CM, Rainey WE (2012) Effect of KCNJ5 mutations on gene expression in aldosterone-producing adenomas and adrenocortical cells. J Clin Endocrinol Metab 97:E1567–E1572
18. Azizan EA, Lam BY, Newhouse SJ, Zhou J, Kuc RE, Clarke J, Happerfield L, Marker A, Hoffman GJ, Brown MJ (2012) Microarray, qPCR, and KCNJ5 sequencing of aldosterone-producing adenomas reveal differences in genotype and phenotype between zona glomerulosa- and zona fasciculata-like tumors. J Clin Endocrinol Metab 97:E819–E829
19. Mulatero P, Tauber P, Zennaro MC, Monticone S, Lang K, Beuschlein F, Fischer E, Tizzani D, Pallauf A, Viola A, Amar L, Williams TA, Strom TM, Graf E, Bandulik S, Penton D, Plouin PF, Warth R, Allolio B, Jeunemaitre X, Veglio F, Reincke M (2012) KCNJ5 mutations in European families with nonglucocorticoid remediable familial hyperaldosteronism. Hypertension 59:235–240
20. Scholl UI, Nelson-Williams C, Yue P, Grekin R, Wyatt RJ, Dillon MJ, Couch R, Hammer LK, Harley FL, Farhi A, Wang WH, Lifton RP (2012) Hypertension with or without adrenal hyperplasia due to different inherited mutations in the potassium channel KCNJ5. Proc Natl Acad Sci U S A 109:2533–2538
21. Charmandari E, Sertedaki A, Kino T, Merakou C, Hoffman DA, Hatch MM, Hurt DE, Lin L, Xekouki P, Stratakis CA, Chrousos GP (2012) A novel point mutation in the KCNJ5 gene causing primary hyperaldosteronism and early-onset autosomal dominant hypertension. J Clin Endocrinol Metab 97:E1532–E1539
22. Oki K, Plonczynski MW, Luis Lam M, Gomez-Sanchez EP, Gomez-Sanchez CE (2012) Potassium channel mutant KCNJ5 T158A expression in HAC-15 cells increases aldosterone synthesis. Endocrinology 153:1774–1782
23. Mulatero P, Williams TA, Monticone S, Veglio F (2011) Is familial hyperaldosteronism underdiagnosed in hypertensive children? Hypertension 57:1053–1055
24. Mulatero P, Tizzani D, Viola A, Bertello C, Monticone S, Mengozzi G, Schiavone D, Williams TA, Einaudi S, La Grotta A, Rabbia F, Veglio F (2011) Prevalence and characteristics of familial hyperaldosteronism: the PATOGEN study (Primary Aldosteronism in TOrino-GENetic forms). Hypertension 58:797–803
25. Mussa A, Camilla R, Monticone S, Porta F, Tessaris D, Verna F, Mulatero P, Einaudi S (2012) Polyuric-polydipsic syndrome in a pediatric case of non-glucocorticoid remediable familial hyperaldosteronism. Endocr J 59:497–502
26. Bartter FC, Biglieri EG (1958) Primary aldosteronism: clinical staff conference at the National Institutes of Health. Ann Intern Med 48:647–654

27. Greco RG, Carroll JE, Morris DJ, Grekin RJ, Melby JC (1982) Familial hyperaldosteronism, not suppressed by dexamethasone. J Clin Endocrinol Metab 55:1013–1016
28. Mulatero P, di Cella SM, Monticone S, Schiavone D, Manzo M, Mengozzi G, Rabbia F, Terzolo M, Gomez-Sanchez EP, Gomez-Sanchez CE, Veglio F (2012) 18-hydroxycorticosterone, 18-hydroxycortisol, and 18-oxocortisol in the diagnosis of primary aldosteronism and its subtypes. J Clin Endocrinol Metab 97:881–889
29. Amlal H, Krane CM, Chen Q, Soleimani M (2000) Early polyuria and urinary concentrating defect in potassium deprivation. Am J Physiol Renal Physiol 279:F655–F663

Chapter 9
The Aldosterone–Renin Ratio: Role and Problems

Michael Stowasser and Richard Douglas Gordon

Abstract The major role of the aldosterone/renin ratio (ARR) test is in screening hypertensive patients for primary aldosteronism (PA). Although currently the most reliable and popular approach, the value of this screening test depends on an appreciation of factors (such as antihypertensive and other medications, posture, time of day, age, gender, phase of menstrual cycle, diet, presence of hypokalemia, medications, and renal function) which can affect the results, on the care with which either these factors are controlled or their effects taken into account, and on access to reliable and reproducible assays for renin and aldosterone. Even then, physiological day-to-day variability reduces the value of a single estimation, and repeated testing is advisable before deciding whether or not to proceed to further diagnostic work-up. Provided that testing of aldosterone suppressibility is always carried out in order to confirm or exclude the diagnosis, and adrenal venous sampling is employed to differentiate unilateral from bilateral forms, wide application of the ARR can have a major beneficial clinical impact, with improved therapeutic outcomes, including possible cure in those with unilateral disease and improved quality of life.

Keywords Primary aldosteronism-aldosterone • Renin • ARR • Assay methodology

M. Stowasser, M.B.B.S., F.R.A.C.P., Ph.D. (✉)
Endocrine Hypertension Research Centre, University of Queensland
School of Medicine, Princess Alexandra Hospital, Brisbane, QLD 4102, Australia
e-mail: m.stowasser@uq.edu.au

R.D. Gordon, M.B.B.S., M.D., Ph.D., F.R.A.C.P., F.R.C.P.
Endocrine Hypertension Research Centre, University of Queensland
School of Medicine, Greenslopes Hospital, Brisbane, QLD 4120, Australia

P. Hellman (ed.), *Primary Aldosteronism: Molecular Genetics, Endocrinology, and Translational Medicine*, DOI 10.1007/978-1-4939-0509-6_9,

Introduction

The plasma aldosterone/renin ratio (ARR) was introduced as a screening test for primary aldosteronism (PA) in the 1980s [42, 44] after being reported to have the ability to detect PA (including surgically curable forms) in hypertensive patients who would otherwise have been missed because they lacked the biochemical "hallmark" of hypokalemia. Since that time, it has emerged as the most popular form of screening for PA. Its wider application among the hypertensive population to include normokalemic (and not just hypokalemic) patients in the 1990s and beyond [36, 38, 51, 58, 66, 76, 92] was largely responsible for the recognition that PA is much more common than previously suspected and possibly accounts for as many as 5–15 % of hypertensive subjects. Not unexpectedly, this has resulted in a marked increase in the number of ARR tests ordered by treating physicians, prompting a critical need to better understand the strengths and weaknesses of the ARR and the factors that can complicate interpretation of results.

The Rationale Behind the Use of the ARR as a Screening Test for PA

Because PA is characterized by aldosterone production which is excessive in relation to body salt/volume status and relatively autonomous of its chronic regulator, renin–angiotensin II (AII) [17], plasma aldosterone levels in PA are higher than would be normally expected for the prevailing level of renin (which is suppressed) and, as a result, the ARR becomes elevated. In early PA, as an adrenal begins to secrete aldosterone autonomously in addition to the correctly regulated secretion, salt is retained, volume expands, and blood pressure (BP) begins to rise [37]. The increase in volume and BP is detected early by volume and BP sensors, and renin secretion is reduced appropriately. During this period of homeostatic adjustment, the fall in renin would be expected to blunt the rise in plasma aldosterone. As a result, the ARR becomes elevated well before aldosterone levels rise above the normal range, rendering it much more sensitive than plasma aldosterone for detection of PA [37]. It is probably only when renin becomes profoundly suppressed and can be suppressed no further that aldosterone becomes clearly elevated.

Measurement of renin alone (that is, without aldosterone) would permit detection of the great majority of patients with PA as levels are almost invariably low in that condition (provided that potentially confounding influences, such as renin-stimulating medications, are not present). However, this approach lacks specificity as renin levels are also suppressed in other low-renin forms of hypertension including the following:

1. *Liddle's syndrome*, in which genetic mutations of the β and γ subunits of the epithelial sodium channel (ENaC) lead to constitutive channel activation (causing salt retention, hypertension, and potassium loss) by preventing binding of these subunits to a regulatory protein (Nedd4) which normally brings about channel degradation [88];

2. *The syndrome of apparent mineralocorticoid excess* (*SAME*), which can result from a mutated gene or be acquired, for example through carbenoxolone administration for peptic ulcer or by consistent ingestion of licorice. Both forms result in deficiency of 11β-hydroxysteroid dehydrogenase type 2 (11βHSD2) activity, an enzyme which functions to prevent cortisol (1,000-fold higher concentrations than aldosterone) from gaining access to and causing excessive stimulation of the mineralocorticoid receptor in the distal nephron, by converting cortisol to cortisone which has no affinity for the receptor [72].
3. *Hypertensive forms of congenital adrenal hyperplasia*, which are caused by mutations in either the 11β-hydroxylase or the 17α-hydroxylase genes, leading to reductions in plasma cortisol levels, compensatory elevation of adrenocorticotrophin (ACTH), and increased production of the mineralocorticoid deoxycorticosterone (DOC) [47, 89].
4. *Primary glucocorticoid resistance*, which prevents normal feedback inhibition of ACTH secretion by cortisol, leading to elevated ACTH and excessive DOC production [6].
5. *Ectopic ACTH production by tumors*, leading to sustained, very high levels of DOC and cortisol, the latter having significant mineralocorticoid activity after exhausting HSD2 conversion to cortisone [87].
6. *DOC-secreting tumors* [45].
7. *Mutations of the mineralocorticoid receptor gene* which cause a modest constitutive activation of the receptor and also permit progesterone and spironolactone to act as agonists rather than antagonists, so that hypertension may be exacerbated during pregnancy and in response to spironolactone treatment [28].
8. *The syndrome of familial hypertension and hyperkalemia with normal glomerular filtration rate* (*FHH*) [31], a salt-sensitive form of hypertension associated with mutations in genes (including *WNK1, WNK4, CUL3*, and *KLHL3*) encoding proteins which regulate the thiazide-sensitive sodium chloride cotransporter in the distal nephron [10, 90]. Unlike PA, aldosterone levels are chronically suppressed (as a result of chronic suppression of renin/AII) in all these salt-dependent, low-renin forms of hypertension with the exception of FHH, in which chronically elevated plasma potassium levels can lead to variable aldosterone levels, but renin is consistently suppressed in the untreated state.
9. *Hypertension in the presence of significantly reduced renal glomerular function* leading to reduced production of renin and sodium retention suppressing renin production.

Hypokalemia was once regarded as the hallmark of PA. However, since screening of normokalemic hypertensives for PA using the ARR became popular, the majority of newly diagnosed PA patients these days have milder forms of PA and are normokalemic. In the natural history of PA development, appearance of hypokalemia is usually delayed and is therefore absent except in those with severe forms (very high plasma aldosterone levels) and in those taking potassium-losing diuretics such as thiazides. Some factors influencing its appearance include the dietary salt load reaching the distal nephron, dietary potassium, and sensitivity of the collecting duct to aldosterone.

Confounders and Limitations to the Use of the ARR

Although the ARR is widely regarded as the most reliable method for screening for PA currently available, like any biochemical screening test false positives and negatives can occur [75]. This is partly because renin is not the sole normal regulator of aldosterone production and plasma levels, and renin and aldosterone do not always move in parallel. Potassium and ACTH are also important regulators of aldosterone production, and they move independently of renin. As well, changes in hepatic blood flow such as occur when upright posture replaces recumbency affect metabolic degradation and hence plasma aldosterone levels. Furthermore, because plasma renin activity (PRA) and the concentration of the "direct active renin" enzyme (DRC) respond differently to certain stimuli, the method used to measure renin can significantly influence the ARR result. Such factors need to be taken into account and controlled for where possible in order to minimize the rate of false-positive and false-negative ratios and thereby maximize the utility of the ARR.

Effects of Posture

Following assumption of upright posture, the resulting translocation of blood into the lower limbs is associated with a rise in plasma aldosterone [85]. This occurs partly due to an increase in renin, released in response to a fall in renal perfusion pressure and an increase in sympathetic output and beta adrenergic receptor stimulation [32], and from the reduction in metabolic clearance of aldosterone that occurs due to reduced hepatic blood flow [8, 61]. Because the effect of reduced hepatic clearance is more rapid, the rise in aldosterone levels measured before and shortly (less than 1 h) after assuming upright posture may not demonstrate close correlation with the rise in renin. Better correlation between changes in aldosterone and renin levels would be expected to occur in studies which use a longer period (2–4 h) of ambulation.

Most centers use an upright sample for ARR testing, usually while seated for 5–15 min. Performance of the ARR in the upright (versus recumbent) position is less likely to miss patients with PA. This is because the majority of patients with PA are AII responsive (AII-R), meaning that their aldosterone levels rise in response to rising renin–AII and thus to upright posture: this includes all patients with AII-R aldosterone-producing adenoma (APA), which makes up at least 50 % of APAs in our experience and most (at least 70 %) with bilateral adrenal hyperplasia [23, 35, 56, 78]. Furthermore, although aldosterone levels in the AII-unresponsive (AII-U) forms (which include AII-U APA, familial hyperaldosteronism type I, and the remaining up to 30 % of bilateral adrenal hyperplasia) fail to rise in response to upright posture [23, 35, 56, 78], upright levels are similar to those of patients with AII-R forms (whose recumbent levels are usually much lower), and upright ARRs appear to be sufficiently sensitive.

Effects of Time of Day

Aldosterone and renin levels obtained midmorning from seated patients will tend to be higher than those measured in the afternoon [33, 86] because the stimulatory effect of upright posture on these levels is greater at that time of day [40]. In patients with PA, renin levels are chronically suppressed and aldosterone levels are strongly influenced by ACTH [48], which follows a striking circadian pattern with the highest levels around 0800 h and falling rapidly thereafter [60]. Their ARR levels are therefore more likely to be elevated during the morning than the afternoon [33].

Age-Related Effects

In the elderly, gradually reducing renal function leads to a fall in renin levels [18], but the accompanying fall in aldosterone levels is less marked, leading to the frequent occurrence of false-positive ratios.

Gender Differences

As illustrated in Fig. 9.1, estrogen stimulates production of the renin substrate angiotensinogen [20, 29]. The resulting rising angiotensin levels lead, by negative feedback on the juxtaglomerular apparatus, to falls in renin release and in DRC. Because the influences of rising substrate and falling renin enzyme levels on product (angiotensin I) formation counteract each other, PRA (which measures generation of angiotensin I) remains relatively stable [25]. Falling DRC will tend to raise ARR, whereas stable PRA will not. Progesterone, secreted during the second half (luteal phase) of an ovulatory menstrual cycle, has mineralocorticoid-antagonist activity [62] and can cause natriuresis, lowering plasma volume and resulting in a compensatory increase in plasma renin and aldosterone. Fluctuations in estrogen and progesterone during the menstrual cycle thus have the potential to complicate interpretation of the ARR.

Fommei and co-workers [26] suggested that a rise in plasma aldosterone in the luteal phase of the menstrual cycle may have implications for screening criteria for PA, for example if plasma aldosterone below a certain level is thought to exclude PA [91]. Pizzolo et al. [64] reported elevated ARR (using DRC) levels to be more prevalent in hypertensive women than men (13.6 % versus 2.3 %), but seldom associated with confirmed PA.

We measured the ARR in 19 normal, ovulating women at three time points in the menstrual cycle and compared it with single measurements in 21 normal males of similar age [3]. In each subject renin was measured as both DRC and PRA and the results compared. ARRs in males were significantly lower than those of females,

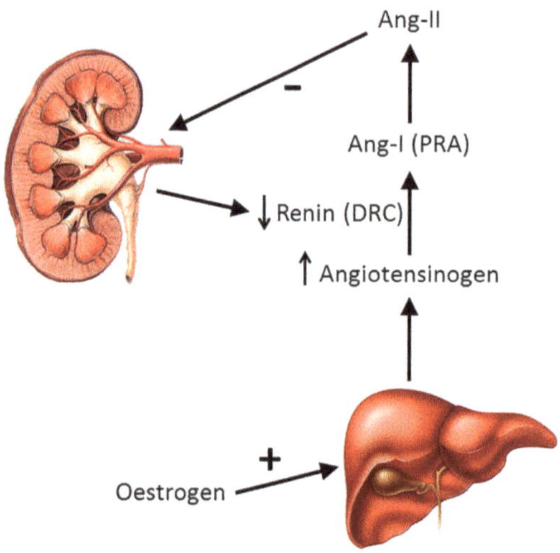

Fig. 9.1 Effects of estrogen on renin, showing differential influences on levels when measured as plasma renin activity [PRA, which measures the generation of angiotensin I (Ang-I)] versus direct renin concentration (DRC, which measures the plasma concentration of active renin enzyme). Estrogen stimulates production of the renin substrate angiotensinogen by the liver. The resulting rising angiotensin I and II (Ang-II) levels lead, by negative feedback on the juxtaglomerular apparatus, to falls in renin release and in DRC. The influences of rising substrate and falling renin enzyme levels on product (Ang-I) formation counteract each other, so that PRA remains relatively stable. As a result, the aldosterone/renin ratio tends to rise in response to estrogen when renin is measured as DRC but not when measured as PRA

regardless of renin assay method, and therefore possibly so well down in the currently accepted normal range that a significant increase associated with developing PA would not be recognized, and represent a false negative. In the females, ARR levels were the lowest (and closest to those of males) during the menses and follicular phase and were the highest during the luteal phase, but the difference only reached significance when DRC (and not when PRA) was used. Two women had luteal ARRs that were falsely elevated using DRC but normal using PRA. These observations may help to explain the higher incidence of false-positive ARRs in hypertensive women than men and suggest that PRA may be preferable to DRC in the determination of ARR, at least in women. They also argue for the development of new reference ranges which take into account gender and sex hormone levels [3].

Effects of Dietary Sodium Intake

Sensitivity of the ratio is likely to be improved if patients maintain a liberal dietary salt intake prior to testing. This is because habitual dietary salt restriction raises renin and aldosterone levels, and because the ARR is more dependent on renin than aldosterone [55], this has the potential to lower the ARR in patients with PA [32, 80]. Conversely, occasional false positives might conceivably arise in patients without PA who consume very large amounts of salt [32, 80]. Although in one study manipulation of dietary salt intake in normotensive subjects, while altering aldosterone and renin levels as expected, did not appear to have a substantial effect on the ARR [49], the relevance of this finding to hypertensives is uncertain and deserving of further study.

Effects of Plasma Potassium Level

Severe, uncorrected hypokalemia can lower aldosterone secretion in PA [15] and therefore has the potential to be associated with false-negative ratios [32, 80]. It is therefore probably safest to assume that a normal ARR should not exclude a diagnosis of PA until measured after correcting hypokalemia with supplemental slow-release potassium chloride tablets. The presence of hypokalemia, however, might not be appreciated if care is not taken during sample collection to avoid false elevations of potassium levels [13, 21]. Common contributors to this include fist clenching (which drives potassium out of the muscles and into the blood), failure to release the torniquet while blood is being collected, the use of vacutainers™ (which can cause hemolysis) rather than syringes, "difficult" sampling (which also causes hemolysis), failure to separate the plasma from the cells within 30 min of blood collection (which allows potassium to leave the red cells as their metabolism slows down), and measurement of potassium in serum rather than plasma (which results in higher levels due to release of potassium from the cells during clotting) [13, 21].

Medications Potentially Causing False-Positive Ratios

Beta-adrenergic blocking medications raise the ARR [2]. Blockade of beta adrenoceptor-mediated stimulation of renin production by juxtaglomerular cells brings about a profound suppression of renin levels [30, 63]. Although aldosterone levels also fall, this is to a lesser degree, possibly because of the continuing stimulatory action of potassium and ACTH, and the ratio therefore rises. Methyldopa [63] and clonidine [52] can have a similar effect by reducing central sympathetic outflow. Nonsteroidal anti-inflammatory agents suppress renin levels by inducing renal sodium and water retention and by suppressing renal prostaglandins which normally stimulate renin release. At the same time they promote retention of potassium leading to stimulation of aldosterone production and further elevation of the ARR [54]. Whether the effects of these agents are sufficient to raise the ARR above the arbitrary cutoff point for PA and thereby cause false-positive test results has been questioned [69, 91], but our own experience has been that falsely elevated ratios are not uncommon in patients receiving these drugs, and our approach is to withdraw them where possible and to repeat the ratio before deciding whether to proceed to confirmatory suppression testing.

For reasons similar to those explained above (see subsection entitled "Gender"), patients receiving oral contraceptive agents and other estrogen-containing preparations may demonstrate falsely elevated ratios when measurements of DRC are used rather than PRA because the increased hepatic production of angiotensinogen, induced by estrogen, results in increased negative feedback by angiotensin-suppressing active renin production [20, 29, 71]. This usually prevents PRA from rising significantly but will lead to suppressed DRC and increased aldosterone/DRC ratio. Statistically significant elevations of ARR using DRC but not PRA were observed following the administration of the combined oral contraceptive preparation ethinylestradiol plus drospirenone (EE + D) [4]. In 3 of the 17 normotensive healthy women studied, aldosterone/DRC ARR values exceeded the upper limit of the normal range 3 weeks after commencing the treatment. Because drospirenone has mineralocorticoid antagonist properties, rises in both renin and aldosterone were expected. The rise in ARR when calculated using DRC presumably reflected an effect of the estrogenic component of EE + D. On the other hand, treatment with subdermal etonogestrel (a progestin-only contraceptive preparation) in 15 other normotensive healthy females was not associated with significant changes in ARR calculated by DRC or PRA [4]. Use of PRA may be preferable to DRC when screening women for PA by ARR measurement without ceasing estrogen-containing oral contraceptive agents.

Medications Potentially Causing False-Negative Ratios

False-negative ratios may be encountered in patients taking medications that stimulate renin production. These include all diuretics [32, 93] including potassium-sparing diuretics such as spironolactone, eplerenone, amiloride, and triamterene, which all induce volume contraction and sympathetic nervous system stimulation. Dihydropyridine calcium channel antagonists briskly stimulate renin [14, 57], probably through reflex sympathetic stimulation as blood pressure falls, natriuretic effects, and direct stimulation of calcium-dependent renin regulatory pathways. Angiotensin-converting enzyme (ACE) inhibitors [57] and AII receptor blockers (ARBs) [57] interfere with negative feedback of AII on renin production and can markedly elevate renin to levels well above normal.

Medication-induced reduction in aldosterone synthesis may also contribute to the generation of false-negative ratios. This can occur with potassium-wasting diuretics such as thiazides which increase renal potassium losses leading to lowering of plasma potassium levels. Dihydropyridine calcium antagonists can reduce aldosterone production by interfering with intracellular, calcium-dependent steps in biosynthesis [5].

ACE inhibitors and ARBs would also be expected to inhibit aldosterone production in patients with AII-R forms of PA [7], and this has been confirmed for the early stages of treatment (up to 1 year), but often is lost later on, with rebounding high levels of aldosterone. The effects of ACE inhibitors and ARBs on the ARR are usually to cause false negatives but are unpredictable and should be replaced when employing ARR to exclude PA.

We recently measured aldosterone, PRA, and DRC levels in normotensive, depressed male patients commencing treatment with either of the selective serotonin reuptake inhibitors (SSRIs) sertraline ($n=12$) or escitalopram ($n=14$) [1]. For both SSRIs, treatment was associated with rises in aldosterone, PRA, and DRC. Because renin rose to a greater degree, the ARR fell significantly in both treatment groups, whether calculated using PRA or DRC. Treatment with SSRIs therefore appears to have the potential to cause false negatives among patients with PA. Further studies involving hypertensive patients are required to address this question.

Effects of Renin Inhibitors

Renin inhibitors have complex effects on renin levels, which depend on how renin is measured [16]. Put simply, these agents are likely to raise the ARR (and cause false positives) if renin is measured as PRA and lower it (causing false negatives) if measured as DRC.

Where Medications Cannot Be Withdrawn

In cases where a potentially interfering medication cannot be withdrawn, useful information can still be obtained by taking into account its known effects when interpreting the ARR result. For example, a raised ratio in patients receiving a diuretic, ACE inhibitor, angiotensin receptor blocker, dihydropyridine calcium blocker, or SSRI antidepressant would make PA very likely, whereas a normal ARR in the presence of beta-blocker treatment or an estrogen-containing oral contraceptive agent would make the diagnosis very unlikely.

Effects of Coexisting Conditions

Conditions which result in stimulation of previously suppressed renin, such as pregnancy [39], renal artery stenosis [79], and malignant hypertension [9, 46, 59], may render ratios falsely negative in patients with PA. False-positive ratios may occur in patients with renal impairment [53], in which renin levels tend to fall as a result of reduced renin secretory mass and also salt and water retention, while any associated hyperkalemia tends to elevate aldosterone. As mentioned above (see section entitled "The Rationale Behind the Use of the ARR as a Screening Test for PA"), false-positive ratios occur in the syndrome of familial hypertension and hyperkalemia with normal glomerular filtration rate (FHH, otherwise known as Gordon syndrome), in which a primary defect in renal tubular function results in excessive resorption of not only sodium (leading to hypertension and renin suppression) but also potassium (causing chronic hyperkalemia, which counteracts suppression of aldosterone) [34].

Falsely Elevated Ratios in the Context of Very Low Renin Levels

Another limitation of the ARR is that, in the presence of very low renin levels (for example, at PRA values of ≤0.1 ng/mL/h), the ARR may be elevated even when plasma aldosterone is also very low (for example, 4 ng/dL or 120 pmol/L) and clearly not consistent with PA. In order to avoid this problem, some investigators include a minimum plasma aldosterone concentration (for example >15 ng/dL or 410 pmol/L) within the screening criteria. In our own experience, however, this approach would have led many of our patients with PA to have been missed because their plasma aldosterone levels fell below this cutoff level [76]. Of 125 patients who underwent removal of APAs within the Endocrine Hypertension Research Center in Brisbane between 2001 and 2010 (inclusive), 20 (16 %) had upright midmorning plasma aldosterone levels of <15 ng/dL and 5 (4 %) had levels <10 ng/dL (278 pmol/L). Because of this, our approach is to proceed with diagnostic work-up for PA in all patients with elevated ARR other than those whose plasma aldosterone concentration is below the level used to define normal suppression during confirmatory fludrocortisone suppression testing (that is, 6 ng/dL or 165 pmol/L). In those patients, we will periodically repeat the ARR and consider, from time to time, further diagnostic work-up depending on the clinical scenario and patient's wishes [74]. We recognize, however, that opinions remain divided on this issue and that the risk of missing APA at plasma aldosterone levels of <10 ng/dL is low.

The Importance of Assay Methodology

Highly reproducible assays are essential for the diagnosis and management of PA. Although the ARR appears to be more dependent on renin than aldosterone [55], accurate measurement of both is required for reliable ARR results. Further, reliable aldosterone quantification is critical during subsequent suppression testing (in which the definitive confirmation or exclusion of PA is dependent on the aldosterone level) and adrenal venous sampling (the results of which largely determine whether a patient is a candidate for unilateral adrenalectomy or, alternatively, treatment with aldosterone antagonist medication) [32, 80].

Aldosterone Assays

The current mainstay for measuring aldosterone is by antibody-based methods [12, 19, 22, 43, 50]. Immunoassays demonstrate varying selectivity and poor interlaboratory reproducibility requiring each laboratory to establish its own reference range for the diagnosis of PA [65]. For example, Schirpenbach et al. [68] reported a two- to threefold difference in aldosterone concentrations measured by four currently used methods. Such discrepancies in aldosterone measurement between laboratories suggest a need for improved aldosterone measurement for both screening and confirmation of PA [33, 77].

Gas chromatography-mass spectrometry has been used to measure aldosterone in biological fluids [11, 70, 73]. While this technique is considered a reference method that provides both accurate results and excellent specificity, these methods in general require extensive sample preparation including chemical derivatization. The lack of automation and complexity of sample preparation have relegated gas chromatography-mass spectrometry to specialist clinical laboratories and is not used in routine clinical services. However, high-performance liquid chromatography-tandem mass spectrometry (HPLC/MS/MS) is a powerful analytical technique that is becoming increasingly used in the clinical setting [82]. HPLC/MS/MS offers the opportunity to provide more reliable measurement of aldosterone than immunoassays [27]. In the wake of concerns raised about currently available immunoassay methodology [68, 77], we developed a high-throughput mass spectrometric method of measuring aldosterone which has proven to be highly reliable and reproducible [83]. This technology also has the ability to simultaneously measure multiple steroids [41, 84]. Wide adoption of such methodology therefore has the potential to improve diagnostic accuracy and optimize clinical outcomes, a great money-saver in the long run. However, for many it may be out of financial reach until the assay becomes more price competitive and widely available. Thus this approach is currently limited to specialized laboratories.

Renin Assays

Concerns also relate to the faster, more convenient methods of directly measuring active renin [24, 33] using immunometric techniques and automated machinery which have widely been adopted in large, busy laboratories in recent years. These include unreliability and poor reproducibility, particular at the low end of the reference range which is particularly relevant to the work-up of patients suspected of or confirmed as having PA. Furthermore, as described above, measurements of DRC, unlike PRA, do not take into account circulating levels of endogenous substrate and are therefore affected by factors such as endogenously or exogenously administered estrogen. Efforts are under way to develop high-throughput assays of angiotensin I (PRA) using mass spectrometry, and results are awaited with great interest.

Because of the critical role of validated assay techniques and the innate variability of both aldosterone and renin, it is important that management decisions not be

Table 9.1 A suggested approach for measurement of the aldosterone/renin ratio (ARR)

(A) *Before ARR measurement*
(1) Correct hypokalemia—avoid factitious rises in plasma potassium by ensuring that blood is collected slowly using a syringe and needle (avoid vacutainers™), avoiding fist clenching during collection, waiting for ≥10 s after torniquet released (if used), and ensuring separation of plasma from cells within 30 min
(2) Encourage patient to liberalize sodium intake
(3) Withdraw medications, where possible, which significantly affect the ARR:
(a) At least 2 weeks before blood collection for beta-blockers, clonidine, methyldopa, nonsteroidal anti-inflammatory drugs, ACE inhibitors, ARBs, dihydropyridine calcium blockers
(b) At least 4 weeks for diuretics—both potassium sparing (e.g., spironolactone, eplerenone, amiloride, and triamterene) and potassium wasting
(4) Where necessary to maintain hypertension control, commence other antihypertensive medications which have lesser effects on the ARR (verapamil slow-release ± hydralazine, and prazosin or doxazosin)
(5) Estrogen-containing oral contraceptive agents may lower renin concentration and cause false-positive ARR when DRC (rather than PRA) is measured. Do not withdraw unless confident of alternative, effective contraception
(B) *Conditions for collection of blood*
(1) Midmorning, after patient ambulant for at least 2 h, seated for 5–15 min
(2) Careful collection technique avoiding stasis and hemolysis [see (A) (1) above]
(C) *Factors to take into account when interpreting results*
(1) Age—in patients over 65 years, renin can be lowered more than aldosterone by age alone, leading to a raised ARR
(2) Gender—ARR higher in females; and phase of menstrual cycle—risk of false positives during luteal phase, but only if calculated using DRC rather than PRA
(3) Time of day, recent diet, posture, and length of time in that posture
(4) All medications
(5) Method of blood collection including any difficulty
(6) Level of potassium
(7) Level of creatinine (renal failure can lead to false-positive ARR)
(8) Assay methodology—could there be a problem?

ACE angiotensin-converting enzyme, *ARBs* angiotensin II receptor blockers, *DRC* direct renin concentration, *PRA* plasma renin activity based on a single ratio. Before deciding that PA is highly likely or highly unlikely, the ratio should be repeated until confident that the ARR is raised, meanwhile adjusting medications and conditions of collection if indicated. The next step, a definitive test involving salt loading, is not entirely risk free in patients with severe hypertension or compromised cardiac or renal function.

A Suggested Approach to Measurement of the ARR

The approach used by the Endocrine Hypertension Research Centre at Greenslopes and Princess Alexandra Hospitals, Brisbane [32, 78, 80] (Table 9.1), attempts to address the above considerations by avoiding, where possible, factors which may confound the ARR or at least taking their effects into account. This approach has resulted in detection of large numbers of patients with PA, including those with surgically correctable forms (which make up around a third of patients in our experience) who have been either cured or had hypertension markedly improved following laparoscopic adrenalectomy, associated with marked improvements in quality of life [67, 78, 81].

References

1. Ahmed AH, Calvird M, Gordon RD, Taylor PJ, Ward G, Pimenta E, Young R, Stowasser M (2011) Effects of two selective serotonin reuptake inhibitor antidepressants, sertraline and escitalopram, on aldosterone/renin ratio in normotensive depressed male patients. J Clin Endocrinol Metab 96(4):1039–1045
2. Ahmed AH, Gordon RD, Taylor P, Ward G, Pimenta E, Stowasser M (2010) Effect of atenolol on aldosterone/renin ratio calculated by both plasma renin activity and direct renin concentration in healthy male volunteers. J Clin Endocrinol Metab 95(7):3201–3206
3. Ahmed AH, Gordon RD, Taylor PJ, Ward G, Pimenta E, Stowasser M (2011) Are women more at risk of false-positive primary aldosteronism screening and unnecessary suppression testing than men? J Clin Endocrinol Metab 96(2):E340–E346
4. Ahmed AH, Gordon RD, Taylor PJ, Ward G, Pimenta E, Stowasser M (2011) Effect of contraceptives on aldosterone/renin ratio may vary according to the components of contraceptive, renin assay method, and possibly route of administration. J Clin Endocrinol Metab 96(6):1797–1804
5. Anderson GH Jr, Howland T, Domschek R, Streeten DH (1986) Effect of sodium balance and calcium channel-blocking drugs on plasma aldosterone responses to infusion of angiotensin II in normal subjects and patients with essential hypertension. J Clin Endocrinol Metab 63(5):1126–1135
6. Arai K, Chrousos GP (1995) Syndromes of glucocorticoid and mineralocorticoid resistance. Steroids 60(1):173–179
7. Atkinson AB, Morton JJ, Brown JJ, Davies DL, Fraser R, Kelly P, Leckie B, Lever AF, Robertson JI (1980) Captopril in clinical hypertension. Changes in components of renin-angiotensin system and in body composition in relation to fall in blood pressure with a note on measurement of angiotensin II during converting enzyme inhibition. Br Heart J 44(3):290–296

8. Balikian HM, Brodie AH, Dale SL, Melby JC, Tait JF (1968) Effect of posture on the metabolic clearance rate, plasma concentration and blood production rate of aldosterone in man. J Clin Endocrinol Metab 28(11):1630–1640
9. Beevers DG, Brown JJ, Ferriss JB, Fraser R, Lever AF, Robertson JI, Tree M (1976) Renal abnormalities and vascular complications in primary hyperaldosteronism. Evidence on tertiary hyperaldosteronism. Q J Med 45(179):401–410
10. Boyden LM, Choi M, Choate KA, Nelson-Williams CJ, Farhi A, Toka HR, Tikhonova IR, Bjornson R, Mane SM, Colussi G, Lebel M, Gordon RD, Semmekrot BA, Poujol A, Valimaki MJ, De FME, Sanjad SA, Gutkin M, Karet FE, Tucci JR, Stockigt JR, Keppler-Noreuil KM, Porter CC, Anand SK, Whiteford ML, Davis ID, Dewar SB, Bettinelli A, Fadrowski JJ, Belsha CW, Hunley TE, Nelson RD, Trachtman H, Cole TR, Pinsk M, Bockenhauer D, Shenoy M, Vaidyanathan P, Foreman JW, Rasoulpour M, Thameem F, Al-Shahrouri HZ, Radhakrishnan J, Gharavi AG, Goilav B, Lifton RP (2012) Mutations in kelch-like 3 and cullin 3 cause hypertension and electrolyte abnormalities. Nature 482(7383):98–102
11. Breuer H, Siekmann L (1975) Mass fragmentography as reference method in clinical steroid assay. J Steroid Biochem 6(5):685–688
12. Brochu M, Fethiere J, Roy M, Ong H, De Lean A (1989) Highly sensitive and rapid radioimmunoassay for aldosterone in plasma and cell culture medium. Clin Biochem 22(4): 289–292
13. Brown JJ, Chinn RH, Davies DL, Fraser R, Lever AF, Rae RJ, Robertson JI (1970) Falsely high plasma potassium values in patients with hyperaldosteronism. Br Med J 2(5700):18–20
14. Brown MJ, Hopper RV (1999) Calcium-channel blockade can mask the diagnosis of Conn's syndrome. Postgrad Med J 75(882):235–236
15. Cain JP, Tuck ML, Williams GH, Dluhy RG, Rosenoff SH (1972) The regulation of aldosterone secretion in primary aldosteronism. Am J Med 53(5):627–637
16. Campbell DJ, Nussberger J, Stowasser M, Danser AH, Morganti A, Frandsen E, Ménard J (2009) Activity assays and immunoassays for plasma renin and prorenin: information provided and precautions necessary for accurate measurement. Clin Chem 55(5):867–877
17. Conn JW (1966) The evolution of primary aldosteronism: 1954–1967. Harvey Lect 62: 257–291
18. Crane MG, Harris JJ (1976) Effect of aging on renin activity and aldosterone excretion. J Lab Clin Med 87(6):947–959
19. Demers LM, Sampson E, Hayes AH Jr (1976) Plasma and urinary aldosterone measurement in healthy subjects with a radioimmunoassay kit not requiring chromatography. Clin Biochem 9(5):243–246
20. Derkx FH, Steunkel C, Schalekamp MP, Visser W, Huisveld IH, Schalekamp MA (1986) Immunoreactive renin, prorenin, and enzymatically active renin in plasma during pregnancy and in women taking oral contraceptives. J Clin Endocrinol Metab 63(4):1008–1015
21. Don BR, Sebastian A, Cheitlin M, Christiansen M, Schambelan M (1990) Pseudohyperkalemia caused by fist clenching during phlebotomy. N Engl J Med 322(18):1290–1292
22. Ekins RP, Newman GB, Piyasena R, Banks P, Slater JD (1972) The radioimmunoassay of aldosterone in serum and urine: theoretical and practical aspects. J Steroid Biochem 3(3): 289–304
23. Espiner EA, Ross DG, Yandle TG, Richards AM, Hunt PJ (2003) Predicting surgically remedial primary aldosteronism: role of adrenal scanning, posture testing, and adrenal vein sampling. J Clin Endocrinol Metab 88(8):3637–3644
24. Ferrari P, Shaw SG, Nicod J, Saner E, Nussberger J (2004) Active renin versus plasma renin activity to define aldosterone-to-renin ratio for primary aldosteronism. J Hypertens 22(2): 377–381
25. Fischer M, Baessler A, Schunkert H (2002) Renin angiotensin system and gender differences in the cardiovascular system. Cardiovasc Res 53(3):672–677
26. Fommei E, Ghione S, Ripoli A, Maffei S, Di Cecco P, Iervasi A, Turchi S (2008) The ovarian cycle as a factor of variability in the laboratory screening for primary aldosteronism in women. J Hum Hypertens 23(2):130–135

27. Fredline VF, Taylor PJ, Dodds HM, Johnson AG (1997) A reference method for the analysis of aldosterone in blood by high-performance liquid chromatography-atmospheric pressure chemical ionization-tandem mass spectrometry. Anal Biochem 252(2):308–313
28. Geller DS, Farhi A, Pinkerton N, Fradley M, Moritz M, Spitzer A, Meinke G, Tsai FT, Sigler PB, Lifton RP (2000) Activating mineralocorticoid receptor mutation in hypertension exacerbated by pregnancy. Science 289(5476):119–123
29. Goldhaber SZ, Hennekens CH, Spark RF, Evans DA, Rosner B, Taylor JO, Kass EH (1984) Plasma renin substrate, renin activity, and aldosterone levels in a sample of oral contraceptive users from a community survey. Am Heart J 107(1):119–122
30. Gordon MS, Williams GH, Hollenberg NK (1992) Renal and adrenal responsiveness to angiotensin II: influence of beta adrenergic blockade. Endocr Res 18(2):115–131
31. Gordon RD (1986) Syndrome of hypertension and hyperkalemia with normal glomerular filtration rate. Hypertension 8:93–102
32. Gordon RD (1995) Primary aldosteronism. J Endocrinol Invest 18(7):495–511
33. Gordon RD (2004) The challenge of more robust and reproducible methodology in screening for primary aldosteronism. J Hypertens 22(2):251–255
34. Gordon RD, Geddes RA, Pawsey CG, O'Halloran MW (1970) Hypertension and severe hyperkalaemia associated with suppression of renin and aldosterone and completely reversed by dietary sodium restriction. Australas Ann Med 19(4):287–294
35. Gordon RD, Gomez-Sanchez CE, Hamlet SM, Tunny TJ, Klemm SA (1987) Angiotensin-responsive aldosterone-producing adenoma masquerades as idiopathic hyperaldosteronism (IHA: adrenal hyperplasia) or low-renin essential hypertension. J Hypertens Suppl 5(5):S103–S106
36. Gordon RD, Klemm SA, Tunny TJ, Stowasser M (1992) Primary aldosteronism: hypertension with a genetic basis. Lancet 340(8812):159–161
37. Gordon RD, Stowasser M, Rutherford JC (2001) Primary aldosteronism: are we diagnosing and operating on too few patients? World J Surg 25(7):941–947
38. Gordon RD, Stowasser M, Tunny TJ, Klemm SA, Rutherford JC (1994) High incidence of primary aldosteronism in 199 patients referred with hypertension. Clin Exp Pharmacol Physiol 21(4):315–318
39. Gordon RD, Tunny TJ (1982) Aldosterone-producing-adenoma (A-P-A): effect of pregnancy. Clin Exp Hypertens A 4(9–10):1685–1693
40. Gordon RD, Wolfe LK, Island DP, Liddle GW (1966) A diurnal rhythm in plasma renin activity in man. J Clin Invest 45(10):1587–1592
41. Guo T, Taylor RL, Singh RJ, Soldin SJ (2006) Simultaneous determination of 12 steroids by isotope dilution liquid chromatography-photospray ionization tandem mass spectrometry. Clin Chim Acta Int J Clin Chem 372(1–2):76–82
42. Hamlet SM, Tunny TJ, Woodland E, Gordon RD (1985) Is aldosterone/renin ratio useful to screen a hypertensive population for primary aldosteronism? Clin Exp Pharmacol Physiol 12(3):249–252
43. Hanquez C, Rajkowski KM, Desfosses B, Cittanova N (1988) A competitive microtitre plate enzyme immunoassay for plasma aldosterone using a monoclonal antibody. J Steroid Biochem 31(6):939–945
44. Hiramatsu K, Yamada T, Yukimura Y, Komiya I, Ichikawa K, Ishihara M, Nagata H, Izumiyama T (1981) A screening test to identify aldosterone-producing adenoma by measuring plasma renin activity. Results in hypertensive patients. Arch Intern Med 141(12):1589–1593
45. Irony I, Biglieri EG, Perloff D, Rubinoff H (1987) Pathophysiology of deoxycorticosterone-secreting adrenal tumors. J Clin Endocrinol Metab 65(5):836–840
46. Kaplan NM (1963) Primary aldosteronism with malignant hypertension. N Engl J Med 269:1282–1286
47. Kater CE, Biglieri EG (1994) Disorders of steroid 17 alpha-hydroxylase deficiency. Endocrinol Metab Clin North Am 23(2):341–357
48. Kem DC, Weinberger MH, Gomez-Sanchez C, Kramer NJ, Lerman R, Furuyama S, Nugent CA (1973) Circadian rhythm of plasma aldosterone concentration in patients with primary aldosteronism. J Clin Invest 52(9):2272–2277

49. Kerstens MN, Muller KAC, Volmer M, Koerts J, Sluiter WJ, Dullaart RP (2011) Reference values for aldosterone-renin ratios in normotensive individuals and effect of changes in dietary sodium consumption. Clin Chem 57(11):1607–1611
50. Kubasik NP, Warren K, Sine HE (1979) Evaluation of a new commercial radioassay kit for aldosterone using an iodinated tracer. Clin Biochem 12(2):59–61
51. Loh KC, Koay ES, Khaw MC, Emmanuel SC, Young WF Jr (2000) Prevalence of primary aldosteronism among Asian hypertensive patients in Singapore. J Clin Endocrinol Metab 85(8):2854–2859
52. Manhem P, Paalzow L, Hokfelt B (1982) Plasma clonidine in relation to blood pressure, catecholamines, and renin activity during long-term treatment of hypertension. Clin Pharmacol Ther 31(4):445–451
53. McKenna TJ, Sequeira SJ, Heffernan A, Chambers J, Cunningham S (1991) Diagnosis under random conditions of all disorders of the renin-angiotensin-aldosterone axis, including primary hyperaldosteronism. J Clin Endocrinol Metab 73(5):952–957
54. Mitnick PD, Greenberg A, DeOreo PB, Weiner BM, Coffman TM, Walker BR, Agus ZS, Goldfarb S (1980) Effects of two nonsteroidal anti-inflammatory drugs, indomethacin and oxaprozin, on the kidney. Clin Pharmacol Ther 28(5):680–689
55. Montori VM, Schwartz GL, Chapman AB, Boerwinkle E, Turner ST (2001) Validity of the aldosterone-renin ratio used to screen for primary aldosteronism. Mayo Clin Proc 76(9): 877–882
56. Mulatero P, Bertello C, Rossato D, Mengozzi G, Milan A, Garrone C, Giraudo G, Passarino G, Garabello D, Verhovez A, Rabbia F, Veglio F (2008) Roles of clinical criteria, computed tomography scan, and adrenal vein sampling in differential diagnosis of primary aldosteronism subtypes. J Clin Endocrinol Metab 93(4):1366–1371
57. Mulatero P, Rabbia F, Milan A, Paglieri C, Morello F, Chiandussi L, Veglio F (2002) Drug effects on aldosterone/plasma renin activity ratio in primary aldosteronism. Hypertension 40(6):897–902
58. Mulatero P, Stowasser M, Loh KC, Fardella CE, Gordon RD, Mosso L, Gomez-Sanchez CE, Veglio F, Young WF Jr (2004) Increased diagnosis of primary aldosteronism, including surgically correctable forms, in centers from five continents. J Clin Endocrinol Metab 89(3): 1045–1050
59. Murphy BF, Whitworth JA, Kincaid-Smith P (1985) Malignant hypertension due to an aldosterone producing adrenal adenoma. Clin Exp Hypertens A 7(7):939–950
60. Ney RL, Shimizu N, Nicholson WE, Island DP, Liddle GW (1963) Correlation of plasma acth concentration with adrenocortical response in normal human subjects, surgical patients, and patients with Cushing's disease. J Clin Invest 42:1669–1677
61. Nowaczynski W, Genest J, Kuchel O, Messerli FH, Guthrie GP Jr, Richardson K, Grose J (1977) Age- and posture-related changes in plasma protein binding and metabolism of aldosterone in essential and secondary hypertension. J Lab Clin Med 90(3):475–489
62. Oelkers WK (1996) Effects of estrogens and progestogens on the renin-aldosterone system and blood pressure. Steroids 61(4):166–171
63. Oparil S (1982) Review of therapeutic modalities acting directly via central pathways. Clin Exp Hypertens A 4(4–5):579–593
64. Pizzolo F, Raffaelli R, Memmo A, Chiecchi L, Pavan C, Guarini P, Guidi GC, Franchi M, Corrocher R, Olivieri O (2010) Effects of female sex hormones and contraceptive pill on the diagnostic work-up for primary aldosteronism. J Hypertens 28(1):135–142
65. Plouin PF, Jeunemaitre X (2004) Would wider screening for primary aldosteronism give any health benefits? Eur J Endocrinol 151(3):305–308
66. Rossi GP, Bernini G, Caliumi C, Desideri G, Fabris B, Ferri C, Ganzaroli C, Giacchetti G, Letizia C, Maccario M, Mallamaci F, Mannelli M, Mattarello MJ, Moretti A, Palumbo G, Parenti G, Porteri E, Semplicini A, Rizzoni D, Rossi E, Boscaro M, Pessina AC, Mantero F (2006) A prospective study of the prevalence of primary aldosteronism in 1,125 hypertensive patients. J Am Coll Cardiol 48(11):2293–2300

67. Rutherford JC, Taylor WL, Stowasser M, Gordon RD (1998) Success of surgery for primary aldosteronism judged by residual autonomous aldosterone production. World J Surg 22(12): 1243–1245
68. Schirpenbach C, Seiler L, Maser-Gluth C, Beuschlein F, Reincke M, Bidlingmaier M (2006) Automated chemiluminescence-immunoassay for aldosterone during dynamic testing: comparison to radioimmunoassays with and without extraction steps. Clin Chem 52(9): 1749–1755
69. Seifarth C, Trenkel S, Schobel H, Hahn EG, Hensen J (2002) Influence of antihypertensive medication on aldosterone and renin concentration in the differential diagnosis of essential hypertension and primary aldosteronism. Clin Endocrinol (Oxf) 57(4):457–465
70. Siekmann L (1979) Determination of steroid hormones by the use of isotope dilution–mass spectrometry: a definitive method in clinical chemistry. J Steroid Biochem 11(1A):117–123
71. Steingold KA, Matt DW, DeZiegler D, Sealey JE, Fratkin M, Reznikov S (1991) Comparison of transdermal to oral estradiol administration on hormonal and hepatic parameters in women with premature ovarian failure. J Clin Endocrinol Metab 73(2):275–280
72. Stewart PM, Mason JI (1995) Cortisol to cortisone: glucocorticoid to mineralocorticoid. Steroids 60(1):143–146
73. Stockl D, Reinauer H, Thienpont LM, De Leenheer AP (1991) Determination of aldosterone in human serum by isotope dilution gas chromatography/mass spectrometry using a new heptafluorobutyryl derivative. Biol Mass Spectrom 20(11):657–664
74. Stowasser M, Ahmed AH, Pimenta E, Taylor PJ, Gordon RD (2012) Factors affecting the aldosterone/renin ratio. Horm Metab Res 44(3):170–176
75. Stowasser M, Gordon RD (2004) The aldosterone-renin ratio for screening for primary aldosteronism. Endocrinologist 14:267–276
76. Stowasser M, Gordon RD (2004) Primary aldosteronism-careful investigation is essential and rewarding. Mol Cell Endocrinol 217(1–2):33–39
77. Stowasser M, Gordon RD (2006) Aldosterone assays: an urgent need for improvement. Clin Chem 52(9):1640–1642
78. Stowasser M, Gordon RD, Gunasekera TG, Cowley DC, Ward G, Archibald C, Smithers BM (2003) High rate of detection of primary aldosteronism, including surgically treatable forms, after "non-selective" screening of hypertensive patients. J Hypertens 21(11):2149–2157
79. Stowasser M, Gordon RD, Klemm SA, Tunny TJ (1993) Renin-aldosterone response to dexamethasone in glucocorticoid-suppressible hyperaldosteronism is altered by coexistent renal artery stenosis. J Clin Endocrinol Metab 77(3):800–804
80. Stowasser M, Gordon RD, Rutherford JC, Nikwan NZ, Daunt N, Slater GJ (2001) Diagnosis and management of primary aldosteronism. J Renin Angiotensin Aldosterone Syst 2(3):156–169
81. Sukor N, Kogovsek C, Gordon RD, Robson D, Stowasser M (2010) Improved quality of life, blood pressure, and biochemical status following laparoscopic adrenalectomy for unilateral primary aldosteronism. J Clin Endocrinol Metab 95(3):1360–1364
82. Taylor PJ (2005) High-performance liquid chromatography-mass spectrometry in the clinical laboratory. Ther Drug Monit 27(6):689–693
83. Taylor PJ, Cooper DP, Gordon RD, Stowasser M (2009) Measurement of aldosterone in human plasma by semiautomated HPLC-tandem mass spectrometry. Clin Chem 55(6):1155–1162
84. Taylor PJ, van RSP, Coombes JS, Gordon RD, Stowasser M (2010) Simultaneous measurement of aldosterone and cortisol by high-performance liquid chromatography-tandem mass spectrometry: application to dehydration-rehydration studies. J Chromatogr B Anal Technol Biomed Life Sci 878(15–16):1195–1198
85. Tuck ML, Dluhy RG, Williams GH (1975) Sequential responses of the renin-angiotensin-aldosterone axis to acute postural change: effect of dietary sodium. J Lab Clin Med 86(5): 754–763
86. Vagnucci AH, McDonald RH Jr, Drash AL, Wong AK (1974) Intradiem changes of plasma aldosterone, cortisol, corticosterone and growth hormone in sodium restriction. J Clin Endocrinol Metab 38(5):761–776

87. Walker BR, Campbell JC, Fraser R, Stewart PM, Edwards CR (1992) Mineralocorticoid excess and inhibition of 11 beta-hydroxysteroid dehydrogenase in patients with ectopic ACTH syndrome. Clin Endocrinol 37(6):483–492
88. Warnock DG (2001) Liddle syndrome: genetics and mechanisms of Na+ channel defects. Am J Med Sci 322(6):302–307
89. White PC (2001) Steroid 11 beta-hydroxylase deficiency and related disorders. Endocrinol Metab Clin North Am 30(1):61–79, vi
90. Wilson FH, Disse-Nicodeme S, Choate KA, Ishikawa K, Nelson-Williams C, Desitter I, Gunel M, Milford DV, Lipkin GW, Achard JM, Feely MP, Dussol B, Berland Y, Unwin RJ, Mayan H, Simon DB, Farfel Z, Jeunemaitre X, Lifton RP (2001) Human hypertension caused by mutations in WNK kinases. Science 293(5532):1107–1112
91. Young WF (2007) Primary aldosteronism: renaissance of a syndrome. Clin Endocrinol (Oxf) 66(5):607–618
92. Young WF Jr (1999) Primary aldosteronism: a common and curable form of hypertension. Cardiol Rev 7(4):207–214
93. Young WFJ (1997) Primary aldosteronism: update on diagnosis and treatment. Endocrinologist 7:213–221

Chapter 10
Confirmatory Testing for Primary Aldosteronism

Matthias Haase, Matthias Gruber, Xing Gao, Oliver Vonend, and Holger S. Willenberg

Abstract To minimize the influence of medication, potassium, angiotensin 2, and corticotropin, because mechanisms of aldosterone escape have been described, and to increase specificity in the diagnostic process, confirmatory testing is necessary in cases suspected to have primary aldosteronism.

There are different approaches to demonstrate that aldosterone is secreted autonomously, including the proof of insufficient suppression of aldosterone secretion or demonstration of a strong suppression of renin.

Nevertheless, all confirmatory tests have pros and cons and sensitivities or specificities are less than 100 %. Therefore, the confirmation of primary aldosteronism is based on a positive screening test and a positive confirmation test but also on details from the case history and or the patient examination. In addition, a typical postinterventional course with reversal of symptoms and signs characteristic of primary aldosteronism help to document the diagnosis.

M. Haase
Department of Endocrinology and Diabetes, Heinrich-Heine University, Duesseldorf, Germany

Department of Medicine III, Technical University, Dresden, Germany

M. Gruber
Department of Medicine III, Technical University, Dresden, Germany

X. Gao
Department of Nephrology, Heinrich-Heine University, Duesseldorf, Germany

O. Vonend
Department of Nephrology, German Clinic of Diagnosticsy, Wiesbaden, Germany

H.S. Willenberg, M.D., Ph.D. (✉)
Division of Endocrinology and Metabolism, University of Rostock, Rostock, Germany

Department of Endocrinology and Diabetes, University Hospital Duesseldorf, Moorenstraße 5, Düsseldorf 40225, Germany
e-mail: holger.willenberg@uni-duesseldorf.de

P. Hellman (ed.), *Primary Aldosteronism: Molecular Genetics, Endocrinology, and Translational Medicine*, DOI 10.1007/978-1-4939-0509-6_10,

Keywords Hypertension • Adrenal • Aldosterone • Fludrocortisone • Sodium • Saline • Captopril • Urine • Dexamethasone • Cortisol

Introduction

Confirmatory testing is mandatory in patients with suspected primary aldosteronism [11]. Main reasons for this rationale include that the influence of medication be minimized; that secretion of aldosterone is controlled by a number of factors, including potassium, angiotensin 2, and corticotropin; and that mechanisms of aldosterone escape have been described [8, 44].

There are different approaches to prove that aldosterone secretion occurs independently of these factors. While a number of tests aim at showing non-suppression of aldosterone secretion, other interventions investigate how strong renin secretion or renin activity is suppressed by the aldosterone action and the negative feedback. In addition, there are tests that try to show that some observations are different in patients with aldosteronomas.

There were efforts to employ endocrine function tests to distinguish different subtypes of primary aldosteronism, including unilateral disease as in aldosterone-producing adenomas and bilateral disease as in bilateral adrenal hyperplasia. However, most of the tests described below do not have the power to differentiate between unilateral or bilateral disease. There are several reasons, and some are mentioned under the corresponding subheadings.

For all tests used to investigate into the physiology of aldosterone secretion, conditions must apply to minimize the influence of ACTH, medication, and other conditions to interfere with the renin- and angiotensin-mediated aldosterone release. To respect the circadian rhythm, all tests should be performed in the morning. In addition, there should be no signs for infection or stress.

In all patients, renin should be low (suppressed). It is not quite clear how low renin needs to be to ensure aldosterone levels against the influence of angiotensin. However, most patients with PA should have plasma renin concentrations below 5 ng/l [29, 46].

Use of glucocorticoids, direct renin inhibitors, mineralocorticoid receptor antagonists, inhibitors of the epithelial sodium channel, or even other diuretics are not allowed as medication. Also, certain progestins, antidepressants, and medication interfering with CYP3A4 activity should be avoided. A guideline provides information on this matter [11].

On the other hand, the more autonomous and unopposed aldosterone secretion occurs, the more suppressed is renin and angiotensin and the less does medication interfere with the salt, water, and volume regulation. In addition, a recent study pointed out that there is probably no need for extensive medication switching in all patients anyway, except for aldosterone antagonists, thiazides, and loop diuretics [39].

However, a problem that really matters when it comes down to cutoff values is the quality of assays employed. Frequently, certain values are quickly adopted from studies while there is a substantial inter-assay variation [37, 38].

Of note, all confirmatory tests have pros and cons and sensitivities or specificities in a range between 80 and 95 %. Therefore, the confirmation of primary aldosteronism is based on a positive screening test and a positive confirmation test but also on details from the case history and or the patient examination. In addition, a typical postinterventional course with reversal of symptoms and signs characteristic of primary aldosteronism document the diagnosis.

Non-suppression of Aldosterone

Fludrocortisone Suppression Test

Principle

Fludrocortisone, 9α-fluoro-cortisol, is a mineralocorticoid receptor agonist and affects salt, water, and volume homeostasis as aldosterone does. The oral administration of fludrocortisone under the condition of a high-salt diet will therefore lead to sodium retention → stimulation of thirst and adiuretin/aquaporin-2 → water retention → hypervolemia and → suppression of renin (Fig. 10.1, Panel A). As a consequence of hypervolemia, endogenous aldosterone secretion is sufficiently downregulated in normal persons or patients with essential hypertension while in patients with primary aldosteronism it is not (Fig. 10.1, Panel A).

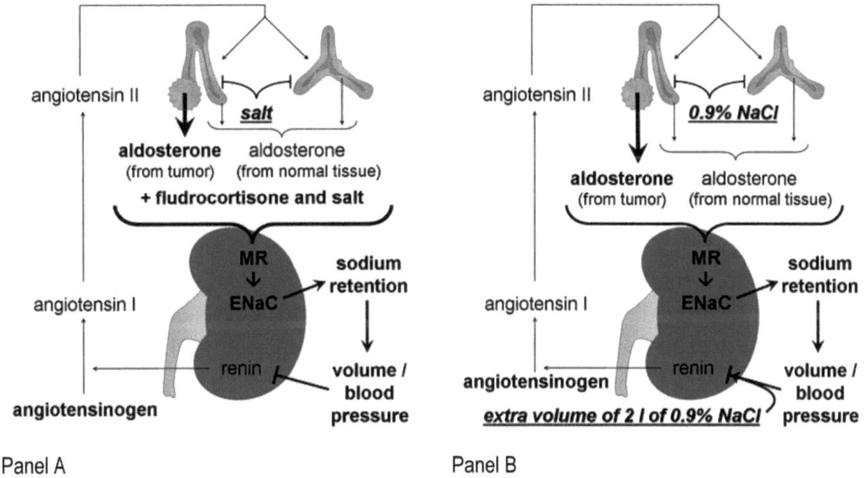

Fig. 10.1 This figure shows the principles of the fludrocortisone suppression test (Panel **a**) and the saline infusion test (Panel **b**)

Protocol

Patients receive 0.1 mg fludrocortisone acetate every 6 h along with potassium chloride or citrate (40 mmol solutions) every 6–8 h (depending on serum potassium values) and a high-salt diet for four full days. If necessary, slow-release sodium chloride supplements (30 mmol) can be given three times daily with meals. It is aimed at serum potassium values of 4 mmol/l and a sodium excretion rate of 3 mmol/kg body weight (min. 200 mmol per day). Blood for aldosterone, renin, and cortisol measurements is sampled after these 4 days around 10 AM (on day 5). Blood for cortisol is also sampled between 7 and 8 AM to ensure a decline between early and late morning time points (exclusion of false-positive aldosterone values due to stress and corticotropin influence). While some centers perform this test on an outpatient basis, the Brisbane group prefers an inpatient setting [41].

This test can be combined with the determination of urinary aldosterone (metabolite) excretion.

Discussion

PA is excluded when aldosterone concentrations drop below 50 ng/l and the diagnosis of PA is safely made when post-FST blood concentrations exceed 60 ng/l [11]. A number of studies applied and/or confirmed this cutoff for plasma/serum aldosterone concentrations, amongst them Gordon and colleagues [14], Fardella et al. [10], Stowasser et al. [41], Mulatero et al. [28, 30], and Willenberg et al. [46].

It is important to note that there is no study showing that after 4 days of fludrocortisone application, the maximum extend of aldosterone suppression was achieved. In this regard, it was not shown that side effects may not develop anymore after cessation of fludrocortisone acetate. The experience of the Düsseldorf group suggests that 3 out of 77 patients (4 %) experience side effects such as left heart failure that may occur in patients with or without PA [46]. Higher doses of fludrocortisone may result in a still higher frequency of cardiac side effects [22].

Although this test may render false-positive results in patients with heart failure (insufficient "transfer of venous volume to arterial volume"), it seems to be more sensitive than the saline infusion test [13, 46]. In 2009, it was shown that primary aldosteronism is excluded when aldosterone levels drop below 80 ng/l (225 pmol/l) after 4 days or below 110 ng/l (305 pmol/l) after 3 days of fludrocortisone treatment (4×100 µg per day) while salt intake does not seem to play a major role [43].

In order to prevent an influence of stress and corticotropin on adrenal aldosterone release, a version of the FST was published that combines the FST with the low-dose overnight dexamethasone suppression test, whereby 1 mg of dexamethasone is given at midnight on day 4 [16]. This test suppresses aldosterone blood concentrations below 25 ng/l (74 pmol/l) in normal individuals.

Saline Infusion Test

Principle

The saline infusion test (SIT) leads to acute volume expansion and is followed by suppression of renin and, consequently, aldosterone when secretion of aldosterone does not occur autonomously or in response to potassium or corticotropin (Fig. 10.1, Panel B). In addition, with the knowledge of unselective electrolyte handling by mutated KCNJ5 potassium pores or loss-of-function ATPase sodium–potassium channels in aldosteronomas, application of sodium in the form of saline may have a direct stimulating effect onto *zona glomerulosa* cells [4, 7, 46].

Protocol

The test should be performed after a period of supine position overnight, but it is also possible to be performed in an outpatient setting. It is then started after a period of minimal 30 min of supine test and blood will be drawn for measurement of aldosterone, cortisol, renin, sodium, and potassium in the morning. Then 2 L of 0.9 % sodium chloride is infused over a time period of 4 h (500 ml per hour). During the infusion blood pressure and heart rate should be controlled in cases of heart failure at least every 30 min. At the end of the test, blood sampling for the measurement of the above mentioned parameters is repeated. During the test the patient is not allowed to stand up, except for miction. Patients should be motivated to remain lying during the last 2 h.

Discussion

The SIT is easy to perform and a practical procedure in an outpatient setting. In experienced hands, the rate of side effects is low when patients are carefully examined for possible contraindications, e.g., cardiac insufficiency and exacerbated arterial hypertension, before testing. In addition, the application of a saluretic agent immediately after the test may be an option to circumvent acute heart failure.

There are several reported cutoffs for a normal suppression of aldosterone at the end of the saline infusion. Mulatero et al. found that plasma aldosterone concentrations below 50 ng/l (138 pmol/l) rule out primary aldosteronism (specificity 88 %, sensitivity 90 %; [28]). This study basically confirmed former findings [17, 18]. However, in 1994, a discussion started that a considerable number of patients with PA are missed with SIT at such cutoff values [13]. In the PAPY study, cutoff values for the plasma aldosterone after saline infusion of 67.5 ng/l (181 pmol/) for aldosterone-producing adenomas and 69.1 ng/l (192 pmol/l) for idiopathic hyperaldosteronism were the results with the best compromise between sensitivity and specificity that were 75 and 83 %, respectively [34]. Likewise, in another study, Giacchetti et al. found a cutoff for serum aldosterone of 70 ng/l (194 pmol/l) to come with a specificity of 100 % and a sensitivity of 88 % [12]. Furthermore, work of the Munich group rather confirmed the rather low cutoff of 51 ng/l (141 pmol/l) to have a good performance in the differentiation between hypokalemic primary aldosteronism and essential hypertension (sensitivity 91 %, specificity 90 %). However, this test may not be appropriate to clearly differentiate between normokalemic primary aldosteronism and essential hypertension (sensitivity 57 %, specificity 90 %; [37, 38]). Interestingly, in this study the participants did not need to stop the antihypertensive medication, except for spironolactone, and the investigators found a similar decrease in aldosterone after saline infusion in the patients with essential hypertension and normal controls.

In comparison with the fludrocortisone suppression test, the study of Mulatero et al. found not much difference in the performance of the SIT for the detection of primary aldosteronism [28]. However, this study demonstrated a correct diagnosis of PA in 88 % of hypertensive patients only when compared to the FST. A recently published study confirmed the divergent results produced by the SIT in comparison to the FST [46]. Interestingly, the FST seemed to be more sensitive than the SIT of which the latter showed the best compromise between exclusion and confirmation of PA at a cutoff value for serum aldosterone of 31.5 ng/l (87 pmol/l), rendering a sensitivity of 82 % and a specificity of 92 % [46]. Interestingly, in this study, it was shown that a substantial number of patients with aldosterone-producing adenomas and hypokalemic hyperaldosteronism did suppress below the cutoff of 50 ng/l (138 pmol/l) suggesting that a continuum exists between essential hypertension over normokalemic hyperaldosteronismus to clear-cut aldosterone-producing adenoma with hypokalemic hypertension. A consequence may be that it makes sense to strictly control other factors of aldosterone release, including potassium or corticotropin, which can partly be achieved by the administration of dexamethasone (1 mg the night before). This procedure, however, leads to even lower cutoff values as reported by Pappa et al. that are as low as 24 ng/l (66 pmol/l) [32].

In recognition of different published cutoffs, the Endocrine Society suggested to exclude primary aldosteronism at concentrations below 50 ng/l (138 pmol/l) and to make the diagnosis of primary aldosteronism when aldosterone values are above 100 ng/l (277 pmol/l) after 4 h of saline infusion. Plasma aldosterone concentrations between 50 and 100 ng/l (138–277 pmol/l) may be consistent with a borderline situation [11]. However, depending on the assay in use, even lower cutoff values have to be considered.

Oral Saline Load/Urinary Aldosterone (Metabolite) Excretion

Principle

Tetrahydroaldosterone (THA) and aldosterone-18-glucuronide (A18G) are aldosterone metabolites that are produced within the liver and excreted through the kidneys along with free aldosterone (free A) into the urine. Therefore, high serum concentrations of aldosterone do more or less result in higher urinary levels of aldosterone

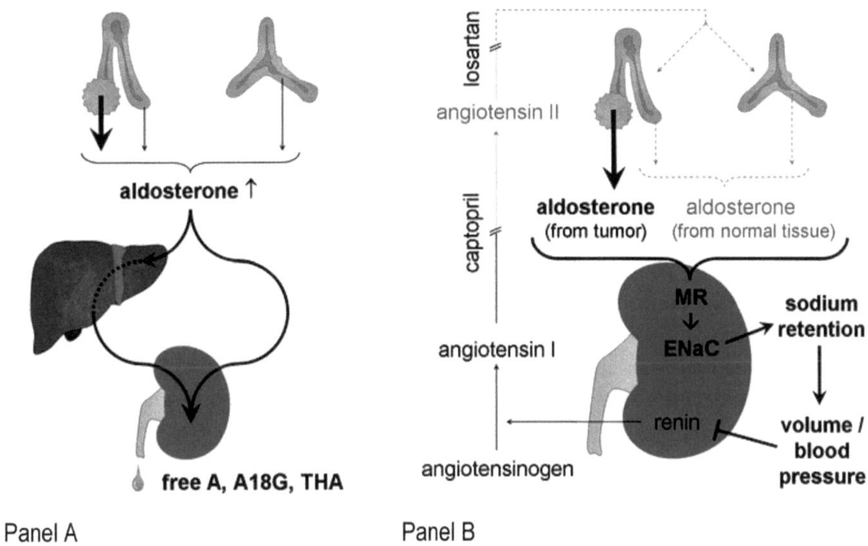

Fig. 10.2 This figure summarizes the principle of aldosterone (metabolite) excretion into urine (Panel **a**) and of the captopril and losartan tests (Panel **b**). Panel **a**, aldosterone is secreted as free aldosterone (free A) and aldosterone-18-glucuronide (A18G), both of which can be assessed by determination of aldosterone before and after complete hydrolysis. In addition, tetrahydroaldosterone is secreted into the urine and can be determined. Panel **b**, captopril inhibits the conversion of angiotensin I into angiotensin II and losartan the association of angiotensin II to its type 1 receptor which normally results in a decline in aldosterone secretion

and its metabolites (Fig. 10.2, Panel A). Measurement of urinary aldosterone (metabolite) concentrations can be done using chromatographic methods with mass spectrometry or by competitive radioimmunoassays [19, 48, 49].

Protocol

The analysis of aldosterone secretion in a 24-h urinary specimen should be performed in the context of a (minimum) 3-day high-salt diet and controlled by the measurement of sodium concentration in the urine. Aldosterone concentrations of >12–14 μg per day in combination with urinary sodium concentrations above 200–250 mmol per day are highly suggestive for autonomous aldosterone secretion [5, 50]. A prerequisite for the interpretation of results, however, is the demonstration of renin suppression.

Discussion

Some studies have shown a high sensitivity and specificity for the analysis of tetrahydroaldosterone for the diagnosis of primary aldosteronism [1]. However, other authors have observed a high overlap of the urine concentrations of these metabolites between patients with essential hypertension and primary aldosteronism [37, 38].

Attempts to overcome the problem of overlap included the correction of urinary aldosterone secretion for plasma renin concentrations or other indices of mineralocorticoid excess, such as the SUSPPUP ratio, and resulted in an increase in specificity up to 100 % [3]. Also, the analysis of urinary THA and A18G per gram creatinine may still have a high specificity (but a low sensitivity) for the diagnosis of primary hyperaldosteronism with the following cutoffs, 126 μg THA/g creatinine or 19.7 μg A18G/g creatinine [37, 38].

The excretion of THA was also studied before and after 3 days of fludrocortisone treatment (300 μg per day) and seemed to be autonomous when it remained higher than 79 % of the control value [24].

18-hydroxy-cortisol (18OH-F) and 18-oxo-cortisol (18oxo-F) are products of adrenal steroidogenesis and reflect the metabolization of cortisol in cells derived from the *zona glomerulosa*, including cells in aldosterone-producing tumors. Detection of these metabolites in urine samples can also be done by immunoassays [26]. Interestingly, patients that suffer from primary aldosteronism show significantly higher concentrations of 18OH-F and 18oxo-F in 24-h urine samples as compared to patients with essential hypertension [27]. The highest levels of these two metabolites have been observed in subjects with glucocorticoid-remediable aldosteronism [27] and cortisol-co-secreting aldosterone-producing adenomas [45]. Since urinary 18OH-F and 18oxo-F concentrations correlate, the sole measurement of urinary 18OH-F may be sufficient in the diagnostic routine and a cutoff of $\leq$130 μg per day for the exclusion of primary aldosteronism has been proposed [27]. However, measurement of 18OH-F and 18oxo-F should not be the determining criteria in the diagnosis of primary aldosteronism since, at present, the data is based on a limited number of patients.

Interestingly, mutations causing primary adosteronism or adrenal tumor development seem to result in specific (urinary) steroid profiles and are currently under investigation.

Suppression of Renin and Non-suppression of Aldosterone

Captopril Challenge Test and Losartan Challenge Test

Principle

Captopril inhibits the conversion of angiotensin I into angiotensin II and losartan the association of angiotensin II to its type 1 receptor which normally results in a decline in aldosterone production and in the stimulation of renin (Fig. 10.2, Panel B). In the case of autonomous aldosterone secretion, blood concentrations of aldosterone do not fall below a certain cutoff and renin will not be stimulated sufficiently.

Protocol (CCT)

Patients remain in a quiescent position throughout the test (lying or sitting). After 30 or 60 min of rest, blood is drawn for basal measurements and patients receive 25–50 mg captopril, for example four crushed 12.5 mg tablets. After another 1 h or after 2 h, blood is again sampled for renin, aldosterone, and cortisol. This test is judged to confirm primary aldosteronism when

- Aldosterone drops less than 30 % of the basal value [36]
- Aldosterone remains higher than 85–120 ng/l [2, 6]
- Aldosterone-to-renin ratio remains higher than 30–50 ng/dl:ng/ml/h [25, 35]

Protocol (LCT)

Instead of captopril, 50 mg of losartan can be given after 1 h of initial rest. Blood is drawn after 2 h [47] or 4 h [12] and primary aldosteronism confirmed if

- Aldosterone-to-renin ratio remains higher than 35 ng/dl:ng/ml/h and the absolute aldosterone remains higher than 100 ng/l [47]
- Aldosterone-to-renin ratio remains higher than 40 ng/dl:ng/ml/h [12]

Discussion

As the above given protocols show there are substantial test variations. In addition, different assays were used. Frequently, assay specifications and even units of measurements were not clearly stated in the papers. Sometimes, interpretations seem to be a matter of tradition rather than of evaluation. Also these tests seem to give too many false-positive or false-negative results [29]. Therefore, captopril challenge test (CCT) and losartan challenge test (LCT) are totally dependent on local experiences.

Nonetheless, the advantage of these tests may be that hypervolemia is not aggravated in patients with hyperaldosteronism. In addition, the CCT seems to perform better in patients with a good sodium load [34].

Postural Test (PT)

Principle

Renin is released with the transition from the supine position to the upright position, and this leads to increase of angiotensin II concentrations in the blood. The negative feedback onto renin secretion and renin activity leads to a decrease in angiotensin II

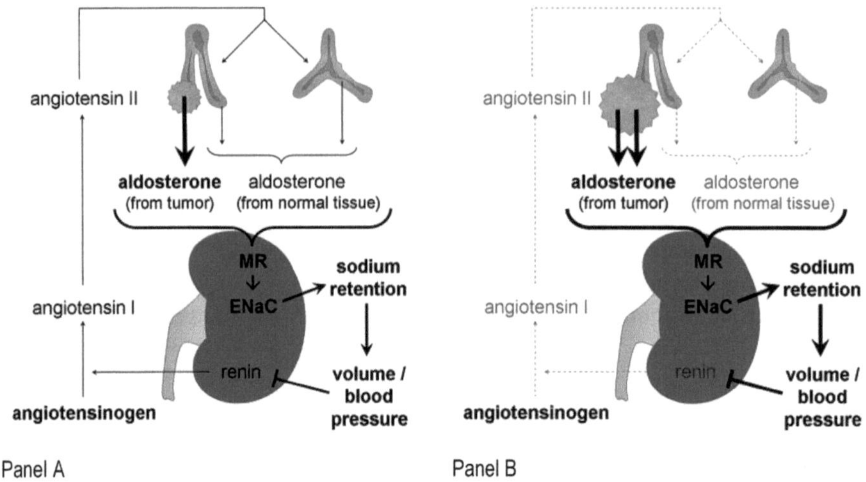

Fig. 10.3 This sketch summarizes the influence of an aldosterone-producing adenoma on the increase in sodium retention, volume expansion, and rise in blood pressure. While small adenomas still allow for an increase in renin activity and generation of angiotensin II during upright posture (Panel **a**), larger adrenal tumors and higher aldosterone secretion rates do not (Panel **b**)

levels and aldosterone secretion from normal *zona glomerulosa* cells. The upright posture results in a lower arterial volume and stimulation of renin secretion in normal individuals, while in primary aldosteronism, salt-mediated hypervolemia cannot be overcome by standing and renin remains suppressed (Fig. 10.3).

Protocol

The patients should sleep overnight constantly for at least 4 h in supine position before testing. Aldosterone and renin concentrations should be measured. Blood sampling should be performed in supine position early in the morning and after 4 h of movement in an upright position. Cortisol measurements are also necessary to exclude a stress-related influence of corticotropin.

Discussion

The posture test can be used to study the volume load and the extend of renin suppression that is less profound in idiopathic (bilateral) forms of aldosteronism (IHA) as compared to definite aldosteronomas. Therefore, the PT has been employed in the differential diagnosis of PA, more specifically to distinguish unilateral from bilateral disease, and is accepted by the Endocrine Society of Japan [31].

The original idea of the posture test is to study the response to angiotensin II [33]. Preceding reports have suggested that IHA is considered to be responsive to angiotensin II, whereas 60 % of definite aldosteronomas secrete aldosterone independently of angiotensin II. It could be shown that in patients with unilateral disease, aldosterone remains constant or even drops "paradoxically" during the time course of the day. This can be explained by the circadian rhythm and the responsiveness of aldosteronomas to corticotropin. If unilateral disease is supported by the results of imaging studies, a fall in both aldosterone and cortisol during PT is very suggestive of a unilateral aldosteronoma so that therapeutic steps can be taken without adrenal venous sampling [9]. However, 30–40 % of visible aldosteronomas were also observed to be responsive to angiotensin II because in this fraction of patients, blood aldosterone concentrations have increased as in patients with IHA [15]. As a result, the sensitivity and specificity of the PT are reduced substantially [30]. A prospective study has shown that the sensitivity of PT is rather low and therefore not useful in the differentiation of PA [20].

An alternative explanation for the reduced performance of the PT was provided recently by the Düsseldorf group: the suppression of renin and angiotensin by small (invisible on imaging) aldosterone-producing tumors may be less severe than the suppression induced by large adrenal adenomas (visible on imaging) that are characterized by a higher rate of aldosterone production [46].

Whether the performance of the PT can be increased is currently under investigation. So far, it seems that the reversed postural test comes with a better sensitivity than the conventional version of the test [42].

Other Tests

Dexamethasone Suppression Test

The dexamethasone suppression test (4 doses of 0.5 mg of dexamethasone for 2 days, followed by 4 doses of 2.0 mg of dexamethasone for 2 days) was described by Liddle [21]. Different variants were employed to screen for glucocorticoid-remediable aldosteronism (GRA or familial hyperaldosteronism type 1). If genetic testing is not established or available, an aldosterone level below 40 ng/l indicates the presence of GRA when patients were given 4×0.5 mg of dexamethasone for 2 days minimum, rather than three full days [23].

This test should not follow immediately the fludrocortisone suppression test to preclude false-positive test results.

Corticotropin Stimulation Test

It was reported that the corticotropin stimulation test can be employed to distinguish patients with an aldosterone-producing adenoma from patients with bilateral disease because aldosterone is stimulated much stronger in patients with an aldosteronoma than in patients with IHA [40]. Again, this phenomenon may also be explained alternatively as stated in Sect. 3.2 since the influence of corticotropin increases relatively to the influence of renin/angiotensin when the latter system is inhibited by hypervolemia. Therefore, this test cannot be used as a confirmatory test per se. On the other hand, adrenal venous sampling may be a test to be used also for confirmation since clear demonstration of unilateral aldosterone secretion would be proof for the presence of an aldosterone-producing adenoma.

References

1. Abdelhamid S, Blomer R, Hommel G, Haack D, Lewicka S, Fiegel P, Krumme B (2003) Urinary tetrahydroaldosterone as a screening method for primary aldosteronism: a comparative study. Am J Hypertens 16:522–530
2. Agharazii M, Douville P, Grose JH, Lebel M (2001) Captopril suppression versus salt loading in confirming primary aldosteronism. Hypertension 37:1440–1443
3. Balas M, Zosin I, Maser-Gluth C, Hermsen D, Cupisti K, Schott M, Schinner S, Knoefel WT, Scherbaum WA, Willenberg HS (2010) Indicators of mineralocorticoid excess in the evaluation of primary aldosteronism. Hypertens Res 33:850–856
4. Beuschlein F, Boulkroun S, Osswald A, Wieland T, Nielsen HN, Lichtenauer UD, Penton D, Schack VR, Amar L, Fischer E, Walther A, Tauber P, Schwarzmayr T, Diener S, Graf E, Allolio B, Samson-Couterie B, Benecke A, Quinkler M, Fallo F, Plouin PF, Mantero F, Meitinger T, Mulatero P, Jeunemaitre X, Warth R, Vilsen B, Zennaro MC, Strom TM, Reincke M (2013) Somatic mutations in ATP1A1 and ATP2B3 lead to aldosterone-producing adenomas and secondary hypertension. Nat Genet 45(4):440–444
5. Bravo EL, Tarazi RC, Dustan HP, Fouad FM, Textor SC, Gifford RW, Vidt DG (1983) The changing clinical spectrum of primary aldosteronism. Am J Med 74:641–651
6. Castro OL, Yu X, Kem DC (2002) Diagnostic value of the post-captopril test in primary aldosteronism. Hypertension 39:935–938
7. Choi M, Scholl UI, Yue P, Björklund P, Zhao B, Nelson-Williams C, Ji W, Cho Y, Patel A, Men CJ, Lolis E, Wisgerhof MV, Geller DS, Mane S, Hellman P, Westin G, Åkerström G, Wang W, Carling T, Lifton RP (2011) K+ channel mutations in adrenal aldosterone-producing adenomas and hereditary hypertension. Science 331:768–772
8. Ehrhart-Bornstein M, Hinson JP, Bornstein SR, Scherbaum WA, Vinson GP (1998) Intraadrenal interactions in the regulation of adrenocortical steroidogenesis. Endocr Rev 19:101–143
9. Espiner EA, Ross DG, Yandle TG, Richards AM, Hunt PJ (2003) Predicting surgically remedial primary aldosteronism: role of adrenal scanning, posture testing and adrenal vein sampling. J Clin Endocrinol Metab 88:3637–3644
10. Fardella CE, Mosso L, Gómez-Sánchez C, Cortés P, Soto J, Gómez L, Pinto M, Huete A, Oestreicher E, Foradori A, Montero J (2000) Primary hyperaldosteronism in essential hypertensives: prevalence, biochemical profile, and molecular biology. J Clin Endocrinol Metab 85:1863–1867
11. Funder JW, Carey RM, Fardella C, Gomez-Sanchez CE, Mantero F, Stowasser M, Young WF Jr, Montori VM (2008) Case detection, diagnosis, and treatment of patients with primary aldosteronism: an endocrine society clinical practice guideline. J Clin Endocrinol Metab 93: 3266–3281
12. Giacchetti G, Ronconi V, Lucarelli G, Boscaro M, Mantero F (2006) Analysis of screening and confirmatory tests in the diagnosis of primary aldosteronism: need for a standardized protocol. J Hypertens 24:737–745
13. Gordon RD (1994) Mineralocorticoid hypertension. Lancet 23(344):240–243
14. Gordon RD (1995) Primary aldosteronism. J Endocrinol Invest 18:495–511
15. Gordon RD, Laragh JH, Funder JW (2005) Low renin hypertensive states: perspectives, unsolved problems, future research. Trends Endocrinol Metab 16:108–113

16. Gouli A, Kaltsas G, Tzonou A, Markou A, Androulakis II, Ragkou D, Vamvakidis K, Zografos G, Kontogeorgos G, Chrousos GP, Piaditis G (2011) High prevalence of autonomous aldosterone secretion among patients with essential hypertension. Eur J Clin Invest 41:1227–1236
17. Holland OB, Brown H, Kuhnert L, Fairchild C, Risk M, Gomez Sanchez CE (1984) Further evaluation of saline infusion for the diagnosis of primary aldosteronism. Hypertension 6:717–723
18. Kem DC, Weinberger MH, Mayes DM, Nugent CA (1971) Saline suppression of plasma aldosterone in hypertension. Arch Intern Med 128:380–386
19. Krone N, Hughes BA, Lavery GG, Stewart PM, Arlt W, Shackleton CH (2010) Gas chromatography/mass spectrometry (GC/MS) remains a pre-eminent discovery tool in clinical steroid investigations even in the era of fast liquid chromatography tandem mass spectrometry (LC/MS/MS). J Steroid Biochem Mol Biol 121:496–504
20. Lau JH, Sze WC, Reznek RH, Matson M, Sahdev A, Carpenter R, Berney DM, Akker SA, Chew SL, Grossman AB, Monson JP, Drake WM (2012) A prospective evaluation of postural stimulation testing, computed tomography and adrenal vein sampling in the differential diagnosis of primary aldosteronism. Clin Endocrinol 76:182–188
21. Liddle GW (1960) Tests of pituitary-adrenal suppressibility in the diagnosis of Cushing's syndrome. J Clin Endocrinol Metab 20:1539–1560
22. Lim PO, Farquharson CA, Shiels P, Jung RT, Strithers AD, MacDonald TM (2001) Adverse cardiac effects of salt with fludrocortisone in hypertension. Hypertension 37:856–861
23. Litchfield WR, New MI, Coolidge C, Lifton RP, Dluhy RG (1997) Evaluation of the dexamethasone suppression test for the diagnosis of glucocorticoid-remediable aldosteronism. J Clin Endocrinol Metab 82:3570–3573
24. Lund JO, Nielsen MD (1980) Fludrocortisone suppression test in normal subjects, in patients with essential hypertension and in patients with various forms of aldosteronism. Acta Endocrinol (Copenh) 93:100–107
25. Lyons DF, Kem DC, Brown RD, Hanson CS, Carollo ML (1983) Single dose captopril as a diagnostic test for primary aldosteronism. J Clin Endocrinol Metab 57:892–896
26. Morra di Cella S, Veglio F, Mulatero P, Christensen V, Aycock K, Zhu Z, Gomez-Sanchez EP, Gomez-Sanchez CE (2002) A time-resolved fluoroimmunoassay for 18-oxocortisol and 18-hydroxycortisol. Development of a monoclonal antibody to 18-oxocortisol. J Steroid Biochem Mol Biol 82:83–88
27. Mulatero P, di Cella SM, Monticone S, Schiavone D, Manzo M, Mengozzi G, Rabbia F, Terzolo M, Gomez-Sanchez EP, Gomez-Sanchez CE, Veglio F (2012) 18-hydroxycorticosterone, 18-hydroxycortisol, and 18-oxocortisol in the diagnosis of primary aldosteronism and its subtypes. J Clin Endocrinol Metab 97:881–889
28. Mulatero P, Milan A, Fallo F, Regolisti G, Pizzolo F, Fardella C, Mosso L, Marafetti L, Veglio F, Maccario M (2006) Comparison of confirmatory tests for the diagnosis of primary aldosteronism. J Clin Endocrinol Metab 91:2618–2623
29. Mulatero P, Monticone S, Bertello C, Mengozzi G, Tizzani D, Iannaccone A, Veglio F (2010) Confirmatory tests in the diagnosis of primary aldosteronism. Horm Metab Res 42:406–410
30. Mulatero P, Stowasser M, Loh KC, Fardella CE, Gordon RD, Mosso L, Gomez-Sanchez CE, Veglio F, Young WF Jr (2004) Increased diagnosis of primary aldosteronism, including surgically correctable forms, in centers from five continents. J Clin Endocrinol Metab 89:1045–1050
31. Nishikawa T, Omura M, Satoh F, Shibata H, Takahashi K, Tamura N, Tanabe A (2011) Guidelines for the diagnosis and treatment of primary aldosteronism -The Japan Endocrine Society 2009. Endocr J 58:711–721
32. Pappa T, Papanastasiou L, Kaltsas G, Markou A, Tsounas P, Androulakis I, Tsiavos V, Zografos G, Vamvakidis K, Samara C, Piaditis G (2012) Pattern of adrenal hormonal secretion in patients with adrenal adenomas: the relevance of aldosterone in arterial hypertension. J Clin Endocrinol Metab 97:E537–E545
33. Phillips JL, Walther MM, Pezzullo JC, Rayford W, Choyke PL, Berman AA, Linehan WM, Doppman JL, Gill JR Jr (2000) Predictive value of preoperative tests in discriminating bilateral adrenal hyperplasia from aldosterone-producing adrenal adenoma. J Clin Endocrinol Metab 85:4526–4533

34. Rossi GP, Belfiore A, Bernini G, Desideri G, Fabris B, Ferri C, Giacchetti G, Letizia C, Maccario M, Mallamaci F, Mannelli M, Montemurro D, Palumbo G, Rizzoni D, Rossi E, Semplicini A, Agabiti-Rosei E, Pessina AC (2007) Mantero F; PAPY Study Investigators. Prospective evaluation of the saline infusion test for excluding primary aldosteronism due to aldosterone-producing adenoma. J Hypertens 25:1433–1442
35. Rossi GP, Bernini G, Caliumi C, Desideri G, Fabris B, Ferri C, Ganzaroli C, Giacchetti G, Letizia C, Maccario M, Mallamaci F, Mannelli M, Mattarello MJ, Moretti A, Palumbo G, Parenti G, Porteri E, Semplicini A, Rizzoni D, Rossi E, Boscaro M, Pessina AC (2006) Mantero F; PAPY Study Investigators. A prospective study of the prevalence of primary aldosteronism in 1,125 hypertensive patients. J Am Coll Cardiol 48:2293–2300
36. Rossi E, Regolisti G, Negro A, Sani C, Davoli S, Perazzoli F (2002) High prevalence of primary aldosteronism using postcaptopril plasma aldosterone to renin ratio as a screening test among Italian hypertensives. Am J Hypertens 15:896–902
37. Schirpenbach C, Seiler L, Maser-Gluth C, Beuschlein F, Reincke M, Bidlingmaier M (2006) Automated chemiluminescence-immunoassay for aldosterone during dynamic testing: comparison to radioimmunoassays with and without extraction steps. Clin Chem 52:1749–1755
38. Schirpenbach C, Seiler L, Maser-Gluth C, Rüdiger F, Nickel C, Beuschlein F, Reincke M (2006) Confirmatory testing in normokalaemic primary aldosteronism: the value of the saline infusion test and urinary aldosterone metabolites. Eur J Endocrinol 154:865–873
39. Solar M, Malirova E, Ballon M, Pelouch R, Ceral J (2012) Confirmatory testing in primary aldosteronism: extensive medication switching is not needed in all patients. Eur J Endocrinol 166:679–686
40. Sonoyama T, Sone M, Miyashita K, Tamura N, Yamahara K, Park K, Oyamada N, Taura D, Inuzuka M, Kojima K, Honda K, Fukunaga Y, Kanamoto N, Miura M, Yasoda A, Arai H, Itoh H, Nakao K (2011) Significance of adrenocorticotropin stimulation test in the diagnosis of an aldosterone-producing adenoma. J Clin Endocrinol Metab 96:2771–2778
41. Stowasser M, Gordon RD, Gunasekera TG, Cowley DC, Ward G, Archibald C, Smithers BM (2003) High rate of detection of primary aldosteronism, including surgically treatable forms, after 'non-selective' screening of hypertensive patients. J Hypertens 21:2149–2157
42. Weickert MO, Schöfl-Siegert B, Arafat AM, Pfeiffer AF, Möhlig M, Schöfl C (2009) A reverse postural test as a screening tool for aldosterone-producing adenoma: a pilot study. Endocrine 36:75–82
43. Westerdahl C, Bergenfelz A, Larsson J, Nerbrand C, Valdemarsson S, Wihl A, Isaksson A (2009) Re-evaluation of the fludrocortisone test: duration, NaCl supplementation and cut-off limits for aldosterone. Scand J Clin Lab Invest 69:234–241
44. Willenberg HS, Schinner S, Ansurudeen I (2008) New mechanisms to control aldosterone synthesis. Horm Metab Res 40:435–441
45. Willenberg HS, Späth M, Maser-Gluth C, Engers R, Anlauf M, Dekomien G, Schott M, Schinner S, Cupisti K, Scherbaum WA (2010) Sporadic solitary aldosterone- and cortisol-cosecreting adenomas—endocrine function tests, histological and genetic findings in a subtype of primary aldosteronism. Hypertens Res 33:467–472
46. Willenberg HS, Vonend O, Schott M, Gao X, Blondin D, Saleh A, Rump LC, Scherbaum WA (2012) Comparison of the saline infusion test and the fludrocortisone suppression test in the diagnosis of primary aldosteronism. Horm Metab Res 44:527–532
47. Wu VC, Chang HW, Liu KL, Lin YH, Chueh SC, Lin WC, Ho YL, Huang JW, Chiang CK, Yang SY, Chen YM, Wang SM, Huang KH, Hsieh BS, Wu KD, TAIPAI Study Group (2009) Primary aldosteronism: diagnostic accuracy of the losartan and captopril tests. Am J Hypertens 22:821–827
48. Wudy SA, Hartmann MF (2004) Gas chromatography–mass spectrometry profiling of steroids in times of molecular biology. Horm Metab Res 36:415–422
49. Schäfer A, Faulstich H, Vecsei P, Hobler H (1974) A solid phase radio immunoassay for urine aldosterone using antibodies linked to nylon nets. FEBS Lett 48:230–234
50. Young WF Jr (2002) Primary aldosteronism: management issues. Ann N Y Acad Sci 970:61–76

Chapter 11
Radiological and Radionuclide Imaging of Adrenocortical Tumours

Anders Sundin

Abstract Because of the increasing use of cross-sectional imaging, mainly computed tomography (CT), adrenal tumours are frequently detected in patients who undergo imaging for other reasons than adrenal disease. These incidentally depicted adrenal lesions, "incidentalomas," comprise a wide variety of different tumour entities. In a minor portion of these patients, biochemical screening reveals a functional tumour and further diagnostic work-up and therapy need to be performed according to the type of hormonal overproduction. In patients without a cancer history almost all adrenal incidentalomas are benign which is in contrast to patients with a known extra-adrenal malignancy who frequently harbour adrenal metastases. Most of the adrenal lesions can be characterised by CT and magnetic resonance imaging based on their morphological appearance and/or by attenuation/signal characteristics consistent with the content of microscopic (cytoplasmatic) or macroscopic fat. A significant number of adrenal lesions can, however, not be easily determined and require radiological follow-up of tumour size in order to exclude that the tumour is malignant or necessitate further work-up by functional imaging methods or biopsy. Non-invasive characterisation by functional radionuclide imaging with scintigraphy and positron emission tomography (PET) is therefore an important adjunct. The most commonly used PET tracer, [^{18}F]FDG, is useful to differ benign from malignant lesions and, before the surgical decision, to establish whether an adrenal metastasis is the only lesion or, in case of disseminated disease, to confirm that non-surgical treatment instead should be chosen. 18-FDG-PET is also useful in pheochromocytoma and ACC. The enzyme inhibitor ^{11}C-metomidate has been developed as a PET tracer for adrenal imaging to differ adrenocortical from non-adrenocortical tumours. ^{11}C-metomidate-PET is currently also tried to diagnose Conn adenomas in primary aldosteronism, but further development is needed before the method can be established for this purpose.

A. Sundin (✉)
Department of Radiology, Oncology and Radiation Science, Uppsala University, Akademiska sjukhuset ing 70 1 tr, Uppsala 751 85, Sweden
e-mail: anders.sundin@radiol.uu.se

P. Hellman (ed.), *Primary Aldosteronism: Molecular Genetics, Endocrinology, and Translational Medicine*, DOI 10.1007/978-1-4939-0509-6_11,

Keywords Adrenal incidentaloma • Adrenal adenoma • Conn adenoma • Positron emission tomography • 18FDG • 11C-metomidate • Computed tomography • Magnetic resonance imaging

Introduction

Since the introduction of spiral, or helical, computed tomography (CT) and of multidetector CT (MDCT) the use of CT has increased considerably. Adrenal tumours are found at image reading in many patients who are referred for CT of the thorax and/or abdomen for reasons unrelated to adrenal disease. These so-called incidentalomas increase with age and are found in approximately 5 % of CT examinations that include the adrenal region [1]. Incidentalomas are also detected by magnetic resonance imaging (MRI) and ultrasonography (US) [2]. The work-up of the patient with an incidentaloma should aim at establishing whether the incidentaloma is hormonally active or not and if the lesion is benign or malignant. The biochemical work-up is usually performed by an endocrinologist, and the imaging characterisation is a task for the radiologist. In patients without a cancer history, malignant incidentalomas are very rare. By contrast, patients with cancer, or those who have previously undergone treatment for cancer, have a high risk that the incidentaloma represents an adrenal metastasis. The reported incidence of adrenal metastases in incidentaloma patients is, however, very varying in the literature [3–5].

As opposed to the patients with incidentaloma, those who present with clinical symptoms from adrenal disease and therefore undergo imaging are rare.

Imaging Techniques

Computed Tomography (CT)

Computed tomography is the basic modality for imaging and characterisation of adrenal tumours and is usually the method by which the incidentaloma was initially detected. In modern CT scanners, a large number of detectors are arranged in parallel rows (MDCT) and by use of the rapidly rotating X-ray tube (0.5–1 s per rotation), typically more than one hundred ½ to 1 mm sections are produced per second. With this fast scanning, there are rarely problems with breathing artefacts and an MDCT examination of both the abdomen and the thorax can usually be performed during one breath-hold. Because modern MDCT scanners produce 1 mm or sub-mm images, these are by default reformatted to produce high-spatial-resolution two-dimensional (2D) coronal and sagittal multiplanar reformatted (MPR) image volumes. For adrenal imaging, these MPRs are valuable and should always be viewed to avoid interpretation errors. For example, what may initially be considered as an adrenal tumour in the transversal plane may in the MPRs be found to represent a horizontally orientated limb of the adrenal.

Dual-energy CT is a recent technique, whereby the CT examination simultaneously is performed at two different tube voltages, for example 80 and 140 kV. This can be achieved either by using two separate X-ray tubes, by switching between two different voltages during exposure with one tube, or by detector-related techniques.

Dual-energy CT may for example be used for tissue characterisation including adrenal incidentalomas although this is not yet an established clinical procedure [6, 7].

The current fast CT scanners also allow for better use of intravenous iodine-based contrast media. The organs and tissues of interest may be examined according to optimised protocols in various contrast-enhancement phases. A prerequisite for optimised injection protocols is a power injector, preferably with two heads, to allow contrast medium injection followed by a saline bolus. By rinsing the brachial, brachio-cephal and subclavian veins with a saline chaser, the contrast medium lodged in these vessels may instead be used for contrast enhancement. Also, image artefacts related to the high contrast medium concentrations in the veins in the upper thorax may be avoided. Early scanning, approximately ½ minute after contrast medium injection starts, visualises the arteries (early arterial phase or CT angiography) and is rarely used for adrenal imaging. Occasionally it is helpful for the imaging work-up before surgical resection of large adrenal tumours, for example an adrenocortical cancer (ACC), when arterial anatomy sometimes needs to be assessed. Optionally, the vascular anatomy can by post-processing also be displayed in three-dimensional (3D) image volumes (maximum intensity projection, MIP) and by using volume-rendering technique (VRT). These 3D volumes may be rotated to facilitate image interpretation. In the late arterial phase (or portal-venous inflow phase), some 10–15 s later, the small arterial branches are contrast enhanced, and this is the best phase to depict hypervascular lesions for example hypervascular liver metastases. Pheochromocytomas are fairly frequently hypervascular and show a pronounced contrast enhancement in this phase. In the venous (or portal-venous) phase, approximately 60–90 s after injection starts, the contrast medium has circulated through the capillaries and into the venous system, including the portal vein to enhance the liver. In the venous phase, the vessels and the parenchymal organs are contrast-enhanced and hypovascular lesions are best delineated. A late or a delayed excretion phase, several minutes after injection starts, is useful in adrenal and renal imaging and sometimes also for CT of the liver. For calculation of the contrast medium washout from adrenal tumours this delayed phase is usually performed at 15 min.

Magnetic Resonance Imaging

Because of the better soft tissue contrast, MRI generally performs better than CT for many imaging applications. A drawback is that MRI is not as readily available as is CT, and in centres with limited access to MRI, the method is mainly used as a problem-solving tool. For adrenal imaging MRI has a role for tumour characterisation and for follow-up in young patients to decrease the radiation dose.

The intravenous gadolinium (Gd)-based MRI contrast media are extracellular agents, similar to the iodine-based contrast media for CT, and the various contrast-enhancement phases are the same. This is executed by repeated MRI acquisition after Gd contrast injection, the so-called dynamical contrast-enhanced (DCE) MRI. Thus, repeated MRI acquisitions allow for MR angiography (MRA), a late arterial phase for imaging of hypervascular lesions and a venous contrast-enhancement phase to delineate those who are hypovascular. When MRI is performed in 3D, the image volume may be reconstructed in the transverse, coronal and sagittal planes. For MRI there are also specific contrast media available such as hepatocyte-specific (gadolinium or manganese based) contrast media and superparamagnetic iron oxide particles that are instead taken up by the Kupffer cells of the reticuloendothelial system. Modern MRI is usually performed using a 1.5 Tesla (T) magnet, but currently also MRI at 3T is becoming available. The higher field strength of the 3T magnets can be used to either achieve better image resolution or shorten the MRI acquisition. When neither spatial resolution nor fast acquisition is critical, the higher field strength can be used for a combination of both. In the characterisation of adrenal lesions signal sequences ("in phase" and "out of phase") to detect cytoplasmatic fat are available.

Ultrasonography (US)

Ultrasonography or ultrasound does not expose the patient to radiation, similarly to MRI, and is therefore beneficial in young patients. Currently US can be performed also during intravenous contrast enhancement (CEUS), by using micro bubbles, and is a very sensitive technique. For liver imaging CEUS has been shown to depict very small sub-0.5 cm liver metastases. CEUS is also very valuable to assess previously equivocal liver lesions at CT and MRI, and by dynamical examination over time the lesion may be characterised by its in- and outflow pattern of the contrast medium. US is an excellent method to guide the needle for tumour biopsies, and a US-guided biopsy is generally performed faster than by CT.

For adrenal imaging US is not yet established for diagnosis or follow-up except in connection with biopsy when an adrenal metastasis is suspected. CEUS has, however, been tried to differ benign from malignant tumours, but the reported results are diverse. In some studies CEUS has been shown to be useful [8, 9] and produced similar results as CT and MRI [10], whereas for others the technique has failed to differ the benign from the malignant adrenal tumours [11].

Scintigraphy

By radionuclide imaging methods (scintigraphy, positron emission tomography (PET)) various aspects of biologic function may be imaged (e.g. metabolism, receptor density, enzyme function, blood flow) as opposed to conventional radiological methods to image morphology-anatomy. The molecules, the biological function of which is imaged by scintigraphy, are labelled with a gamma-emitting radionuclide to produce a tracer preparation. Common gamma emitter uses in nuclear medicine are ^{99m}Tc, ^{123}I and ^{111}In. ^{99m}Tc is conveniently eluded from a generator in the nuclear medicine department and used for labelling. Most molecules that are used to produce tracers for scintigraphy are delivered as labelling kits to which the radionuclide is added. After administration of the tracer, usually intravenously, the patient is placed on the couch of the gamma camera. Scintigraphy by 2D planar imaging is acquired by positioning the detectors in front of and/or behind the patient, and the detectors are stepwise, or slowly continuously, moved along the patient to cover the anatomical area of interest. By single-photon emission computed tomography (SPECT) 3D imaging is acquired by stepwise moving the detector heads around the patient in a circular fashion to produce transverse images. These images are regularly reformatted in also the coronal and sagittal plane. The resulting 2D planar and 3D SPECT images are greyscale or colour coded to represent radioactivity concentration. New gamma cameras for SPECT also comprise a CT scanner in the same gantry (SPECT/CT). Because most SPECT/CT examinations are performed in nuclear medicine departments, the CT protocols generally do not include intravenous contrast enhancement and are performed at a low radiation dose. The SPECT/CT examinations are evaluated in a computer workstation, and three image volumes are displayed: SPECT, CT and a software SPECT/CT overlay or fusion of the two to facilitate anatomical correlation of the SPECT findings.

Positron Emission Tomography/Computed Tomography

The positron-emitting radionuclides are generally produced in a low-energy cyclotron, and their half-lives are usually short. For ^{18}F the half-life is 110 min, for ^{68}Ga 68 min and for ^{11}C 20 min. In practice ^{18}F may be transported within approximately a 2-h radius from a cyclotron site to a PET unit without their own PET tracer production. A PET camera resembles a CT scanner, with a patient couch and a gantry, which holds tens of thousands of detectors, arranged in rings. The detector axial range is approximately 15–20 cm, and the patient is therefore stepwise moved through the gantry and examined about 3 min per "bed position, typically to include the abdomen, thorax and neck". Standalone PET scanners have become rare, and currently PET is regularly performed together with CT in PET/CT hybrid scanners. The CT examination is usually performed after the PET acquisition. [^{18}F]fluoro-deoxy-glucose ([^{18}F]FDG) is the most commonly used PET tracer and is predominately applied in oncologic imaging because malignant tumour accumulates [^{18}F]FDG to a higher extent than most normal tissues. [^{18}F]FDG is usually administered 1 h before examination, but with ^{11}C-labelled tracers scanning is started earlier after injection. Unlike the gamma camera, the detectors in the PET camera indirectly register the positron emissions. The emitted positron within a few millimetres collides with an electron upon which both are annihilated and converted into two high-energy (511 keV) photons.

These travel in opposite directions and simultaneously (within a few nanoseconds) reach the detector rings, and the line of decay is registered. By collecting all decays during the acquisition, transversal images representing radioactivity concentration (Bq/mL) are reconstructed. Since not all the photons reach the detectors because of attenuation in the tissues, the PET acquisition data are corrected for attenuation by using the CT examination performed in the same imaging session. The PET/CT examination is evaluated using a computer workstation by viewing PET, CT and the PET/CT fusion. The CT examination, thus, supplies an excellent anatomical map to correlate the PET findings and vice versa. Optimally, the CT should be performed as a fully diagnostic examination by using a radiological protocol including intravenous contrast enhancement. Unfortunately, some centres still use an un-enhanced low-radiation-dose CT protocol whereby the full potential of the technique is not employed. Only when a fully diagnostic CT examination has recently been performed, within the last few weeks, one can refrain from i.v. contrast enhancement in connection with PET/CT. The attenuation-corrected PET images are regularly recalculated to provide images of standardised uptake values (SUVs) whereby the radioactivity concentration data in the images (Bq/mL) are divided by the ratio between the injected dose (Bq) and the patient's body weight (g). This recalculation is used to normalise the uptake in the patient' various tissues for differences in injected activity and distribution volume.

Adrenocortical Adenoma

CT

Most incidentalomas represent benign cortical nodules, generally referred to as adrenocortical adenomas. As opposed to the macroscopic fat in a myelolipoma, the adrenocortical adenomas have an abundance of *microscopic* cytoplasmatic fat. Approximately 70 % of these lesions may be characterised as benign adenomas by attenuation measurement of the tumour in a non-contrast-enhanced CT examination. The attenuation of the normal parenchymal organs measures approximately 30–70 HU. However, in an adrenocortical adenoma the presence of cytoplasmatic fat (fat attenuation −100 HU) decreases the attenuation of the tumour. A parallel phenomenon is the low hepatic attenuation seen in patients with liver steatosis. In the pre-contrast (native) CT, the attenuation of the incidentaloma is measured in the transversal slice where the tumour is the largest. Low-radiation-dose examinations, for example CT performed for attenuation correction at PET/CT, can, however, not be used since these attenuation measurements cannot be relied on. A circular region of interest (ROI) with a diameter that will cover ¾ to 4/5 of the tumour diameter is placed in the slice, a second and third ROI is placed in the adjacent (cranial and caudal) slices, and the mean of the three measurements is noted. Incidentalomas which at CT appear morphologically benign and measure ≤10 HU in the pre-contrast CT examination can be diagnosed as a benign adrenocortical adenoma with 98–99 % specificity and 65–71 % sensitivity [12, 13]. According to Swedish national guidelines benign adrenocortical adenomas measuring less than 4 cm in transaxial diameter generally require no further imaging or radiological follow-up. The routines in this respect, however, vary in different countries and centres. In order not to misdiagnose a simple cyst (attenuation approximately 0–15 HU) as a benign adrenocortical adenoma, it should, however, be confirmed that the lesion is contrast enhancing.

MRI

MRI is useful in young patients to decrease the radiation dose and in those who cannot receive i.v. iodine-based contrast media because of impaired kidney function or a previous severe adverse reaction. MRI represents an alternative to CT to visualise microscopic fat, occasionally also in incidentalomas with a pre-contrast attenuation >10 HU. MRI of the adrenals is performed to include MRI signal sequences "in phase" and "out of phase" [14, 15]. In a benign adrenocortical adenoma, the protons in the mixture of microscopic fat and water within the cytoplasm will add to the signal intensity (in phase) in the image but will counteract and decrease the signal (out of phase). Other tumour entities do not demonstrate this so-called chemical shift phenomenon, and, similarly to CT, the "lipid-poor adenomas" (benign adrenocortical adenomas with a low concentration of cytoplasmatic fat) will escape characterisation. MRI is also advantageous in young patients for follow-up of the tumour size and allows for a "second chance" to characterise the lesion by "in- and out-of-phase" imaging.

Contrast Medium Washout

Because the initial CT, by which the incidentaloma was diagnosed, usually was performed during intravenous contrast enhancement, a new pre-contrast (native) examination is often needed to allow for attenuation measurements. Examination is also performed during contrast enhancement in the venous phase (90–120 s after injection starts) and a delayed scan at 15 min. As previously pointed out, before a dedicated CT or MRI examination of the adrenals is undertaken, inquiries should be made for any previous CT/MRI of the abdomen/thorax that by showing a morphologically unchanged incidentaloma may make further imaging redundant.

The reason to include delayed scanning in the dedicated protocol for CT of the adrenals is that incidentalomas with morphologically benign appearance, but with a pre-contrast attenuation >10 HU (and therefore cannot be discarded as a benign adrenocortical adenoma), may in addition be characterised regarding their contrast enhancement and washout. The mechanisms for this are not fully understood, but the concept is based on the different characteristics of malignant as opposed to benign tumours. Malignant tumours are known to generally be hypovascular, and the relative volume of the interstitial space is larger than that in normal tissues.

Also, the interstitial pressure is higher in malignant tumours than in normal tissues. These characteristics of malignant tumours will impede their contrast enhancement and delay the contrast medium washout. By contrast, benign adrenal tumours similarly to normal organs and tissues contrast-enhance rapidly and have a fast contrast medium washout. The degree of contrast enhancement and washout is based on the attenuation measurements of the incidentaloma in the pre-contrast (unenhanced, U) CT, contrast-enhanced (enhanced, E) and delayed (D) phases (at 15 min). The "absolute washout" is calculated according to the following expression:

$$\text{Absolute washout} = (\text{E} - \text{D}) / (\text{E} - \text{U})$$

Delayed scanning has in the various published studies been performed mainly at 10 and 15 min and different "cut-off" values have been applied for the resulting quotient. In the daily clinical setting, calculation of the "absolute washout" is usually based on a 15-min delayed examination and a quotient >0.6 indicates that the adrenal tumour probably represents a benign adrenocortical adenoma. A quotient <0.6 conversely indicates that the lesion may be malignant. The sensitivity to differ malignant from benign incidentalomas is mean 88 (range 86–89 %) and the specificity mean 93 (range 87–96 %) [16–19].

A general problem for incidentaloma characterisation, as previously pointed out, is that the initial CT customarily was performed without a pre-contrast scan. However, in case the incidentaloma is revealed while the patient is still in the CT scanner, a delayed phase may be added at 15 min and a "relative washout" can be calculated according to the following expression:

$$\text{Relative washout} = (\text{E} - \text{D}) / \text{E}$$

At a threshold value of 0.4 the sensitivity is mean 87 (range 82–95 %) and the specificity mean 95 (range 92–100 %) [16–18].

When interpreting the results of pre-contrast attenuation measurements and those of contrast medium washout calculations it is important to realise that these measurements may not always be reliable. Variations in the attenuation measurements may depend on technical parameters such as partial volume effects, especially with small incidentalomas and particularly when no thin (1–3 mm) slices are available. Also, there are operator-dependent factors to consider, mainly the size of the ROI that is chosen for the attenuation measurement, relative to the tumour diameter and how the ROI is positioned within the incidentaloma. Also, factors related to maintenance, for example the routines for calibration of the CT scanner, are of importance to acquire reliable attenuation measurements.

Impact of Washout

There are also varying routines in different departments as to how the results of washout measurements are used for the patient management. In some departments, a morphologically benign but previously uncharacterised incidentaloma (pre-contrast attenuation >10 HU) with an absolute washout >0.6 may be discarded as benign with no need for further imaging [12]. Other centres, for instance that of the author, instead advise radiological follow-up by CT or MRI to measure the tumour size in order to confirm or rule out the malignant nature of an incidentaloma with a pre-contrast attenuation >10 HU. In this routine the result of the “absolute washout” merely indicates how soon the follow-up should be performed after the time point when the incidentaloma was first detected. With an “absolute washout” <0.6, follow-up at 3 months is recommended and >0.6 at 6 months. If the incidentaloma is unchanged in morphological appearance and size, the final CT/MRI is performed at 1 year, before the patient is discarded. The final biochemical follow-up is performed at 2 years.

Radionuclide Imaging

Imaging of the vast majority of adrenal incidentalomas is adequately managed by CT and MRI. For some of these tumours, further imaging characterisation is, however, needed. For these patients there are several radionuclide imaging (molecular imaging, nuclear medicine imaging) techniques available.

^{131}I-Norcholesterol (NP-59) Scintigraphy

^{131}I-norcholesterol (NP-59) was previously primarily used for scintigraphy including SPECT for preoperative localisation of aldosterone-secreting adrenocortical tumours (Conn adenomas) in primary hyperaldosteronism [20]. The tracer is, however, no longer available in most European countries since the production of the tracer has been ended. The technique was mainly used in specialised centres and had several drawbacks, for instance a high radiation dose to the patient, limited spatial resolution of SPECT making small tumours difficult to visualise, the need for thyroid blocking and repeated imaging.

Positron Emission Tomography of Adrenal Tumours

PET with [^{18}F]FDG) has developed as a powerful molecular imaging technique, mainly in oncological patients, and is today regularly combined with CT (PET/CT) to also acquire a morphological reference to the functional image findings and vice versa. The use of [^{18}F]FDG for oncological PET/CT is based on its accumulation to a higher extent in malignant compared to benign tumours and most normal tissues, except the brain. There is also a high accumulation of [^{18}F]FDG in kidney since it is excreted into the urine, and high radioactivity concentrations are found in the urinary collective system and bladder. [^{18}F]FDG-PET/CT is mainly used in oncology for tumour characterisation, staging, detection of current disease and therapy monitoring and is well established in lung cancer, lymphoma, colorectal cancer and melanoma. The high clinical impact of [^{18}F]FDG-PET and PET/CT has been reported for many different tumour types in a large number of studies and reviews [21–23].

^{11}C-Metomidate-PET for Characterisation of Adrenal Tumours

Metomidate and etomidate are inhibitors of the CYP11B enzymes 11β-hydroxylase (CYP11B1, P45011β) and aldosterone synthase (CYP11B2, P450aldo) involved in the synthetic pathways of cortisol and aldosterone, respectively. Both etomidate and metomidate have been labelled with ^{11}C and ^{18}F and used for PET imaging of adrenocortical tumours. ^{11}C-metomidate was chosen as the tracer in the first clinical trial because of its better radiochemical characteristics [24]. In this study, 15 patients with various adrenal tumours underwent ^{11}C-metomidate-PET. All adrenocortical tumours (adenoma, hyperplasia, ACC) showed a high ^{11}C-metomidate uptake and were unequivocally distinguished from the non-adrenocortical lesions (myelolipoma, pheochromocytoma, metastasis, cyst) without tracer uptake.

Two studies have compared PET with ^{11}C-metomidate and [^{18}F]FDG in the same patients [25, 26]. In these reports, the patients (19 and 16, respectively) had various benign and malignant adrenal tumours. All adrenocortical lesions were ^{11}C-metomidate positive, and [^{18}F]FDG-PET detected two-thirds of the malignant tumours in the first group [25]. In the second study, ^{11}C-metomidate-PET distinguished the adrenocortical tumours from the non-adrenocortical lesions and [^{18}F]FDG-PET differed the malignant from the benign tumours [26].

The largest study to date on ^{11}C-metomidate-PET comprised 73 patients with 75 adrenal tumours (adrenocortical adenoma, hyperplasia, pheochromocytoma, ACC, metastasis, various tumours of non-adrenal origin) ranging 1–20 cm in size [27]. Correlation with the histopathological diagnosis showed 89 % sensitivity and 96 % specificity for ^{11}C-metomidate-PET to distinguish adrenocortical from non-adrenocortical lesions. Three small ≤1 cm tumours were false negative. PET measurements of ^{11}C-metomidate uptake (SUV) could not differ the benign from the malignant adrenocortical tumours.

The role of ^{11}C-metomidate-PET in comparison with CT and MRI was tested in a clinical setting for the imaging work-up of 44 adrenal incidentalomas in 38 patients [28]. Morphological imaging proved sufficient for all but a few patients in whom CT and MRI failed to characterise the tumour. ^{11}C-metomidate-PET could add information by defining the adrenocortical or non-adrenocortical origin of these lesions. In the management of patients with incidentaloma ^{11}C-metomidate-PET thus has a marginal role. The method is best employed as a problem-solving tool when CT and MRI fail to characterise the tumour and when time is of essence and follow-up imaging cannot be awaited.

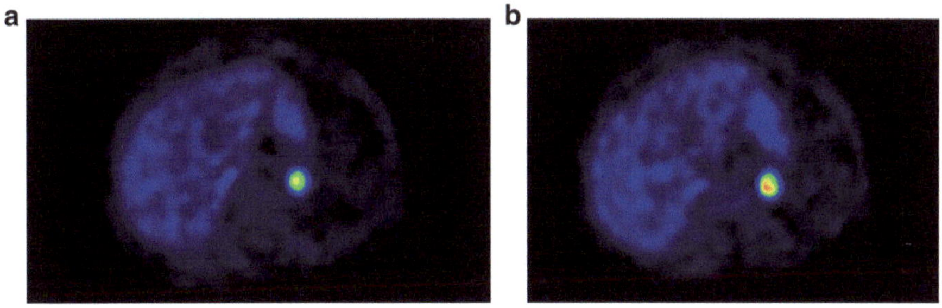

Fig. 11.1 Transaxial ^{11}C-metomidate-PET images of a patient with primary aldosteronism who was examined at baseline (**a**) and after oral administration of 0.5 mg of dexamethasone three times daily for 3 days (**b**). The PET examinations were performed after injection of 10MBq ^{11}C-metomidate per kg body weight. The images show summation of PET data 15–45 min after tracer administration. Comparing the baseline examination (**a**) with the follow-up study b, the maximum ^{11}C-metomidate uptake (standardised uptake value, SUV_{max}) in the Conn tumour (*arrow*) increased by 20 % and the quotient between the uptake in the adenoma and that of the normal contralateral adrenal increased by 30 %

Primary Aldosteronism

Patients with a biochemical diagnosis of primary aldosteronism undergo CT/MRI of the adrenals. A unilateral finding of an adrenal tumour by CT/MRI is, however, generally not sufficient for the surgical decision. In occasional patients the Conn adenoma is located in the contralateral adrenal but is so small that it escapes detection by CT/MRI. Most patients therefore also undergo lateralisation of the Conn adenoma by selective venous sampling and subsequent hormonal analysis. This is a technically challenging procedure, and thorough training is required to succeed to sample blood bilaterally. Preoperative lateralisation is generally needed in order to avoid surgical resection of a non-secreting adenoma.

^{11}C-metomidate-PET has also been evaluated in primary aldosteronism [29, 30]. In a previous study small ≤1 cm adrenocortical adenomas were missed by ^{11}C-metomidate-PET because of a similar tracer uptake in tumours and normal adrenal. Therefore nine patients with small Conn adenomas (average 1.7 cm; range 1–2.5 cm) were examined and then re-examined after 3 days of per oral dexamethasone medication. For matters of comparison, two patients with non-functioning adrenocortical adenomas were included into the study. It was hypothesised that corticoid treatment decreases ACTH secretion and thereby the 11-beta-hydroxylase activity in normal adrenal parenchyma but not in Conn adenomas. The tumour visibility was, however, similar in both examinations [29]. Neither did principal compartment analysis (PCA) improve the image contrast. PCA was applied in a cohort of seven patients who underwent ^{11}C-metomidate-PET before and after dexamethasone treatment according to the same protocol [30]. By contrast, by pre-medication with a higher dose of per oral cortisone, it was possible for another group to increase the adenoma-to-normal adrenal ratio by mean 25 ± 5 % and by ^{11}C-metomidate PET/CT visualise sub-centimeter adenomas (Fig. 11.1a, b).

In 25 patients with PA and lateralisation by adrenal venous sampling to the side of the adenoma, the tumour SUVmax was higher (mean 21.7) than in normal adrenal (mean 13.8). However, this difference was absent in ten patients without lateralisation. The authors concluded that ^{11}C-metomidate PET/CT is a sensitive and specific non-invasive alternative to adrenal venous sampling in PA [31].

^{123}I-Metomidate-SPECT

An iodinated tracer [^{123}I]-iodometomidate has been developed for SPECT [32]. This is advantageous because the SPECT systems are more generally available than PET/CT scanners. Conveniently, the long half-life of ^{123}I allows for distribution of [^{123}I]-iodometomidate to centres without their own tracer production. In addition, the longer half-life of ^{123}I, as compared to 11C, allows for imaging at later time points. Imaging can be performed 4–6 h after [^{123}I]-iodometomidate injection, but the best tumour-to-background ratios were found at 24 h. A drawback is that the spatial resolution of SPECT is inferior to that of PET (1–1.5 cm versus 0.5 cm). The binding properties of [^{123}I]-iodometomidate are comparable to those of metomidate and etomidate in vitro, and preclinical and clinical evaluation has demonstrated high and specific uptake of [^{123}I]-iodometomidate in normal adrenals, adrenocortical tumours and distant ACC metastases. Similarly to ^{11}C-metomidate-PET, [^{123}I]-iodometomidate-SPECT cannot differ adrenocortical adenoma from ACC, unless metastases also are detected.

References

1. Hammarstedt L, Muth A, Wängberg B, Björneld L, Sigurjónsdóttir HA, Götherström G, Almqvist E, Widell H, Carlsson S, Ander S, Hellström M (2010) Adrenal Study Group of Western Sweden. Adrenal lesion frequency: A prospective, cross-sectional CT study in a defined region, including systematic re-evaluation. Acta Radiol 51:1149–1156
2. Mantero F, Terzolo M, Arnaldi G, Osella G, Masini AM, Alì A, Giovagnetti M, Opocher G, Angeli A (2000) A survey on adrenal incidentaloma in Italy. Study Group on Adrenal Tumors of the Italian Society of Endocrinology. J Clin Endocrinol Metab 85:637–644
3. Abrams HL, Spiro R, Goldstein N (1950) Metastases in carcinoma; analysis of 1000 autopsied cases. Cancer 3:74–85
4. Copeland PM (1983) The incidentally discovered adrenal mass. Ann Intern Med 98:940–945
5. Hammarstedt L, Muth A, Sigurjónsdóttir HÁ, Almqvist E, Wängberg B, Hellström M (2012) Adrenal Study Group of Western Sweden. Adrenal lesions in patients with extra-adrenal malignancy—benign or malignant? Acta Oncol 51:215–221
6. Gnannt R, Fischer M, Goetti R, Karlo C, Leschka S, Alkadhi H (2012) Dual-energy CT for characterization of the incidental adrenal mass: preliminary observations. AJR Am J Roentgenol 198:138–144
7. Gupta RT, Ho LM, Marin D, Boll DT, Barnhart HX, Nelson RC (2010) Dual-energy CT for characterization of adrenal nodules: initial experience. AJR Am J Roentgenol 194:1479–1483
8. Mostbeck G (2011) CEUS of adrenal mass lesions–the break-through? Ultraschall Med 32:437–439

9. Friedrich-Rust M, Glasemann T, Polta A, Eichler K, Holzer K, Kriener S, Herrmann E, Nierhoff J, Bon D, Bechstein WO, Vogl T, Zeuzem S, Bojunga J (2011) Differentiation between benign and malignant adrenal mass using contrast-enhanced ultrasound. Ultraschall Med 32:460–471
10. Friedrich-Rust M, Schneider G, Bohle RM, Herrmann E, Sarrazin C, Zeuzem S, Bojunga J (2008) Contrast-enhanced sonography of adrenal masses: differentiation of adenomas and nonadenomatous lesions. AJR Am J Roentgenol 191:1852–1860
11. Dietrich CF, Ignee A, Barreiros AP, Schreiber-Dietrich D, Sienz M, Bojunga J, Braden B (2010) Contrast-enhanced ultrasound for imaging of adrenal masses. Ultraschall Med 31:163–168
12. Boland GW, Lee MJ, Gazelle GS, Halpern EF, McNicholas MM, Mueller PR (1998) Characterization of adrenal masses using unenhanced CT: an analysis of the CT literature. AJR Am J Roentgenol 171:201–204
13. Ozcan Kara P, Kara T, Kara Gedik G, Kara F, Sahin O, Ceylan Gunay E, Sari O (2011) The role of fluorodeoxyglucose-positron emission tomography/computed tomography in differentiating between benign and malignant adrenal lesions. Nucl Med Commun 32:106–112
14. Korobkin M, Lombardi TJ, Aisen AM, Francis IR, Quint LE, Dunnick NR, Londy F, Shapiro B, Gross MD, Thompson NW (1995) Characterization of adrenal masses with chemical shift and gadolinium-enhanced MR imaging. Radiology 197:411–418
15. Korobkin M, Giordano TJ, Brodeur FJ, Francis IR, Siegelman ES, Quint LE, Dunnick NR, Heiken JP, Wang HH (1996) Adrenal adenomas: relationship between histologic lipid and CT and MR findings. Radiology 200:743–747
16. Korobkin M, Brodeur FJ, Francis IR, Quint LE, Dunnick NR, Londy F (1998) CT time-attenuation washout curves of adrenal adenomas and nonadenomas. AJR Am J Roentgenol 170:747–752
17. Caoili EM, Korobkin M, Francis IR, Cohan RH, Dunnick NR (2000) Delayed enhanced CT of lipid-poor adrenal adenomas. AJR Am J Roentgenol 175:1411–1415
18. Caoili EM, Korobkin M, Francis IR, Cohan RH, Platt JF, Dunnick NR, Raghupathi KI (2002) Adrenal masses: characterization with combined unenhanced and delayed enhanced CT. Radiology 222:629–633
19. Kebapci M, Kaya T, Gurbuz E, Adapinar B, Kebapci N, Demirustu C (2003) Differentiation of adrenal adenomas (lipid rich and lipid poor) from nonadenomas by use of washout characteristics on delayed enhanced CT. Abdom Imaging 28:709–715
20. Volpe C, Enberg U, Sjögren A, Wahrenberg H, Jacobsson H, Törring O, Hamberger B, Thorén M (2008) The role of adrenal scintigraphy in the preoperative management of primary aldosteronism. Scand J Surg 97:248–253
21. Gambhir SS, Czernin J, Schwimmer J, Silverman DH, Coleman RE, Phelps ME (2001) A tabulated summary of the FDG PET literature. J Nucl Med 42(5 Suppl):1S–93S
22. Reske SN, Kotzerke J (2001) FDG-PET for clinical use. Results of the 3rd German Interdisciplinary Consensus Conference, "Onko-PET III", 21 July and 19 September 2000. Eur J Nucl Med 28:1707–1723
23. von Schulthess GK, Steinert HC, Hany TF (2006) Integrated PET/CT: current applications and future directions. Radiology 238:405–422
24. Bergström M, Juhlin C, Bonasera TA, Sundin A, Rastad J, Akerström G, Långström B (2000) PET imaging of adrenal cortical tumors with the 11beta-hydroxylase tracer 11C-metomidate. J Nucl Med 41:275–282
25. Minn H, Salonen A, Friberg J, Roivainen A, Viljanen T, Långsjö J, Salmi J, Välimäki M, Någren K, Nuutila P (2004) Imaging of adrenal incidentalomas with PET using (11) C-metomidate and (18)F-FDG. J Nucl Med 45:972–979
26. Zettinig G, Mitterhauser M, Wadsak W, Becherer A, Pirich C, Vierhapper H, Niederle B, Dudczak R, Kletter K (2004) Positron emission tomography imaging of adrenal masses: (18) F-fluorodeoxyglucose and the 11beta-hydroxylase tracer (11)C-metomidate. Eur J Nucl Med Mol Imaging 31:1224–1230
27. Hennings J, Lindhe O, Bergström M, Långström B, Sundin A, Hellman P (2006) [11C] metomidate positron emission tomography of adrenocortical tumors in correlation with histopathological findings. J Clin Endocrinol Metab 91:1410–1414

28. Hennings J, Hellman P, Ahlström H, Sundin A (2009) Computed tomography, magnetic resonance imaging and 11C-metomidate positron emission tomography for evaluation of adrenal incidentalomas. Eur J Radiol 69:314–2
29. Hennings J, Sundin A, Hägg A (2010) Hellman P 11C-metomidate positron emission tomography after dexamethasone suppression for detection of small adrenocortical adenomas in primary aldosteronism. Langenbecks Arch Surg 395:963–967
30. Razifar P, Hennings J, Monazzam A, Hellman P, Långström B, Sundin A (2009) Masked volume wise Principal Component Analysis of small adrenocortical tumours in dynamic [11C]-metomidate Positron Emission Tomography. BMC Med Imaging 9:6
31. Burton TJ, Mackenzie IS, Balan K, Koo B, Bird N, Soloviev DV, Azizan EA, Aigbirhio F, Gurnell M, Brown MJ (2012) Evaluation of the sensitivity and specificity of (11)C-metomidate positron emission tomography (PET)-CT for lateralizing aldosterone secretion by Conn's adenomas. J Clin Endocrinol Metab 97:100–109
32. Hahner S, Stuermer A, Kreissl M, Reiners C, Fassnacht M, Haenscheid H, Beuschlein F, Zink M, Lang K, Allolio B, Schirbel A (2008) [123 I]Iodometomidate for molecular imaging of adrenocortical cytochrome P450 family 11B enzymes. J Clin Endocrinol Metab 93:2358–2365

Chapter 12
Aldosterone and Cardiovascular Diseases

Andreas Tomasschitz and Stefan Pilz

Abstract In the past, dysregulations of aldosterone secretion as well as aldosterone-related genomic and non-genomic effects have been recognized to play an important role in the development and progression of cardiovascular diseases (CVDs) beside of the renin–angiotensin system. Growing evidence suggest that aldosterone significantly contributes to cardiovascular damage even in the absence of primary aldosteronism and independent of arterial blood pressure. This phenomenon led to the concept of relative aldosterone excess; several studies in humans and animals consistently documented a profound role of aldosterone in mediating arterial hypertension, vascular damage, myocardial dysfunction, kidney and metabolic diseases. The interplay between (1) aldosterone and angiotensin 2; (2) aldosterone and calcium regulatory endocrine systems; and (3) aldosterone and salt intake are key research fields of aldosterone-mediated target organ damage. In addition, novel treatment strategies to block aldosterone in addition to the classical mineralocorticoid receptor blockade are upcoming.

Keywords Aldosterone • Cardiovascular disease (CVD) • Angiotensin II • Cardiovascular risk • Heart failure

A. Tomasschitz (✉)
Department of Cardiology, Medical University of Graz,
Auenbruggerplatz 15, Graz 8036, Austria

Specialist Clinic for Rehabilitation PV Bad Aussee, Bad Aussee, Austria
e-mail: andreas.tomaschitz@gmx.at

S. Pilz, M.D., Ph.D.
Division of Endocrinology and Metabolism, Department of Internal Medicine,
Medical University of Graz, Graz, Austria

P. Hellman (ed.), *Primary Aldosteronism: Molecular Genetics, Endocrinology, and Translational Medicine*, DOI 10.1007/978-1-4939-0509-6_12,

Introduction

Ischemic heart disease is globally the most important cause of premature death [1]. The renin–angiotensin–(aldosterone) system (RA(A)S) has essential implications for the development of cardiovascular diseases (CVDs).

In the past, dysregulation of aldosterone secretion as well as aldosterone-related genomic and non-genomic effects have been recognized to play an important role in the development and progression of cardiovascular, renal, and metabolic diseases beside of angiotensin II.

Primary aldosteronism (PA) has been defined as aldosterone production, which is inappropriately high, relatively autonomous from the RAS, and non-suppressible by sodium loading [2]. Arterial hypertension due to absolute aldosterone excess (PA) has been initially considered as a benign form of disease with low risk of organ complications. More recent epidemiological studies suggested that the chronic exposure to absolutely elevated aldosterone levels is however related to blood pressure (BP) independent target organ damage.

Growing evidence suggest that aldosterone significantly contributes to cardiovascular damage even in the absence of PA. This phenomenon led to the concept of relative aldosterone excess.

Several interventional studies in patients with heart failure (HF) demonstrated that the benefit of mineralocorticoid receptor (MR) blockade to reduce CVD outcomes occurs independent of prevailing BP levels - even in patients with aldosterone levels "within the physiological range" [3–5]. The spectrum of (relative and absolute) aldosterone excess ranges from hyperaldosteronism in the setting of HF to low-renin hypertension (LREH) and finally PA due to bilateral adrenal hyperplasia or aldosterone producing adenoma. The continuum of aldosterone excess restricts the application of cutoffs for aldosterone levels, such as the use of the aldosterone to renin ratio (ARR) to screen for PA, in order to accurately indicate "absolute aldosterone excess" [6, 7].

This chapter will summarize the current knowledge about (1) the mechanistic background of aldosterone-mediated cardiovascular damage in different settings; (2) the clinical evidence pointing to aldosterone as a mediator of CVD, (3) the utility of aldosterone as a biomarker for detecting CVD and related diseases; and (4) the evidence of aldosterone—"blocking" treatment strategies.

For this purpose, a literature search focusing on available experimental and clinical data was performed in the electronic database MEDLINE via PubMed.

Regulation of Aldosterone Secretion

The transport of cholesterol to the inner mitochondrial membrane (for conversion to pregnenolone) by the steroidogenic acute regulatory protein (StAR) protein and the conversion of 11-deoxycorticosterone to aldosterone by aldosterone synthase (encoded by the CYP11B2 gene) are the two major rate-limiting steps of adrenal aldosterone synthesis [8, 9]. Aldosterone synthesis is mainly regulated by extracellular potassium concentration and angiotensin II. Both potassium and angiotensin II increase the intracellular calcium content through calcium release from intracellular stores and via calcium influx through T- and L-type Ca^{2+} channels [10–12]. There is however evidence that several further factors, such as ACTH, non-esterified fatty acids, lipoproteins, and parathyroid hormone (PTH), participate in the regulation of aldosterone synthesis [13–16]. Doi et al. documented that aldosterone synthesis is additionally regulated by cryptochrome genes Cry1 and Cry2—core elements of the circadian clock [17]. Moreover, increased sympathetic activity and dietary salt intake modulate the sensitivity of the adrenal gland to angiotensin II [18]. This is in line with the finding from the Framingham Offspring Study that urinary sodium is the strongest determinant (R^2: 10 %) of circulating aldosterone [19].

Somatic mutations, e.g., in the KCNJ5 gene, which encodes the G-protein-activated inward rectifier K^+ channel 4 (GIRK4), have been recently found in aldosterone producing adenomas and are implicated to increase CYP11B2 gene expression contributing to the development of absolute aldosterone excess [20].

Several studies pointed to a potentially relevant aldosterone synthesis outside the adrenal glands, e.g., in the vasculature [21]. Silvestre et al. documented CYP11B2 transcription in the rat heart [22]. In humans, cardiac CYP11B2 expression was particularly observed in pathological circumstances. The dimension and pathological consequences of cardiovascular aldosterone synthesis remains however to be elucidated in further studies.

Patho-Physiology of Aldosterone Action

Aldosterone contributes to cardiovascular damage (1) directly via genomic and non-genomic effects and (2) indirectly via mediating the development and progression of arterial hypertension, metabolic diseases and renal dysfunction, which are related to an increased cardiovascular risk [23].

Genomic Aldosterone-Mediated Effects

Given that the MR has also been identified in non-epithelial tissues, such as vascular smooth muscle cells (VSMC), endothelial cells (EC), macrophages, adipocytes, and cardiomyocytes, the classic view that aldosterone acts exclusively on transport epithelial cells has been broadened to include cells other than transport epithelia within the kidney [24].

In its classical "genomic" action, aldosterone binds to the MR and regulates gene transcription of the epithelial sodium channel (ENaC) in the distal renal tubulus promoting sodium retention [25]. Binding of aldosterone to the MR induces the expression of several further genes involved in sodium/potassium regulation including Na^+/K^--ATPase and the renal outer medullary K^+-channel (ROMK) [26–28].

Inappropriately elevated aldosterone levels exert proinflammatory, profibrotic, proliferative, and proarrhythmogenic effects on the cardiovascular system.

Experimental and observational studies documented aldosterone-induced upregulation of various modulators involved in the pathophysiology of target organ damage: transforming growth factor β (TGF-β), adhesion molecules (VCAM-1, ICAM-1, and selectins), plasminogen activator inhibitor-1 (PAI-1), nuclear factor-kappa B (NF κ B), osteopontin, placental growth factor, metallothioneins, connective tissue growth factor, etc. [29, 30]. In addition, aldosterone promotes oxidative stress via activating the NADPH oxidase and via decreasing the expression of glucose-6-phosphate dehydrogenase [31, 32].

Dietary salt intake is a central regulator of adrenal aldosterone synthesis and modulator of aldosterone-related effects and of the adrenal sensitivity to angiotensin II response [7, 18]. This is in line with the findings of Fliser et al., who postulated the existence of background pacemakers, possibly dietary salt intake and/or ACTH, for the regulation of aldosterone secretion independent of the RAS [33].

Accumulating evidence suggests a modulatory role of epigenetic mechanisms on adrenal aldosterone secretion. The link between fetal insults and epigenetic modification of genes of the RAAS and the ensuing alterations of gene expression in adult life might contribute to the development of hypertension and CVD [34].

Non-genomic Aldosterone-Mediated Effects

Rapid non-genomic aldosterone-mediated effects are related to the development of ventricular hypertrophy and apoptosis of cardiac myocytes, vasoconstriction and vasodilatation (depending on the bioavailability of NO), and renal injury [35–38].

Mechanistic studies did not consistently document an involvement of the MR in mediating non-genomic effects. Accordingly, not all non-genomic effects are affected by MR-blockade. Several authors proposed the existence of an alternative "aldosterone receptor." Grossmann et al. suggested the involvement of MR-dependent and MR-independent pathways in inducing rapid non-genomic effects [39]. In VSCMs non-genomic aldosterone effects were in part linked to the GPR30-coupled signaling pathway [40].

Aldosterone-induced rapid signaling cascades involve (1) ERK1/2-activation leading to modulation of cell growth [41]; (2) the p38 MAP kinase subfamily, which participate in cell differentiation, apoptosis and cell cycle progression [42]; (3) the activation of the protein kinase D 1 (PKD1) leading to cell proliferation [41]; (4) increased reactive oxygen species (ROS) generation through NADPH oxidase-dependent mechanisms [43]; (5) pronounced expression of collagens in fibroblasts; (6) modulation of microRNA expression in various tissues (e.g., miR-23a and MiR-208b) [44, 45]; (7) regulation of Na+/H+exchanger (NHE) 1–9 activities, which modulate intracellular pH [46]; and (8) regulation of urinary acidification by regulating H+-ATPase activity, etc. [47]. Rapid non-genomic aldosterone-mediated effects further imbed the activation of extracellular signal regulated kinase (EGFR), mediated by the non-receptor tyrosine kinase—Src

Importantly, many cross talk mechanisms restrict a clear delineation between genomic and non-genomic aldosterone-mediated effects.

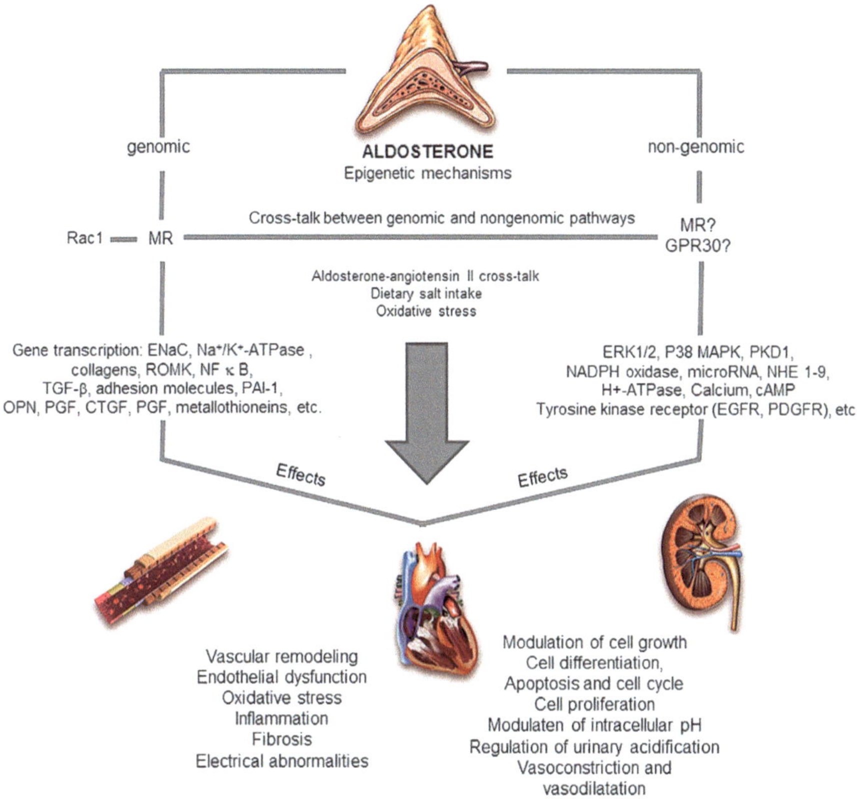

Fig. 12.1 Genomic and non-genomic aldosterone-mediated effects

Figure 12.1 provides an overview about aldosterone-mediated genomic and non-genomic effects.

Cross talk Between Aldosterone and Angiotensin II

Mechanistic studies pointed to several routes of a cross talk between genomic and non-genomic aldosterone-related effects and components of the RAS. In particular, the cross talk between aldosterone and the pathways regulated by angiotensin II might potentiate target organ damage induced by the RAAS [48, 49]. It has been suggested that this cross talk depends on the non-receptor tyrosine kinase c-Src, and on receptor tyrosine kinases, EGFR and PDGFR, and results in activation of MAP kinases and cell growth, migration, and inflammation [50].

The cross talk between aldosterone and angiotensin II is strengthened by studies in rat cardiomyocytes revealing an upregulation of angiotensin converting enzyme (ACE) by raised aldosterone levels [51]. Subsequently, elevated angiotensin II levels in turn stimulated aldosterone synthesis. In humans, aldosterone upregulated angiotensin II receptors in VSMCs and potentiated the vasoconstrictor effect of angiotensin II in coronary arteries [52]. Aldosterone–MR interaction pronounced angiotensin II-induced activation of the NADPH oxidase in the cardiovascular system [53]. Accordingly, MR antagonism decreased gene expression of the angiotensin II type 1 receptor, ACE, and endothelin-1 in non-infarcted myocardial tissue [54].

Recently, de Almeida et al. showed that NO modulates the cross talk between aldosterone and Ang-(1–7), which amplifies $Ca^{(2+)}$ signals in cardiomyocytes [55].

MR Activation by Aldosterone and Glucocorticoids

Funder et al. suggested that in the absence of 11β-hydroxysteroid dehydrogenase type 2 (11β-HSD2), which prevents binding of glucocorticoids (GCs) to the MR, cortisol is bound to for example cardiac MRs in a tonic inhibitory mode and prevents activation of the MR by aldosterone. In cell types with low or no 11β-HSD2 activity, such as in cardiomyocytes or VSMCs, GCs might activate the MR particularly in the setting of an increased ROS generation [56]. Funder et al. proposed that NADH act as a transcriptional repressor of GC/MRs. Alterations of the NAD/NADH ratio however will result in GC-related MR activation—presumably in addition to aldosterone [56]. This hypothesis was strengthened by findings in animals [57]. Studies noted that the aldosterone–MR interaction might be similarly pronounced in the setting of increased ROS-generation [58]. Indeed, in rats with myocardial ischemia both aldosterone and cortisol respectively increased infarct size and apoptosis index, which was prevented by spironolactone [56].

These findings added fuel to the debate about a varying degree of 11β-HSD2 expression in different tissues and the resulting degree of aldosterone and cortisol-mediated MR activation.

In addition, it should stressed that (1) the MR-aldosterone complex is more stable and 200-fold more active than the GC-MR complex [59]; (2) the elicited signaling pathways of GCs and aldosterone might vary substantially; and (3) the expression levels of the MR might differ depending on for example environment factors [60]. Novel evidence points to a ligand-independent activation of the MR, e.g., mediated by GTPase Rac1 [61].

Clinical Evidence for Aldosterone-Related Cardiovascular Risk

Cardiovascular Risk Related to Primary Aldosteronism

In 2012 James Funder wrote: "So while essential hypertension (EH) is a cardiovascular risk factor, this is very much magnified in PA [62]."

In fact, the risk of cardiovascular events in patients with PA is increased compared to in otherwise similar patients with essential hypertension (EH). PA has been related to the development and progression arterial hypertension, severe target organ damage and increased cardiovascular mortality [63–66].

Cardiovascular complications occurred in 14–35 % of patients with absolute aldosterone excess [65, 67, 68]. Data from the German Conn's registry, inaugurated in 2006, confirmed that cardiovascular mortality is the main cause of death in PA (50 % versus 34 % in hypertensive controls; $P<0.05$) [69].

In the German Conn's Registry, the prevalence of atrial fibrillation and cardiovascular events (angina pectoris, myocardial infarction, chronic cardiac insufficiency, coronary angioplasty) was 7.1 % and 16.3 %, respectively. Angina pectoris and chronic cardiac insufficiency were significantly more prevalent in hypokalemic PA (9.0 vs. 2.1 %, $P<0.001$; 5.5 vs. 2.1 %, $P<0.01$), indicating a stronger impact on CVD health with increasing severity of aldosterone excess [70]. Takeda et al. documented a significantly higher incidence of cerebral hemorrhage in the patients with aldosterone producing adenoma (APA) when compared to the EH patients [67]. A large recent study in 459 patients with PA revealed a significantly higher prevalence of CAD (adjusted odds ratio, 1.9), nonfatal MI (adjusted odds ratio, 2.6), HF (adjusted odds ratio, 2.9), and atrial fibrillation (adjusted odds ratio, 5.0) compared to EH [71].

LV hypertrophy is a major independent risk factor of HF, sudden cardiac death (SCD) and CVD mortality in humans [72]. Higher left ventricular (LV) wall thickness, LV mass index as well as longer PQ interval were found in patients with PA compared to EH [73]. In patients with PA LV end-diastolic dimension index was significantly larger than in EH with and without LV hypertrophy [74]. Freel et al. demonstrated a significant increase in the frequency of noninfarct late gadolinium enhancement (70 %) and higher pulse wave velocity in PA when compared with EH subjects (13 %; $P<0.0001$) but with no difference in LV mass independent of BP [75]. PA patients treated with adrenalectomy or MR blockade showed a comparable decrease of LV mass after 3 and 7 years follow up [76].

In the large PAPY Study Rossi et al. reported a significantly higher LV mass in PA compared to EH patients (27.1 % versus 16.2 %; $P=0.020$), despite similar BP values [77]. After a median follow-up of 3 years BP declined ($P<0.0001$ versus baseline) to similar values in adrenalectomized ($135\pm15/83\pm9$ mmHg) and medically treated PA ($133\pm11/83\pm7$ mmHg), compared to EH ($139\pm15/86\pm9$ mmHg) patients. In accordance to the above findings, Stehr et al. found higher levels of malondialdehyde (MDA) and amino terminal propeptides of type I (PINP) in patients with PA compared to EH. These data suggest increased oxidative stress and myocardial fibrosis as pivotal mechanisms leading to CVD damage and LV hypertrophy in patients with PA [78].

Pimenta et al. recently reported that in patients with PA higher dietary salt intake (reflected by 24-h urinary sodium) independently predicts LV wall thickness and LV mass among the patients with PA but not in patients with EH. This finding underlines the importance of salt excess for potentiating deleterious effects in the setting of inappropriately elevated aldosterone levels [79].

Recent studies added the knowledge that PA promotes an abnormal pattern of LV filling in parallel to ventricular hypertrophy [80]. With this in line, both the E wave flow velocity integral and the E/A integral ratio respectively were lower, and atrial contribution to LV filling was higher in PA patients compared with essential hypertensives [81].

Evidence suggests that aldosterone excess even promotes pulmonary vascular disease independent LV function and pulmonary capillary wedge pressure in addition to increased arterial wall stiffness, carotid intima–media thickness and carotid plaques [82, 83]. Patients with PA had significantly higher intima–media thickness in the common carotid artery than EH patients and controls independent of age and 24-h systolic BP [84]. Bernini et al. documented a greater intima–media thickness and higher femoral pulse wave velocity as well as a higher aortic augmentation index in PA patients compared to matched hypertensives [85]. The media–lumen ratio of small arteries from fat tissue of consecutive aldosterone-producing adenoma patients significantly predicted the BP response to adrenalectomy [86].

Tunica media to internal lumen ratio of small resistance arteries derived from biopsy of gluteal fat tissue was significantly increased in PA and in essential hypertension compared with normotensive controls. In addition, total collagen and type III vascular collagen were significantly greater in PA compared to essential hypertensives [87]. The TAIPAI Study Group reported an inverse correlation between the number of circulating endothelial progenitor cells and plasma aldosterone concentration, arterial stiffness and serum high-sensitivity C-reactive protein levels. High-dose aldosterone attenuated endothelial progenitor cells proliferation and angiogenesis in vitro. Interestingly, the preoperative number of endothelial progenitor cells predicted the curability of hypertension after adrenalectomy [88]. Adrenalectomy of PA patients resulted in significantly decreased carotid intima–media thickness and lower brachial-ankle pulse wave velocity levels [89].

After medical (MR blocker) or surgical (adrenalectomy) treatment of PA, the cardiovascular outcome for patients with PA was significantly improved and comparable to EH patients [65]. Surgical therapy was suggested to cure hypertension in up to 50 % and improve BP in the remainder of patients with PA [2, 90]. Cardiovascular outcome was comparable in PA patients treated with adrenalectomy vs. MR blockade [65, 91]. However, one study noted a significant decrease of LV wall thickness and mass in patients treated with adrenalectomy of an aldosterone-producing tumor, but not in those with medical therapy after 1 year of follow-up [81]. In patients with PA treatment with low-dose spironolactone for 1 year significantly decreased systolic and diastolic BP and reduced LV mass index [92]. Changes in systolic BP and pretreatment aldosterone levels are suggested as independent predictors of LV mass changes after treatment [76].

Several issues regarding diagnosing and treating PA are still unresolved [7]. Although observational and interventional studies strongly indicate a (partially) reversible CVD risk related to PA it still unknown whether (1) the diagnostic workup in PA patients significantly improves cardiovascular outcome compared to aldosterone–(MR) blockade in patients with "elevated ARR levels" without prior detection of PA; and (2) whether adrenalectomy improves cardiovascular outcome compared to aldosterone–(MR) blockade in PA already diagnosed with PA. A more differentiated look between cardiovascular outcome of patients with aldosterone producing adenoma, bilateral adrenal hyperplasia and patients with LREH should elucidate the relationship between aldosterone excess and cardiovascular risk. In particular, in regard of lacking evidence for an improved outcome of patients with PA, particularly in those with bilateral adrenal hyperplasia and low renin essential hypertension (LREH), interventional studies are urgently warranted to compare different diagnostic strategies and treatment regimen within the broad continuum of aldosterone excess.

Cardiovascular Risk Related to "Relative Aldosterone Excess"

Several observational studies consistently documented a robust relationship between elevated aldosterone levels and increased CVD morbidity and mortality independent of the presence of PA. It is therefore increasingly recognized that, even in the absence of absolute aldosterone excess, a relative excess of aldosterone, i.e., aldosterone concentrations within the "normal range" but inappropriately elevated in regard to for example dietary salt intake plays an eminent role in the pathogenesis of CVDs [93].

In patients referred to coronary angiography circulating aldosterone levels "within the physiological range" were related to increased risk of cardiovascular mortality independent of LV function and further established CVD risk factors [94]. In addition, aldosterone-related CVD morbidity and mortality is strongly linked to a decreased kidney function [95]. Further observational studies in different CVD risk groups, e.g., in patients with ST elevation acute myocardial infarction, in stable CAD patients, in female nursing home residents, and in hemodialysis patients, consistently documented a strong relationship between circulating aldosterone levels and risk of CVD morbidity/mortality [96–100].

Epidemiological investigations documented significant associations between urinary aldosterone excretion and cardiovascular risk. Increased urinary aldosterone levels were related to a dysfunctional subcutaneous adipose tissue, increased LV mass index, severity of sleep apnea syndrome, insulin resistance, and resistant hypertension [101–105]. Novel evidence points to a eminent role of aldosterone in modulating CV aging processes in humans: plasma aldosterone levels are inversely related to telomere length of white blood cells [106].

Aldosterone and Arterial Hypertension

Primary Aldosteronism, Relative Aldosterone Excess, and Arterial Hypertension: Clinical Evidence

Aldosterone plays a key role in homeostatic control and maintenance of arterial BP by regulating extracellular volume, vascular tone, and cardiac output [23].

Increasing severity of arterial hypertension is paralleled by a rising prevalence of PA, which is therefore considered as the most common curable form of arterial hypertension [107, 108]. PA, comprising two main subtypes, aldosterone producing adenoma (APA; unilateral disease) and bilateral adrenal hyperplasia (idiopathic aldosteronism (IHA)), may be found in 3–32 % of hypertensive patients [109–113]. However, the true prevalence of PA in the setting of arterial hypertension is still a subject of great controversy [114–116].

There is an ongoing discussion whether previously diagnosed cases of absolute aldosterone excess are true PA or the upper end of a continuum with inappropriately elevated aldosterone levels, high volume state and low renin secretion. Adlin et al. recently revealed that LREH might be present in 31 % of patients with untreated hypertension [117]. Indirect support for a major role of the aldosterone in modulating BP is the observation that two-thirds of patients with refractory hypertension have a low renin status and can be treated effectively with an MR blocker [118]. LREH and IHA were proposed to represent two ends of a continuum with a relative excess of aldosterone for a given level of renin [119, 120]. Accordingly, similar variations of the CYP11B2 gene have been found in patients with IHA and LREH. Moreover, in LREH as well as in patients with idiopathic PA with bilateral adrenal hyperplasia, an increased adrenal sensitivity to angiotensin II has been revealed, which strengthens a common pathophysiological background of these entities.

The bimodal serum aldosterone distribution in subjects with LREH indicated aldosterone-dependent and aldosterone-independent mechanisms of LREH. Warnock suggested that LREH might be related to increased ENaC activation with subsequent sodium and volume overload resulting in renin suppression, whereas aldosterone levels remain largely within the normal range [121].

Important limitations in our understanding of "aldosterone excess" include the difficulties of identifying a renin level as "low" and of comprehending the mechanisms that drive the activation of the adrenal or extra-adrenal RAAS.

A key finding in the field of aldosterone research was that in normotensive individuals without PA the plasma aldosterone concentration was predictive for the subsequent development of sustained hypertension [19]. Further findings from the community-based Framingham Offspring Study supported a considerable heritability of the ARR reflecting relative aldosterone excess [122]. In a large study of participants at CVD risk inappropriately elevated aldosterone levels exerted a strong effect on BP values and constituted the most important and second-most important predictor of systolic and diastolic BP levels, respectively [123]. In fact, the association between BP and the ARR was evident even at borderline hypertensive BP values, and implies that a varying degree of relative hyperaldosteronism is common among hypertensive patients [123]. Meneton et al. showed that in addition to high plasma aldosterone low renin levels precede the occurrence of hypertension in middle-aged Caucasians [124].

In animal models a modest increased expression of the aldosterone synthase sensitized BP to salt [125]. In this context Connell et al. hypothesized that a long-term increase of aldosterone synthesis from early life resulting from the interaction between genetic and environmental factors, might lead to aldosterone-related hypertension and cardiovascular damage [126].

MR blockers and aldosterone synthase inhibitors, administered as monotherapy or add-on therapy, are efficacious in the treatment of arterial hypertension. In a head-to-head comparison, the MR blocker spironolactone lowered arterial BP as effectively as thiazide diuretics in patients with low renin levels and high aldosterone-to-renin ratio values [127]. In patients with resistant hypertension spironolactone lowered BP levels irrespective of prevailing aldosterone and renin concentrations [128]. Spironolactone, even at very low doses, contributes to the lowering of BP when used as fourth-line, add-on therapy in patients with resistant hypertension [129, 130]. The second generation MR blocker eplerenone effectively reduced BP in patients with arterial hypertension, including LREH, and even in patients with mild to moderate hypertension [131, 132]. Although spironolactone has been never tested in cardiovascular outcome RCTs before, the above mentioned evidence justifies the use of MR blockade as a third- or fourth-line drug for treating arterial hypertension [133].

Important consequences of previous studies might be that relative hyperaldosteronism (1) is recognized as a crucial mediator of arterial hypertension; and (2) the consideration of a wider use of MR blockade, especially when other antihypertensive drugs are insufficient for the control of BP [133]. More research is however needed to better understand the mechanisms controlling aldosterone secretion and to make MR blockade a safe treatment option in hypertensive patients.

Evolutionary Aspects for the Role of Aldosterone in Mediating Arterial Hypertension

The RAAS is the principle volume-regulatory effector in humans. About 400 Ma, the transition of organisms form the ocean to dry land offered challenges regarding the maintenance of the internal environment in a salt scarce environment. Thus, the RAAS probably evolved in Paleozoic times in response to environmental pressures when our early terrestrial ancestors were confronted with low salt availability. Under these conditions, activation of the RAAS would favor renal salt conservation and water retention, thus contributing to maintaining sufficient tissue perfusion in a salt-scarce environment [134].

Homo sapiens emerged around 150,000 years ago [135]. The increased use of salt for food conservation in advanced civilizations provokes a over-driven RAAS, which is inappropriately downregulated and triggers target organ damage [136]. The gap between the primary function of the RAAS in our early ancestral and the completely changed environment in Western societies is a feasible evolutionary reason for the tremendous health burden exerted by CVDs.

Na^+ reabsorption occurring via the epithelial Na^+ channel (ENaC) in distal tubules and cortical colleting ducts is the final renal step of a complex network of regulators of sodium and volume homeostasis. The varying responsiveness of ENaC to aldosterone plays a pivotal role in the pathophysiology of arterial hypertension.

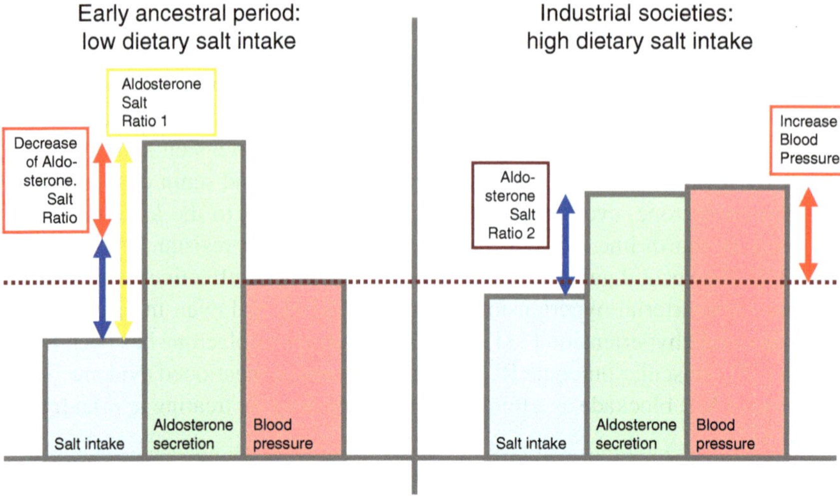

Fig. 12.2 Relative aldosterone excess: inadequate downregulation of aldosterone due to inappropriately high dietary salt intake in modern societies

In fact, the inappropriate adjustment of aldosterone–ENaC activity to high dietary salt intake in modern societies is the central mechanism for the development of salt-sensitive, aldosterone-dependent hypertension [134]. This phenomenon is further confirmed by findings in Yanomama Indians (Venezuela). Yanomama Indians live on extremely low Na^+ intakes (10 mmol per day) and show clearly raised serum aldosterone concentrations (14.7 mmol/l), yet have low BP (mean 102/62 mmHg) [137]. Thus, the "two-hit" concept of aldosterone-mediated BP elevation comprise an increased Na^+ reabsorption and high dietary salt loading together with an inappropriate downward adjustment of aldosterone secretion (Fig. 12.2).

Gomez-Sanchez et al. additionally proposed an important role of centrally acting mineralocorticoids in mediating salt appetite, sympathetic drive, vasopressin release, and finally salt sensitive hypertension [138]. Arterial hypertension caused by centrally acting mineralocorticoids is preventable by MR blockade.

The relationship of dietary salt (sodium) intake and cardiovascular morbidity/mortality has been intensively debated. The American Heart Association recently strongly recommended a dietary sodium intake of less than 1.5 g/day for all Americans. It has been argued that although high sodium intake is related to deleterious effects a low sodium diet in turn results may worsen cardiovascular prognosis [139]. This is at least questionable in regard of mineralocorticoid-related arterial hypertension when considering the low BP levels found in Yanomama Indians despite elevated aldosterone concentration. Alderman and Cohen recently discussed the conflicting results regarding salt-related CVD risk; In humans with average sodium intakes of less than 4.5 g/day, most observational studies found an inverse association of salt intake with outcome; in subjects with average intakes greater than 4.5 g/day, most studies reported direct associations between sodium intake and CVD outcomes [140]. These results indicated a "J-shaped" relationship between sodium and cardiovascular outcomes with higher risk for sodium intakes above and below the range of 2.5–6.0 g/day.

Effects of Aldosterone on the Vasculature

Both ECs and VSMCs are established sites of MR expression and local aldosterone synthesis [21]. Numerous mechanistic studies demonstrated genomic and non-genomic aldosterone-related effects on the vasculature which contributed to functional and structural alterations and the ensuing development of arterial hypertension and CVD. In experimental studies and humans MR activation promoted endothelial dysfunction, systemic vascular resistance, vasoconstriction, and decreased forearm blood flow [58, 141]. MR blockade improved endothelial dependent vasodilatation independent of BP [142]. Lieb et al. found a positive correlation between the ARR and various measures of arterial stiffness [143]. This is in line with a decreased collagen-to-elastin ratio and improved vessel remodeling as well as decreased vascular stiffness due to MR antagonism [144].

Oberleithner et al. impressively demonstrated that the response of the endothelium to small changes of sodium concentration strongly depends on aldosterone [145]. This is supported by the fact that in humans the association of circulating aldosterone with CVD death is strongly linked to prevailing circulating sodium levels [94]. Aldosterone stimulated the insertion of the ENaC in the EC membrane. In addition, CRP promoted the insertion of ENaC in EC membranes and potentiated endothelial stiffness, which was prevented by MR blockade [146]. Recent investigations of ECs cultured in aldosterone-supplemented medium demonstrated an impressive increase of MR and ENaC expression, which was paralleled by an increased cortical stiffness. MR blockade by spironolactone resulted in an improved endothelial function by increasing NO release by 50 % [147].

Decreased NO availability and the increase of ROS-generation, which result in an enhanced production of local vasoconstrictors such as prostacyclin, endothelin, and angiotensin II, are two key mechanisms for aldosterone-induced endothelial dysfunction [148–150]. This is underlined by an increased NOS activity and decreased arterial BP levels after MR blockade in animal models with hypertension [151].

In VSMCs aldosterone modulated intracellular levels of Ca^{2+} and cAMP and induced NHE activity as well as the phosphorylation of different kinases followed by proliferation and inflammation [152–156]. MR activation in human VSMCs and ECs resulted in increased inflammatory gene expression, such as ICAM1, VCAM1, interleukin-16, cytotoxic T-lymphocyte-associated protein, that was followed by leukocyte adhesion to coronary ECs [49, 157].

Kasal et al. identified suppressor T-regulatory lymphocytes (Tregs) as a potential target to prevent aldosterone-induced vascular injury. Aldosterone enhanced macrophage infiltration in the aorta and renal cortex as well as infiltration of the aorta by

T-cells. Tregs in the renal cortex were diminished, while the adoptive transfer of Tregs prevented the adverse vascular and renal effects induced by aldosterone. This finding indicated that immunomodulatory interventions may interfere with aldosterone-induced vascular damage [158].

Aldosterone and Heart Failure

In a landmark investigation Swedberg et al. documented a robust association between elevated aldosterone levels (in the setting of neuroendocrine activation) and increased risk of death in patients with severe HF [159]. Vantrimpont et al. confirmed a positive relationship between circulating aldosterone levels and adverse outcome in patients with LV ejection fraction <40 % at 3 months after myocardial infarction (MI) [160]. Similarly, in patients with acute MI plasma aldosterone emerged as short- and long-term predictor of fatal CVD events [94, 161–163]. In the LURIC study patients with acute coronary syndrome and with either low or high circulating aldosterone levels were at higher risk of fatal cardiovascular events (Fig. 12.3). In the EVEREST trial comprising patients hospitalized for worsening HF (LVEF <40 %) higher baseline serum aldosterone

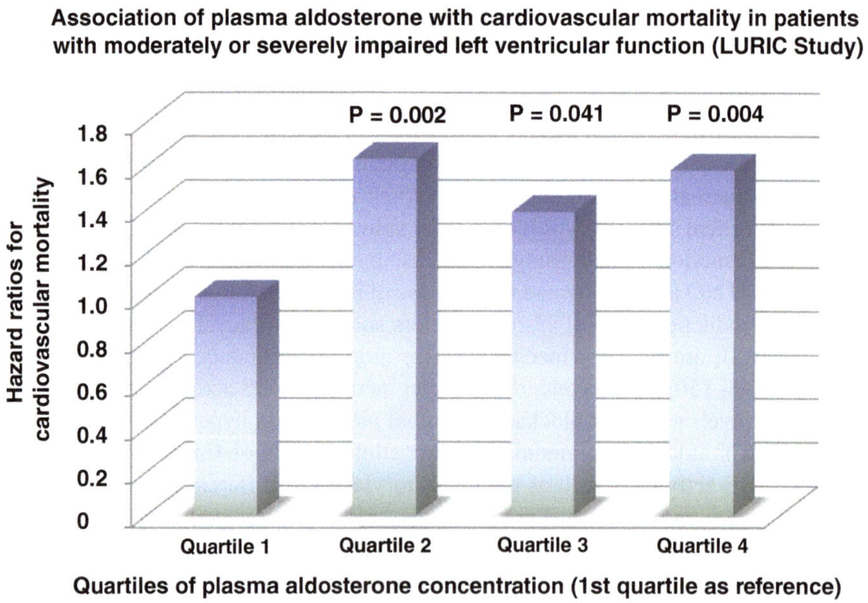

Fig. 12.3 Risk of death due to fatal cardiovascular events in patients with moderately or severely impaired left ventricular function. Findings from the Ludwigshafen Risk and Cardiovascular Health (LURIC) study

levels were associated with an increased risk for all-cause and cardiovascular mortality or HF rehospitalization [164]. These findings concurred with the upregulation of MR expression after acute experimental MI [165]. In patients with acute HF circulating aldosterone levels remained high for almost 10 month after discharge and were strongly associated with all-cause and cardiovascular mortality [164].

In the Framingham Offspring Study relative aldosterone excess reflected by the ARR was positively associated with both concentric/eccentric LV hypertrophy and parameters of extracellular matrix turnover [166]. We reported that in patients with preserved LV function (LVEF > 60 %) circulating aldosterone levels are independently related with echocardiographic parameters of LV structure, particularly in women [167].

The central role of aldosterone in the pathophysiology of HF and related complications has been underlined by findings derived from the landmark studies RALES, EPHESUS, and EMPHASIS-HF [3–5]. In RALES and EPHESUS MR blockade significantly reduced risk of death in patients with severe HF NYHA III/IV and in patients with decreased LV function (EF < 40 %) after acute MI, respectively. A substudy of the EPHESUS trial additionally revealed decreased levels of amino-terminal propeptide of collagen type I (PINP) and PIIINP after 6 months treatment with eplerenone [168]. In the EMPHASIS-HF trial treatment of eplerenone compared to placebo significantly reduced risk of death and of risk of hospitalization in NYHA II patients with a LV ejection fraction <35 %.

In the 4E–LV hypertrophy Study enrolling hypertensive patients with LV hypertrophy eplerenone was as effective as enalapril in regression of LV hypertrophy and BP control [169].

Thus, use of MR blockers are currently recommended in patients with (1) persisting symptoms (NYHA II–IV) and an EF < 35 % despite treatment with an ACE-I (or ARB) and beta-blocker; (2) HF and ventricular arrhythmia in addition to ACE-I/Beta-blocker; (3) as third-line therapy in uncontrolled arterial hypertension; and (4) PA due to bilateral adrenal disease [2, 133, 170].

Caution should be taken in regard of MR-blockade associated risk of hyperkalemia and decline of kidney function. In the EPHESUS trial, however, the incidence of serious hyperkalemia was rather low [4]. In addition short-term increase of potassium after initiating MR-blockade was not related to mortality outcomes. The PEARL-HF study in HF patients revealed that the use of the potassium binder RLY5016 in parallel to spironolactone (25–50 mg/day) prevents MR-related hyperkalemia [171].

Additional evidence suggests that MR blockade by spironolactone might improve CVD outcome in patients with HF and preserved ejection fraction (HFpEF). Interestingly, in states of pressure overload (HFpEF) the myocardium becomes increasingly sensitized to aldosterone excess [172]. In the ALDO-DHF Study Pieske et al. demonstrated that in NYHA II/III patients with HFpEF (LVEF > 50 %) and evidence of diastolic dysfunction spironolactone treatment compared to placebo for 12 months results in decreased diastolic dysfunction, decline of LV mass index and improved neuroendocrine activation [173]. This supports the hypothesis that MR blockade reverses early phases of HF development. More evidence in this field will be gained by the TOPCAT (Treatment Of Preserved Cardiac function HF with an Aldosterone antagonist Trial) Study, which currently evaluates the effect of MR blockade on hard clinical endpoints in patients with HFpEF [174].

Mechanistic experimental studies attempted to shed more light on the mechanisms underlying aldosterone-related myocardial damage. Primarily, aldosterone-mediated changes on the myocardium comprise fibrosis, inflammation, hypertrophy, and apoptosis [175].

Gekle et al. proposed a coincidence model of aldosterone-mediated target organ damage; According to the "two hit" concept a second trigger, such as angiotensin II, salt excess, and/or oxidative stress, is necessary to trigger aldosterone-induced cardiac damage [176].

The increase of aldosterone-related ROS generation is mediated via the multifunctional Ca^{2+}/calmodulin (CaM) dependent protein kinase (CaMKII) [177]. CaMKII is strongly associated with aldosterone-mediated post-MI matrix remodeling and cardiac rupture. The stimulation of cardiac myocyte NHE activity and ensuing ROS generation is one suggested mechanisms of aldosterone-related fibrosis [178].

Aldosterone–MR interaction regulates the expression of various genes, which are deeply involved in pathologic cardiac remodeling, independent of BP regulation: ANP, BNP, TGF-beta, PAI-1, Col I/II, etc. [179]. The upregulation of these genes is prevented by MR-blockade. Latouche et al. detected two novel MR-specific genes which contribute to myocardial matrix remodeling: Adamts1 and SerpinA3 [180]. In addition, aldosterone–MR activation is followed by stimulation of inflammatory mediators such as the chemokine receptor CXCR4 [181].

These findings are in line with reduced pathologic remodeling after an early initiation of MR-blockade in mice with MI [182]. Finally, MR activation of macrophages might play an additional crucial role in mediating cardiac remodeling processes [183].

In rat models of renovascular hypertension and PA Weber and Brilla et al. identified aldosterone (in addition to salt) as major culprit of ventricular hypertrophy [184, 185]. Cardiac hypertrophy was attenuated by MR blockade with spironolactone independent of BP changes [186]. Histological abnormalities related to aldosterone–salt effects were dominated by perivascular fibrosis and acute inflammatory response including the upregulation of ICAM-1, connective tissue growth factor, PAI-1, monocyte chemoattractant molecule-1, TNFa, collagen, and metalloproteinases [29, 187].

In further experimental animal studies with HF following myocardial infarction due to coronary ligation the cardiomyocyte-specific inactivation of the MR gene prevents adverse cardiac remodeling, attenuated pulmonary edema, increased capillary density, and reduced accumulation of extracellular matrix proteins in the surviving LV myocardium [188]. This study supported the importance of the cardiomyocyte MR activation for ischemic HF development. In mice macrophages lacking MR in myeloid cells mimicked the effects of MR blockade and protected against cardiac hypertrophy, fibrosis, and vascular damage caused by L-NAME/angiotensin2 [183].

The cardiomyocyte/coronary vessel-MR-aldosterone cross talk caused coronary dysfunction due to an increased local aldosterone synthesis within myocardial cells [189]. One further pivotal question concerns the balance between MR activation and aldosterone excess. It has been hypothesized that particularly patients with pre-existing cardiovascular damage, e.g., after acute MI, show an increased susceptibility to MR activation and/or an increased sensitivity to basal MR activity.

Inconsistent findings have been however revealed regarding local aldosterone synthesis in cardiomyocytes [22, 190, 191]. It has been speculated that cardiomyocytes produce aldosterone particularly under pathological conditions, which might favor MR activation even in the setting of low cardiac 11β-HSD2 activity. In addition, aldosterone might be delivered from circulation to the heart via inflammatory cells, e.g., via monocytes and macrophages [183].

Sodium and calcium homeostasis are tightly regulated by endocrine systems. Considering that aldosterone excess is paralleled by elevated PTH levels and vice versa, it has been proposed that clinically relevant interactions exist between the RAAS and the vitamin D–PTH axis [15, 192, 193].

Evidence for the interplay between the RAAS and the vitamin D–PTH axis has been gained from animal and human studies; Adrenalectomy results in increased circulating calcium and decreased PTH levels, and parathyroidectomy is followed by decreased calcium, renin, and aldosterone levels [194, 195].

Maniero demonstrated the expression of both type 1 PTH receptors in aldosterone-producing adrenocortical nodules as well as expression of the MR in the nuclei of parathyroid adenoma and even in normal parathyroid cells [196].

Novel evidence indicates that in the setting of high dietary salt intake aldosterone promotes reabsorption of sodium and increases calcium (and magnesium) excretion in the renal distal tubule followed by PTH secretion. This mechanism might explain why the association between circulating aldosterone and PTH levels varied depending on dietary salt intake reflected by 24-h urinary sodium excretion [193].

Considering the wide use of MR antagonists, the above-discussed findings may have significant clinical implications: PTH excess exerts adverse effects on bone health and accumulating evidence indicates that PTH is an independent cardiovascular risk factor. Thus, lowering PTH by MR blockade may have beneficial cardiovascular, renal, and metabolic effects. This is supported by the observation in patients with chronic HF that MR blockade is associated with reduced fracture risk. In patients with PA, treatment with either MR blockers or adrenalectomy does not only normalize elevated PTH levels but is also related to improved bone mineral density and decreased fracture risk [194, 197].

HF is one further clinically relevant setting in which the mutual interplay between sodium and calcium regulating hormones may have detrimental consequences: hyperaldosteronism despite sodium and fluid retention results in further salt retention and renal/fecal calcium/magnesium wasting and subsequent secondary hyperparathyroidism. The PTH-promoted mitochondrial Ca^{2+} excess, e.g., in the myocardium, induces oxidative stress and necrotic cell death which in the long term aggravates HF [198]. PTH tends to increase adrenal aldosterone synthesis, thus triggering a vicious circle of mutually reinforcing hyperaldosteronism and hyperparathyroidisms with the resulting risk of even more target organ damage (Fig. 12.4).

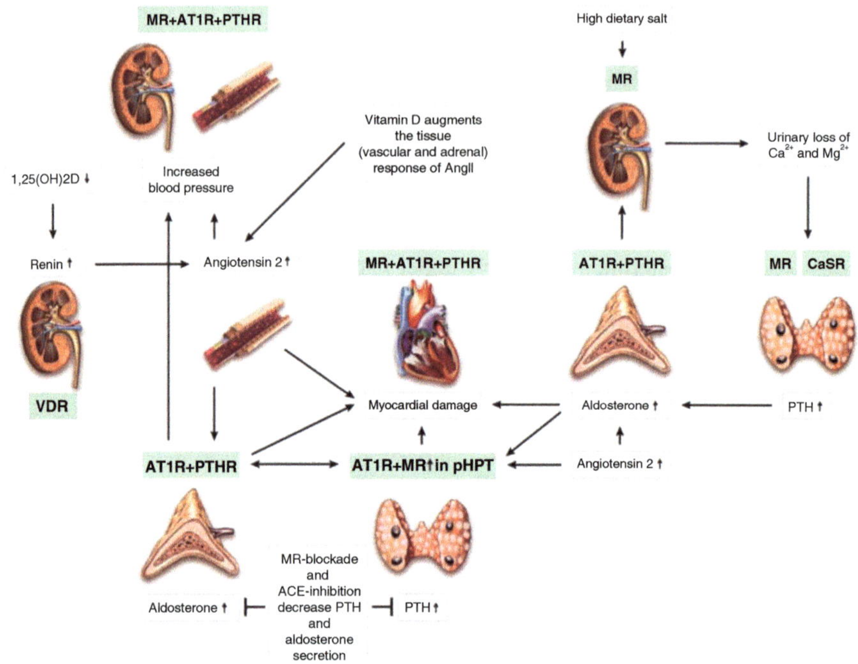

Fig. 12.4 The interplay between calcium and sodium regulatory hormones. Parathyroid hormone (PTH) directly stimulates aldosterone synthesis in zona glomerulosa cells. PTH increases sensitization towards angiotensin 2. PTH contributes to the development of cardiovascular damage via binding to the PTH/PTH-rP receptor, which is expressed in vascular smooth muscle cells and cardiomyocytes. Inappropriately elevated aldosterone secretion in the setting of primary aldosteronism, heart failure, and dietary salt excess results in (1) accelerated renal (and fecal) calcium and magnesium loss and salt/water retention and (2) increased parathyroid hormone (PTH) secretion via activation of calcium sensing receptor and (b) activation of mineralocorticoid receptors (MR) located on chief cells of the parathyroid glands. Aldosterone exerts genomic (by binding to the MR), and non-genomic profibrotic and proinflammatory effects on blood vessels and the myocardium. 1,25(OH)2D (1) modulates renin gene transcription and renin synthesis in the kidney independent of serum calcium and PTH and (2) modifies tissue sensitivity to angiotensin 2. Circulating angiotensin 2 stimulates PTH secretion. The stimulatory effects of both angiotensin 2 and aldosterone are attenuated by ACE inhibition and MR-blockade, respectively. Finally, the vicious circle between angiotensin 2, aldosterone, and PTH might potentiate CV damage. *PTH(R)* parathyroid hormone (receptor), *MR* mineralocorticoid receptor, *AT1R* angiotensin 2 type 1 receptor, *Ang II* angiotensin 2, *VDR* vitamin D receptor, *pHPT* primary hyperparathyroidism, *CaSR* calcium-sensing receptor

Considering the wide use of RAAS blocking agents, the results of ongoing RCTs evaluating the clinical effects of ACE-inhibitors or MR blockers on PTH, bone metabolism, and CVD are awaited with high interest. The Effect of eplerenone on parathyroid hormone (EPATH) Study currently evaluates in patients with primary hyperparathyroidism the effects of MR blockade by eplerenone on PTH levels and cardiovascular risk factors [199].

MR blockade increases aldosterone (and cortisol) levels, which might result in pronounced non-genomic aldosterone-induced effects [200]. Novel treatment strategies to block aldosterone in the setting of HF are upcoming. Aldosterone-synthase inhibitors are a promising therapy option: aldosterone-synthase inhibitor FAD286 significantly improved coronary vascular dysfunction and normalized HF-related myocardial oxidative stress compared to spironolactone [201]. Because of the homology of the enzymes responsible for aldosterone and cortisol synthesis, such blockade is however not specific for aldosterone synthesis and will therefore also suppress cortisol release.

The novel orally active aldosterone synthase inhibitor LCI699 decreased dose-dependently plasma and urine aldosterone concentration by up to 70–80 %. This orally active aldosterone synthase inhibitor also impacted on the GC axis. In a randomized double-blind placebo and active-control phase 2 trial the compound caused significant reduction of systolic BP and ambulatory 24-h-BP [202].

Studies in humans are needed to further evaluate effects of aldosterone synthase inhibition.

Aldosterone, Stroke and Arrhythmia

Background

Aldosterone–MR interaction induced cardiomyocyte ionic remodeling by modulating T-type calcium channel expression, potassium channel expression, L-type calcium channel expression, and ryanodine receptor activities [203–206]. Aldosterone impacted on the control of myocyte calcium signaling, modulation of calcium transients, sarcoplasmatic reticulum diastolic leaks, resulting in an increased risk of arrhythmia due to prolonged repolarization and early after-depolarization [207]. Pro-arrhythmic properties of aldosterone may be further mediated by increased sympathetic drive, decreased heart rate variability, disturbed baroreceptor function, and blunted myocardial norepinephrine uptake [208].

Aldosterone and Atrial Fibrillation

Reil et al. suggested that aldosterone-mediated atrial fibrosis, myocyte hypertrophy, and conduction disturbances result in a higher risk of atrial arrhythmia [209]. Higher levels of circulating aldosterone levels were found patients with chronic atrial fibrillation and rapidly decreased after electric cardioversion [210, 211]. Of note, Li et al. suggested a relationship between CYP11B2 T-344C gene polymorphism and higher AF risk [212].

Spironolactone prevented atrial remodeling and apoptosis in a canine model of atrial fibrillation [213]. In patients with persistent atrial fibrillation use of eplerenone was related to a increased maintenance of sinus rhythm after radiofrequency catheter ablation [214]. In the EMPHASIS-HF Study eplerenone reduced the risk of new onset atrial fibrillation or flutter [215].

Aldosterone and Ventricular Arrhythmia

LV hypertrophy due to pro-fibrotic effects of aldosterone is characterized by a diffuse accumulation of connective tissue accelerating the development of profound ventricular arrhythmia via increased electric inhomogeneity of conduction and impaired gap junction function. Accordingly, in rat ventricular myocytes a normalization of post MI pathological electrical remodeling after MR-blocker therapy was observed [216].

In patients at cardiovascular risk circulating plasma aldosterone levels over a broad range were related to an increased risk for SCD [94]. Accordingly, much of the benefit of MR blockade has been attributed to the reduction of SCD [3, 4]. This is supported by the observation of impressive reduction of ventricular extrasystoles and QT intervals after MR blockade [217]. Recent findings confirmed the eminent role of aldosterone as mediator of ventricular arrhythmia; In patients presenting for primary PCI for STEMI early MR blockade resulted in reductions in rates of life-threatening arrhythmia and cardiac arrest independent of the initial risk profile and HF [218]. Gomez et al. documented a strong correlation between aldosteronemia and risk of cardiac arrhythmia in HF [206].

Aldosterone and Metabolic Disorders

In 1965 JW Conn observed an increased incidence of impaired glucose tolerance in PA [219]. Thereafter, clinical and experimental studies by the majority supported a direct impact of aldosterone on glucose homeostasis independent of changes in circulating potassium levels. Aldosterone excess may have multiple metabolic consequences: at a cellular level aldosterone caused insulin resistance by increasing oxidative stress, attenuating insulin signaling, and thus decreasing glucose transport. Aldosterone also diminished glucose stimulated insulin secretion, both in vivo and in vitro, through a MR-independent mechanism [220].

An association between aldosterone levels and insulin resistance has been reported both in normotensive and hypertensive populations [221, 222]. In normotensive healthy subjects circulating aldosterone levels were related insulin resistance independent of traditional risk factors [222]. Fallo et al. noted in patients with PA a higher prevalence of metabolic syndrome and higher levels of fasting glucose compared to EH patients independent of the type of PA, BP levels, abdominal obesity, body mass index, and lipid levels [223]. This group found in patients with PA in the absence of metabolic syndrome a higher insulin resistance, defined by increased homeostasis model assessment (HOMA index), than in those with LREH. Circulating adiponectin levels were lower in PA than in patients with LREH [224].

Another study implicated a higher prevalence of metabolic disorders in IHA compared with APA patients similar to EH [225]. In the Framingham Offspring Study aldosterone levels was strongly associated with the development of metabolic syndrome [226]. In two German population based studies, circulating aldosterone was independently related to the presence of metabolic syndrome [227].

One study impressively confirmed that patients with PA have greater homeostasis model assessment index ($P<0.05$) and plasma insulin response to an oral glucose load ($P<0.05$) and lower quantitative insulin sensitivity check index ($P<0.01$) than normotensive controls. After PA treatment parameters of insulin sensitivity were restored to normal [228].

Shimamoto et al. found that after adrenalectomy of PA patients, blood glucose levels were significantly decreased and the total insulin levels during 75 g OGTT were significantly increased compared with the normal range [229]. Giachetti et al. found a positive correlation between homeostasis model assessment (HOMA) insulin resistance index and HOMA beta cell and serum aldosterone levels in both patients with aldosterone producing adenoma and bilateral adrenal hyperplasia, respectively [230].

One group reported improved insulin action in patients with PA after adrenalectomy, whereas spironolactone treatment of patients with idiopathic PA did not significantly influence insulin action [231]. No significant associations between insulin sensitivity expressed by the hyperinsulinemic clamp and by the homeostasis model assessment (HOMA) and QUICKI indexes in the patients with insulinoma or PA have been reported by Skrha et al. [232].

In the German Conn's Registry diabetes mellitus was more prevalent in patients with PA ($n=638$) than in 338 matched controls (23 % vs. 10 % in controls) [233]. In contrast, one further large study revealed a lower prevalence of impaired fasting glucose in patients with primary aldosteronism than in matched controls, and the prevalence of hyperglycemia (impaired fasting glucose or diabetes mellitus) and blood levels of glucose and lipids did not differ between cases and controls.

In one further study no significant difference between preoperative and postoperative levels of either fasting plasma glucose or serum lipids in PA patients who underwent adrenalectomy have been observed [234].

Clinical findings regarding lipid metabolism in PA are inconsistent. Most studies did not reveal any differences in the serum lipid profile of patients with PA compared to EH [223, 228, 234, 235]. Inappropriately elevated levels of aldosterone are related to obesity in normotensive and hypertensive populations and BMI (body mass index) is related to circulating aldosterone concentrations in healthy normotensive subjects with dietary salt excess [236–238]. Iacobellis et al. showed that low HDL-cholesterol prevalence was significantly higher in subjects with PA than in EH (73.7 % vs. 17.5 %) [239]. Ronconi et al. suggested that adiponectin gene polymorphisms, e.g., the genotype 276 T/T, is associated with worse metabolic profile in PA

[240]. The Framingham Study failed to document a relation between subcutaneous adipose tissue and plasma aldosterone concentration and ARR levels, respectively, raising doubts whether regional adiposity measures are associated with circulating indicators of the RAAS [241]. This issue needs further investigation. Further studies showed that plasma aldosterone is related to BMI in EH but not in PA [242]. Ishimori et al. did not document changes in fasting plasma glucose and the glucose area under the curve during the oral glucose tolerance test after adrenalectomy although fasting plasma insulin and the insulin area under the curve increased significantly [243].

The inconsistency of reports regarding metabolic disturbances in patients with PA might be due to differences in selection of participants with PA and controls, study conditions and sample size as well in the methods used to evaluate insulin sensitivity. Furthermore, abnormalities of the glucose metabolism in patients with PA and EH might result from common pathogenetic mechanisms [244].

Several different pathogenic mechanisms have been implicated to underlie aldosterone-induced insulin resistance: one important mechanism is the inhibition of transcriptional activity of the insulin receptor gene by aldosterone/MR [245–247]. Aldosterone mediates the degradation of insulin receptor substrate (IRS)-1 and IRS-2 via production of reactive oxygen species (ROS), leading to impaired glucose uptake in adipocytes [248]. Lastra et al. demonstrated that spironolactone improved insulin sensitivity in the rat skeletal muscle [249]. Kraus et al. demonstrated that aldosterone impacts on the insulin-induced glucose uptake in murine brown adipocytes [250].

Various cytokines, such as TNF-a, interleukin 6, adiponectin, and leptin, which are modulated by aldosterone, might play a crucial role in mediating the development and progression of metabolic syndrome [251, 252].

Recent animal studies documented an emerging role of the local as well as the systemic RAAS in the genesis of cardiometabolic abnormalities of visceral adiposity [253]. MRs have been identified in brown adipose tissue. Fat cell-derived factors, adipocytokines, and lipids modulated adrenal aldosterone synthesis [254]. Investigations by Caprio et al. indicated pro-adipogenic effects of aldosterone on human adipocytes [255].

Aldosterone contributed to the differentiation of brown adipose cells and affected energy expenditure [256]. In an adipocyte cell line (3T3-L1), mature adipocytes were isolated from human or mouse adipose tissue and from perivascular fat of obese diabetic mice. Aldosterone synthase was detected in adipocytes both under basal conditions and after exposure to angiotensin; this was associated with increased aldosterone secretion [257].

Rats fed a high-fat diet developed elevated aldosterone levels accompanied by a twofold increase in adrenal aldosterone synthase mRNA expression and zona glomerulosa hypertrophy [258]. Plasma resistin concentration was significantly higher in PA subjects when compared with EH [239]. Flynn et al. reviewed the role of adipocyte-secreted factors in stimulating aldosterone release from the adrenal cortex. Visceral adipocytes stimulated aldosterone release involving both Wnt-signaling pathways and mitogen-activated protein kinases [259].

Aldosterone-mediated gene repression of adiponectin and peroxisome proliferator-activated receptor γ (PPARγ) have been reversed by MR blockade in obese mice models [260, 261].

Aldosterone excess affects glucose uptake through defective expression of glucose transporter 2 and 4 genes in liver and skeletal muscle of adult male rat [262].

In the vasculature aldosterone–MR activation led to an increased production of reactive oxygen species and oxidative stress, resulting in increased insulin resistance [263].

It might be speculated that aldosterone impairs the whole-body insulin-sensitivity acting outside the adipose tissue. This is line with beneficial effects of MR blockers on hepatic steatosis in mice [264]. Conflicting results were however reported in regard of the impact of MR blockers on glucose homeostasis. Some studies reported a worsened glycemic control in hypertensive patients with diabetes after MR blocker treatment [265]. Further studies are warranted in this field.

Cardiovascular Risk Related to Aldosterone-Mediated Kidney Damage

Patients with chronic kidney disease (CKD) are more likely to die of CVD than progress to end-stage kidney failure [266]. Growing evidence supports that aldosterone-mediated effects participate in the development and progression of renal damage and thus linking the increased mortality risk with declining kidney function. This is in line with reports documenting nephroprotective effects of MR antagonists in addition to an RAS blockade-based regimen.

In patients with PA, elevated aldosterone levels are linked to increased renal damage and CVD mortality [267, 268]. Sechi et al. documented a partially reversible renal dysfunction in PA compared to patients with EH [64]. In the PAPY Study 24-h urine albumin excretion and prevalence of microalbuminuria was significantly higher in PA than in EH patients [269]. In 148 patients with PA renal dysfunction and elevated albuminuria were reversible after treatment with eplerenone or spironolactone [270].

It has been further suggested that even in patients not suggestive for PA the association of higher plasma aldosterone concentration with overall CVD mortality and SCD is stronger for patients with lower kidney function [95]. In an observational study in the general Japanese population adverse renal outcome was predicted by higher baseline ARR levels [271]. Similarly in the Framingham Offspring Study baseline aldosterone concentration are significantly associated with the incidence of CKD [272].

In the 4D study Drechsler et al. showed in hemodialyzed patients with type 2 diabetes that both circulating aldosterone and cortisol levels are powerful predictors of SCD—an observation calling for appropriate studies to assess the efficacy of aldosterone targeted intervention in renal patients [99].

A recent randomized small crossover study by Boesby documented that eplerenone as add-on treatment reduced albuminuria independent of arterial BP [273]. In a double-blind randomized placebo controlled crossover study in patients with type 1 diabetes and microalbuminuria spironolactone on top of standard antihypertensive treatment significantly lowered albuminuria by 60 % [274]. In patients with CKD 2/3 on RAS blockade with well controlled BP spironolactone significantly reduced LV mass/index as well as pulse wave velocity [275].

A causal role of aldosterone in renal disease is also plausible in view of past findings of Quinkler et al. in kidney biopsies of patients with renal failure and mild to marked proteinuria: serum aldosterone was correlated negatively with creatinine clearance and positively with renal scarring. In the samples of heavy proteinuric patients the MR was increased fivefold and sgk1 (a key molecule for Na+ reabsorption) 2.5-fold [276].

Apart from kidney protection another target of MR blockade in CKD patients may be the frequent LV-hypertrophy.

Mechanistic studies implicated that aldosterone causes BP independent kidney damage as a result of oxidative and nitrative stress, accompanied by structural and mutagenic DNA damage. Terada et al. found that aldosterone increased expression and activation of SGK1(Serine/threonine-protein kinase); in addition it activated NFκB and caused expression of ICAM-1 (intercellular adhesion molecule-1) and CTGF (connective tissue growth factor) [277]. This effect was abrogated by eplerenone. Activation of SGK1 and NFκB are involved in the progression of aldosterone-induced mesangial fibrosis and inflammation.

Xue et al. documented the existence of a local aldosterone system in the kidney [278]. Local activation of renal cells is obviously important, because Lee et al. showed that activation of the local aldosterone system is involved in the apoptosis of podocytes in streptozotocin treated Sprague–Dawley rats [279]. The levels of the synthase CYP11B2 and of the MR were significantly higher in podocytes of diabetic animals and this was associated with increased apoptosis.

Activation of the MR as well as Rac1 are involved in kidney injury from salt-induced hypertension. The observation that adrenalectomy abrogated salt-induced proteinuria led to the further conclusion that Rac1 is an enhancer of aldosterone-induced MR activation in the kidney—and possibly a future therapeutic target as well [280].

Apart from glomerular effects, aldosterone affects non-glomerular renal structures as well; Fu et al. recently showed that aldosterone affects macula densa function and the resulting tubuloglomerular feedback [281].

Aldosterone should be considered a novel therapeutic renal target in CKD patients with the added potential "off-target" effects on heart and vasculature [282]. The decrease of the glomerular filtration rate often observed after the initiation of MR blockade is presumably the result of reversing hyperfiltration. As a result of recent opinions and findings, in the future aldosterone and the MR may become an additional therapeutic target in CKD. Figure 12.5 provides an overview about aldosterone-related myocardial, vascular, and kidney damage.

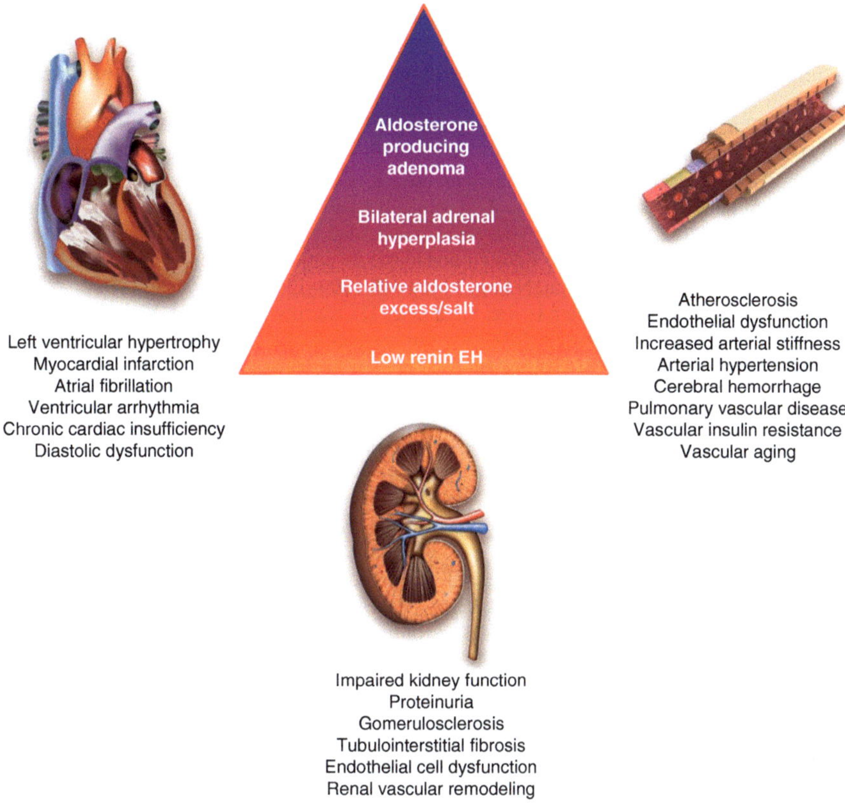

Fig. 12.5 Overview about the aldosterone continuum and related myocardial, vascular, and kidney damage

Acknowledgment The author thanks Dunja Bacinger Tomaschitz and Heinz-Dieter Stangl for their help in providing the artwork.

References

1. Perk J, De Backer G, Gohlke H, Graham I, Reiner Z, Verschuren WM, Albus C, Benlian P, Boysen G, Cifkova R, Deaton C, Ebrahim S, Fisher M, Germano G, Hobbs R, Hoes A, Karadeniz S, Mezzani A, Prescott E, Ryden L, Scherer M, Syvanne M, Scholte OP, Reimer WJ, Vrints C, Wood D, Zamorano JL, Zannad F, Fifth Joint Task Force of the European Society of C, Other Societies on Cardiovascular Disease Prevention in Clinical Practice, European Association for Cardiovascular Practice and Rehabilitation (2012) European Guidelines on cardiovascular disease prevention in clinical practice (version 2012): The Fifth Joint Task Force of the European Society of Cardiology and Other Societies on Cardiovascular Disease Prevention in Clinical Practice (constituted by representatives of nine societies and by invited experts). Atherosclerosis 223:1–68

2. Funder JW, Carey RM, Fardella C, Gomez-Sanchez CE, Mantero F, Stowasser M, Young WF Jr, Montori VM, Endocrine S (2008) Case detection, diagnosis, and treatment of patients with primary aldosteronism: an endocrine society clinical practice guideline. J Clin Endocrinol Metab 93:3266–3281
3. Pitt B, Zannad F, Remme WJ, Cody R, Castaigne A, Perez A, Palensky J, Wittes J (1999) The effect of spironolactone on morbidity and mortality in patients with severe heart failure. Randomized aldactone evaluation study investigators. N Engl J Med 341:709–717
4. Pitt B, Remme W, Zannad F, Neaton J, Martinez F, Roniker B, Bittman R, Hurley S, Kleiman J, Gatlin M (2003) Eplerenone post-acute myocardial infarction heart failure E, survival study I. Eplerenone, a selective aldosterone blocker, in patients with left ventricular dysfunction after myocardial infarction. N Engl J Med 348:1309–1321
5. Zannad F, McMurray JJ, Krum H, van Veldhuisen DJ, Swedberg K, Shi H, Vincent J, Pocock SJ, Pitt B, Group E-HS (2011) Eplerenone in patients with systolic heart failure and mild symptoms. N Engl J Med 364:11–21
6. Kaplan NM (2011) Primary aldosteronism: a contrarian view. Rev Endocr Metab Disord 12:49–52
7. Tomaschitz A, Pilz S (2010) Aldosterone to renin ratio – a reliable screening tool for primary aldosteronism? Horm Metab Res 42:382–391
8. Denner K, Doehmer J, Bernhardt R (1995) Cloning of CYP11B1 and CYP11B2 from normal human adrenal and their functional expression in cos-7 and v79 Chinese hamster cells. Endocr Res 21:443–448
9. Sewer MB, Li D (2013) Regulation of adrenocortical steroid hormone production by rhoa-diaphanous 1 signaling and the cytoskeleton. Mol Cell Endocrinol 371:79–86
10. Boyd JE, Mulrow PJ (1972) Further studies of the influence of potassium upon aldosterone production in the rat. Endocrinology 90:299–301
11. Lotshaw DP (2001) Role of membrane depolarization and T-type Ca2+ channels in angiotensin II and K+ stimulated aldosterone secretion. Mol Cell Endocrinol 175:157–171
12. Spat A, Hunyady L (2004) Control of aldosterone secretion: a model for convergence in cellular signaling pathways. Physiol Rev 84:489–539
13. Davies E, Holloway CD, Ingram MC, Friel EC, Inglis GC, Swan L, Hillis WS, Fraser R, Connell JM (2001) An influence of variation in the aldosterone synthase gene (CYP11B2) on corticosteroid responses to ACTH in normal human subjects. Clin Endocrinol 54:813–817
14. Goodfriend TL, Egan BM (1997) Nonesterified fatty acids in the pathogenesis of hypertension: theory and evidence. Prostaglandins Leukot Essent Fatty Acids 57:57–63
15. Tomaschitz A, Ritz E, Pieske B, Fahrleitner-Pammer A, Kienreich K, Horina JH, Drechsler C, Marz W, Ofner M, Pieber TR, Pilz S (2012) Aldosterone and parathyroid hormone: a precarious couple for cardiovascular disease. Cardiovasc Res 94:10–19
16. Saha S, Schwarz PE, Bergmann S, Bornstein SR, Graessler J, Kopprasch S (2013) Circulating very-low-density lipoprotein from subjects with impaired glucose tolerance accelerates adrenocortical cortisol and aldosterone synthesis. Horm Metab Res 45:169–172
17. Doi M, Takahashi Y, Komatsu R, Yamazaki F, Yamada H, Haraguchi S, Emoto N, Okuno Y, Tsujimoto G, Kanematsu A, Ogawa O, Todo T, Tsutsui K, van der Horst GT, Okamura H (2010) Salt-sensitive hypertension in circadian clock-deficient Cry-null mice involves dysregulated adrenal Hsd3b6. Nat Med 16:67–74
18. Oelkers W, Brown JJ, Fraser R, Lever AF, Morton JJ, Robertson JI (1974) Sensitization of the adrenal cortex to angiotensin II in sodium-deplete man. Circ Res 40:69–77
19. Vasan RS, Evans JC, Larson MG, Wilson PW, Meigs JB, Rifai N, Benjamin EJ, Levy D (2004) Serum aldosterone and the incidence of hypertension in nonhypertensive persons. N Engl J Med 351:33–41
20. Choi M, Scholl UI, Yue P, Bjorklund P, Zhao B, Nelson-Williams C, Ji W, Cho Y, Patel A, Men CJ, Lolis E, Wisgerhof MV, Geller DS, Mane S, Hellman P, Westin G, Akerstrom G, Wang W, Carling T, Lifton RP (2011) K+ channel mutations in adrenal aldosterone-producing adenomas and hereditary hypertension. Science 331:768–772

21. Takeda Y, Miyamori I, Yoneda T, Iki K, Hatakeyama H, Blair IA, Hsieh FY, Takeda R (1995) Production of aldosterone in isolated rat blood vessels. Hypertension 25:170–173
22. Silvestre JS, Robert V, Heymes C, Aupetit-Faisant B, Mouas C, Moalic JM, Swynghedauw B, Delcayre C (1998) Myocardial production of aldosterone and corticosterone in the rat. Physiological regulation. J Biol Chem 273:4883–4891
23. Tomaschitz A, Pilz S, Ritz E, Obermayer-Pietsch B, Pieber TR (2010) Aldosterone and arterial hypertension. Nat Rev Endocrinol 6:83–93
24. Lombes M, Oblin ME, Gasc JM, Baulieu EE, Farman N, Bonvalet JP (1992) Immunohistochemical and biochemical evidence for a cardiovascular mineralocorticoid receptor. Circ Res 71:503–510
25. Arriza JL, Weinberger C, Cerelli G, Glaser TM, Handelin BL, Housman DE, Evans RM (1987) Cloning of human mineralocorticoid receptor complementary DNA: structural and functional kinship with the glucocorticoid receptor. Science 237:268–275
26. Kolla V, Litwack G (2000) Transcriptional regulation of the human Na/K ATPase via the human mineralocorticoid receptor. Mol Cell Biochem 204:35–40
27. Asher C, Wald H, Rossier BC, Garty H (1996) Aldosterone-induced increase in the abundance of Na+ channel subunits. Am J Physiol 271:C605–C611
28. Beesley AH, Hornby D, White SJ (1998) Regulation of distal nephron K+ channels (romk) mRNA expression by aldosterone in rat kidney. J Physiol 509(Pt 3):629–634
29. Marney AM, Brown NJ (2007) Aldosterone and end-organ damage. Clin Sci 113:267–278
30. Tomaschitz A, Pilz S, Ritz E, Grammer T, Amrein K, Merger S, Meinitzer A, Winkelmann BR, Boehm BO, Marz W (2011) Relationship between plasma aldosterone concentration and soluble cellular adhesion molecules in patients referred to coronary angiography. Exp Clin Endocrinol Diabetes 119:649–655
31. Johar S, Cave AC, Narayanapanicker A, Grieve DJ, Shah AM (2006) Aldosterone mediates angiotensin II-induced interstitial cardiac fibrosis via a Nox2-containing NADPH oxidase. FASEB J 20:1546–1548
32. Leopold JA, Dam A, Maron BA, Scribner AW, Liao R, Handy DE, Stanton RC, Pitt B, Loscalzo J (2007) Aldosterone impairs vascular reactivity by decreasing glucose-6-phosphate dehydrogenase activity. Nat Med 13:189–197
33. Fliser D, Veldhuis JD, Dikow R, Schmidt-Gayk H, Ritz E (1998) Effects of acute ace inhibition on pulsatile renin and aldosterone secretion and their synchrony. Hypertension 32:929–934
34. Bogdarina I, Welham S, King PJ, Burns SP, Clark AJ (2007) Epigenetic modification of the renin-angiotensin system in the fetal programming of hypertension. Circ Res 100:520–526
35. Tsybouleva N, Zhang L, Chen S, Patel R, Lutucuta S, Nemoto S, DeFreitas G, Entman M, Carabello BA, Roberts R, Marian AJ (2004) Aldosterone, through novel signaling proteins, is a fundamental molecular bridge between the genetic defect and the cardiac phenotype of hypertrophic cardiomyopathy. Circulation 109:1284–1291
36. Hayashi H, Kobara M, Abe M, Tanaka N, Gouda E, Toba H, Yamada H, Tatsumi T, Nakata T, Matsubara H (2008) Aldosterone nongenomically produces NADPH oxidase-dependent reactive oxygen species and induces myocyte apoptosis. Hypertens Res 31:363–375
37. Uhrenholt TR, Schjerning J, Hansen PB, Norregaard R, Jensen BL, Sorensen GL, Skott O (2003) Rapid inhibition of vasoconstriction in renal afferent arterioles by aldosterone. Circ Res 93:1258–1266
38. Nishiyama A, Abe Y (2006) Molecular mechanisms and therapeutic strategies of chronic renal injury: renoprotective effects of aldosterone blockade. J Pharmacol Sci 100:9–16
39. Grossmann C, Benesic A, Krug AW, Freudinger R, Mildenberger S, Gassner B, Gekle M (2005) Human mineralocorticoid receptor expression renders cells responsive for nongenotropic aldosterone actions. Mol Endocrinol 19:1697–1710
40. Gros R, Ding Q, Sklar LA, Prossnitz EE, Arterburn JB, Chorazyczewski J, Feldman RD (2011) Gpr30 expression is required for the mineralocorticoid receptor-independent rapid vascular effects of aldosterone. Hypertension 57:442–451

41. McEneaney V, Dooley R, Harvey BJ, Thomas W (2010) Protein kinase D stabilizes aldosterone-induced ERK1/2 MAP kinase activation in M1 renal cortical collecting duct cells to promote cell proliferation. J Steroid Biochem Mol Biol 118:18–28
42. Callera GE, Touyz RM, Tostes RC, Yogi A, He Y, Malkinson S, Schiffrin EL (2005) Aldosterone activates vascular p38MAP kinase and NADPH oxidase via c-Src. Hypertension 45:773–779
43. Nakamura T, Kataoka K, Fukuda M, Nako H, Tokutomi Y, Dong YF, Ichijo H, Ogawa H, Kim-Mitsuyama S (2009) Critical role of apoptosis signal-regulating kinase 1 in aldosterone/salt-induced cardiac inflammation and fibrosis. Hypertension 54:544–551
44. Elvira-Matelot E, Zhou XO, Farman N, Beaurain G, Henrion-Caude A, Hadchouel J, Jeunemaitre X (2010) Regulation of WNK1 expression by miR-192 and aldosterone. J Am Soc Nephrol 21:1724–1731
45. Azibani F, Devaux Y, Coutance G, Schlossarek S, Polidano E, Fazal L, Merval R, Carrier L, Solal AC, Chatziantoniou C, Launay JM, Samuel JL, Delcayre C (2012) Aldosterone inhibits the fetal program and increases hypertrophy in the heart of hypertensive mice. PLoS One 7:e38197
46. Winter DC, Schneider MF, O'Sullivan GC, Harvey BJ, Geibel JP (1999) Rapid effects of aldosterone on sodium-hydrogen exchange in isolated colonic crypts. J Membr Biol 170:17–26
47. Leite-Dellova DC, Malnic G, Mello-Aires M (2011) Genomic and nongenomic stimulatory effect of aldosterone on H+-ATPase in proximal S3 segments. Am J Physiol Renal Physiol 300:F682–F691
48. Lemarie CA, Paradis P, Schiffrin EL (2008) New insights on signaling cascades induced by cross-talk between angiotensin II and aldosterone. J Mol Med 86:673–678
49. Jaffe IZ, Mendelsohn ME (2005) Angiotensin II and aldosterone regulate gene transcription via functional mineralocortocoid receptors in human coronary artery smooth muscle cells. Circ Res 96:643–650
50. Rautureau Y, Paradis P, Schiffrin EL (2011) Cross-talk between aldosterone and angiotensin signaling in vascular smooth muscle cells. Steroids 76:834–839
51. Harada E, Yoshimura M, Yasue H, Nakagawa O, Nakagawa M, Harada M, Mizuno Y, Nakayama M, Shimasaki Y, Ito T, Nakamura S, Kuwahara K, Saito Y, Nakao K, Ogawa H (2001) Aldosterone induces angiotensin-converting-enzyme gene expression in cultured neonatal rat cardiocytes. Circulation 104:137–139
52. Chai W, Garrelds IM, de Vries R, Batenburg WW, van Kats JP, Danser AH (2005) Nongenomic effects of aldosterone in the human heart: interaction with angiotensin II. Hypertension 46:701–706
53. Stas S, Whaley-Connell A, Habibi J, Appesh L, Hayden MR, Karuparthi PR, Qazi M, Morris EM, Cooper SA, Link CD, Stump C, Hay M, Ferrario C, Sowers JR (2007) Mineralocorticoid receptor blockade attenuates chronic overexpression of the renin-angiotensin-aldosterone system stimulation of reduced nicotinamide adenine dinucleotide phosphate oxidase and cardiac remodeling. Endocrinology 148:3773–3780
54. Fraccarollo D, Galuppo P, Schmidt I, Ertl G, Bauersachs J (2005) Additive amelioration of left ventricular remodeling and molecular alterations by combined aldosterone and angiotensin receptor blockade after myocardial infarction. Cardiovasc Res 67:97–105
55. de Almeida PW, de Freitas LR, de Morais Gomes ER, Rocha-Resende C, Roman-Campos D, Gondim AN, Gavioli M, Lara A, Parreira A, de Azevedo Nunes SL, Alves MN, Santos SL, Alenina N, Bader M, Resende RR, dos Santos CJ, Souza dos Santos RA, Guatimosim S (2013) Functional cross-talk between aldosterone and angiotensin-(1–7) in ventricular myocytes. Hypertension 61:425–430
56. Mihailidou AS, Le Loan TY, Mardini M, Funder JW (2009) Glucocorticoids activate cardiac mineralocorticoid receptors during experimental myocardial infarction. Hypertension 54:1306–1312
57. Rossier MF, Lenglet S, Vetterli L, Python M, Maturana A (2008) Corticosteroids and redox potential modulate spontaneous contractions in isolated rat ventricular cardiomyocytes. Hypertension 52:721–728

58. Skott O, Uhrenholt TR, Schjerning J, Hansen PB, Rasmussen LE, Jensen BL (2006) Rapid actions of aldosterone in vascular health and disease – friend or foe? Pharmacol Ther 111:495–507
59. Farman N, Rafestin-Oblin ME (2001) Multiple aspects of mineralocorticoid selectivity. Am J Physiol Rhenal Physiol 280:F181–F192
60. Konishi A, Tazawa C, Miki Y, Darnel AD, Suzuki T, Ohta Y, Suzuki T, Tabayashi K, Sasano H (2003) The possible roles of mineralocorticoid receptor and 11beta-hydroxysteroid dehydrogenase type 2 in cardiac fibrosis in the spontaneously hypertensive rat. J Steroid Biochem Mol Biol 85:439–442
61. Shibata S, Nagase M, Yoshida S, Kawarazaki W, Kurihara H, Tanaka H, Miyoshi J, Takai Y, Fujita T (2008) Modification of mineralocorticoid receptor function by Rac1 GTPase: implication in proteinuric kidney disease. Nat Med 14:1370–1376
62. Funder JW (2012) Primary aldosteronism: are we missing the wood for the trees? Horm Metab Res 44:251–253
63. Tanabe A, Naruse M, Naruse K, Hase M, Yoshimoto T, Tanaka M, Seki T, Demura R, Demura H (1997) Left ventricular hypertrophy is more prominent in patients with primary aldosteronism than in patients with other types of secondary hypertension. Hypertension Res 20:85–90
64. Sechi LA, Novello M, Lapenna R, Baroselli S, Nadalini E, Colussi GL, Catena C (2006) Long-term renal outcomes in patients with primary aldosteronism. JAMA 295:2638–2645
65. Catena C, Colussi G, Nadalini E, Chiuch A, Baroselli S, Lapenna R, Sechi LA (2008) Cardiovascular outcomes in patients with primary aldosteronism after treatment. Arch Intern Med 168:80–85
66. Mulatero P, Monticone S, Bertello C, Viola A, Tizzani D, Iannaccone A, Crudo V, Burrello J, Milan A, Rabbia F, Veglio F (2013) Long-term cardio- and cerebro-vascular events in patients with primary aldosteronism. J Clin Endocrinol Metab 98:4826–4833
67. Takeda R, Matsubara T, Miyamori I, Hatakeyama H, Morise T (1995) Vascular complications in patients with aldosterone producing adenoma in Japan: comparative study with essential hypertension. The research committee of disorders of adrenal hormones in Japan. J Endocrinol invest 18:370–373
68. Milliez P, Girerd X, Plouin PF, Blacher J, Safar ME, Mourad JJ (2005) Evidence for an increased rate of cardiovascular events in patients with primary aldosteronism. J Am Coll Cardiol 45:1243–1248
69. Reincke M, Fischer E, Gerum S, Merkle K, Schulz S, Pallauf A, Quinkler M, Hanslik G, Lang K, Hahner S, Allolio B, Meisinger C, Holle R, Beuschlein F, Bidlingmaier M, Endres S (2012) Observational study mortality in treated primary aldosteronism: the German Conn's registry. Hypertension 60:618–624
70. Born-Frontsberg E, Reincke M, Rump LC, Hahner S, Diederich S, Lorenz R, Allolio B, Seufert J, Schirpenbach C, Beuschlein F, Bidlingmaier M, Endres S, Quinkler M, Participants of the German Conn's R (2009) Cardiovascular and cerebrovascular comorbidities of hypokalemic and normokalemic primary aldosteronism: results of the German Conn's Registry. J Clin Endocrinol Metab 94:1125–1130
71. Savard S, Amar L, Plouin PF, Steichen O (2013) Cardiovascular complications associated with primary aldosteronism: a controlled cross-sectional study. Hypertension 62:331–336
72. Levy D, Garrison RJ, Savage DD, Kannel WB, Castelli WP (1990) Prognostic implications of echocardiographically determined left ventricular mass in the Framingham Heart Study. N Engl J Med 322:1561–1566
73. Lee HH, Hung CS, Wu XM, Wu VC, Liu KL, Wang SM, Lin LC, Chen PC, Guo YL, Chueh SC, Lin YH, Ho YL, Wu KD, Taipai SG (2013) Myocardial ultrasound tissue characterization of patients with primary aldosteronism. Ultrasound Med Biol 39:54–61
74. Shigematsu Y, Hamada M, Okayama H, Hara Y, Hayashi Y, Kodama K, Kohara K, Hiwada K (1997) Left ventricular hypertrophy precedes other target-organ damage in primary aldosteronism. Hypertension 29:723–727

75. Freel EM, Mark PB, Weir RA, McQuarrie EP, Allan K, Dargie HJ, McClure JD, Jardine AG, Davies E, Connell JM (2012) Demonstration of blood pressure-independent noninfarct myocardial fibrosis in primary aldosteronism: a cardiac magnetic resonance imaging study. Circ Cardiovasc Imaging 5:740–747
76. Catena C, Colussi GL, Marzano L, Sechi LA (2012) Predictive factors of left ventricular mass changes after treatment of primary aldosteronism. Horm Metab Res 44:188–193
77. Rossi GP, Cesari M, Cuspidi C, Maiolino G, Cicala MV, Bisogni V, Mantero F, Pessina AC (2013) Long-term control of arterial hypertension and regression of left ventricular hypertrophy with treatment of primary aldosteronism. Hypertension 62:62–69
78. Stehr CB, Mellado R, Ocaranza MP, Carvajal CA, Mosso L, Becerra E, Solis M, Garcia L, Lavandero S, Jalil J, Fardella CE (2010) Increased levels of oxidative stress, subclinical inflammation, and myocardial fibrosis markers in primary aldosteronism patients. J Hypertens 28:2120–2126
79. Pimenta E, Gordon RD, Ahmed AH, Cowley D, Leano R, Marwick TH, Stowasser M (2011) Cardiac dimensions are largely determined by dietary salt in patients with primary aldosteronism: results of a case–control study. J Clin Endocrinol Metab 96:2813–2820
80. Catena C, Colussi G, Lapenna R, Nadalini E, Chiuch A, Gianfagna P, Sechi LA (2007) Long-term cardiac effects of adrenalectomy or mineralocorticoid antagonists in patients with primary aldosteronism. Hypertension 50:911–918
81. Rossi GP, Sacchetto A, Visentin P, Canali C, Graniero GR, Palatini P, Pessina AC (1996) Changes in left ventricular anatomy and function in hypertension and primary aldosteronism. Hypertension 27:1039–1045
82. Strauch B, Petrak O, Wichterle D, Zelinka T, Holaj R, Widimsky J Jr (2006) Increased arterial wall stiffness in primary aldosteronism in comparison with essential hypertension. Am J Hypertens 19:909–914
83. Maron BA, Opotowsky AR, Landzberg MJ, Loscalzo J, Waxman AB, Leopold JA (2013) Plasma aldosterone levels are elevated in patients with pulmonary arterial hypertension in the absence of left ventricular heart failure: a pilot study. Eur J Heart Fail 15:277–283
84. Holaj R, Zelinka T, Wichterle D, Petrak O, Strauch B, Widimsky J Jr (2007) Increased intima-media thickness of the common carotid artery in primary aldosteronism in comparison with essential hypertension. J Hypertens 25:1451–1457
85. Bernini G, Galetta F, Franzoni F, Bardini M, Taurino C, Bernardini M, Ghiadoni L, Bernini M, Santoro G, Salvetti A (2008) Arterial stiffness, intima-media thickness and carotid artery fibrosis in patients with primary aldosteronism. J Hypertens 26:2399–2405
86. Rossi GP, Bolognesi M, Rizzoni D, Seccia TM, Piva A, Porteri E, Tiberio GA, Giulini SM, Agabiti-Rosei E, Pessina AC (2008) Vascular remodeling and duration of hypertension predict outcome of adrenalectomy in primary aldosteronism patients. Hypertension 51:1366–1371
87. Rizzoni D, Paiardi S, Rodella L, Porteri E, De Ciuceis C, Rezzani R, Boari GE, Zani F, Miclini M, Tiberio GA, Giulini SM, Rosei CA, Bianchi R, Rosei EA (2006) Changes in extracellular matrix in subcutaneous small resistance arteries of patients with primary aldosteronism. J Clin Endocrinol Metab 91:2638–2642
88. Wu VC, Lo SC, Chen YL, Huang PH, Tsai CT, Liang CJ, Kuo CC, Kuo YS, Lee BC, Wu EL, Lin YH, Sun YY, Lin SL, Chen JW, Lin SJ, Wu KD, Group TS (2011) Endothelial progenitor cells in primary aldosteronism: a biomarker of severity for aldosterone vasculopathy and prognosis. J Clin Endocrinol Metab 96:3175–3183
89. Lin YH, Lin LY, Chen A, Wu XM, Lee JK, Su TC, Wu VC, Chueh SC, Lin WC, Lo MT, Wang PC, Ho YL, Wu KD, Group TS (2012) Adrenalectomy improves increased carotid intima-media thickness and arterial stiffness in patients with aldosterone producing adenoma. Atherosclerosis 221:154–159
90. Rossi GP, Pessina AC, Heagerty AM (2008) Primary aldosteronism: an update on screening, diagnosis and treatment. J Hypertens 26:613–621
91. Sechi LA, Colussi G, Di Fabio A, Catena C (2010) Cardiovascular and renal damage in primary aldosteronism: outcomes after treatment. Am J Hypertens 23:1253–1260

92. Lin YH, Wu XM, Lee HH, Lee JK, Liu YC, Chang HW, Lin CY, Wu VC, Chueh SC, Lin LC, Lo MT, Ho YL, Wu KD, Group TS (2012) Adrenalectomy reverses myocardial fibrosis in patients with primary aldosteronism. J Hypertens 30:1606–1613
93. Tomaschitz A, Pilz S, März W (2011) Arterial hypertension and cardiovascular disease – absolute aldosterone excess is the tip of the iceberg. J Lab Med 35:147–151
94. Tomaschitz A, Pilz S, Ritz E, Meinitzer A, Boehm BO, Marz W (2010) Plasma aldosterone levels are associated with increased cardiovascular mortality: the Ludwigshafen Risk and Cardiovascular Health (LURIC) study. Eur Heart J 31:1237–1247
95. Tomaschitz A, Pilz S, Ritz E, Grammer T, Drechsler C, Boehm BO, Marz W (2011) Association of plasma aldosterone with cardiovascular mortality in patients with low estimated GFR: the Ludwigshafen Risk and Cardiovascular Health (LURIC) study. Am J Kidney Dis 57:403–414
96. Beygui F, Montalescot G, Vicaut E, Rouanet S, Van Belle E, Baulac C, Degrandsart A, Dallongeville J, Investigators O (2009) Aldosterone and long-term outcome after myocardial infarction: a substudy of the french nationwide observatoire sur la prise en charge hospitaliere, l'evolution a un an et les caracteristiques de patients presentant un infarctus du myocarde avec ou sans onde q (opera) study. Am heart J 157:680–687
97. Hillaert MA, Lentjes EG, Kemperman H, van der Graaf Y, Nathoe HM, Beygui F, Montalescot G, Doevendans PA, Wassink AM, van Belle E, Group SS (2013) Aldosterone, atherosclerosis and vascular events in patients with stable coronary artery disease. Int J Cardiol 167: 1929–1935
98. Ivanes F, Susen S, Mouquet F, Pigny P, Cuilleret F, Sautiere K, Collet JP, Beygui F, Hennache B, Ennezat PV, Juthier F, Richard F, Dallongeville J, Hillaert MA, Doevendans PA, Jude B, Bertrand M, Montalescot G, Van Belle E (2012) Aldosterone, mortality, and acute ischaemic events in coronary artery disease patients outside the setting of acute myocardial infarction or heart failure. Eur Heart J 33:191–202
99. Drechsler C, Ritz E, Tomaschitz A, Pilz S, Schonfeld S, Blouin K, Bidlingmaier M, Hammer F, Krane V, Marz W, Allolio B, Fassnacht M, Wanner C (2013) Aldosterone and cortisol affect the risk of sudden cardiac death in haemodialysis patients. Eur Heart J 34:578–587
100. Tomaschitz A, Pilz S, Pieske B, Ritz E, Marz W, Meinitzer A, Dobnig H, Amrein K, Kienreich K, Verheyen N, Kraigher-Krainer E, Drechsler C, Colantonio C, Wagner D, Fahrleitner-Pammer A (2013) Circulating aldosterone and mortality in female nursing home residents. Exp Gerontol 48:313–318
101. Harada E, Mizuno Y, Katoh D, Kashiwagi Y, Morita S, Nakayama Y, Yoshimura M, Masuzaki H, Saito Y, Yasue H (2013) Increased urinary aldosterone excretion is associated with subcutaneous not visceral, adipose tissue area in obese individuals: a possible manifestation of dysfunctional subcutaneous adipose tissue. Clin Endocrinol 79:510–516
102. Jin Y, Kuznetsova T, Maillard M, Richart T, Thijs L, Bochud M, Herregods MC, Burnier M, Fagard R, Staessen JA (2009) Independent relations of left ventricular structure with the 24-hour urinary excretion of sodium and aldosterone. Hypertension 54:489–495
103. Gonzaga CC, Gaddam KK, Ahmed MI, Pimenta E, Thomas SJ, Harding SM, Oparil S, Cofield SS, Calhoun DA (2010) Severity of obstructive sleep apnea is related to aldosterone status in subjects with resistant hypertension. J Clin Sleep Med 6:363–368
104. Freel EM, Tsorlalis IK, Lewsey JD, Latini R, Maggioni AP, Solomon S, Pitt B, Connell JM, McMurray JJ (2009) Aldosterone status associated with insulin resistance in patients with heart failure – data from the aloft study. Heart 95:1920–1924
105. Calhoun DA, Nishizaka MK, Zaman MA, Harding SM (2004) Aldosterone excretion among subjects with resistant hypertension and symptoms of sleep apnea. Chest 125:112–117
106. Benetos A, Gardner JP, Kimura M, Labat C, Nzietchueng R, Dousset B, Zannad F, Lacolley P, Aviv A (2005) Aldosterone and telomere length in white blood cells. J Gerontol A Biol Sci Med Sci 60:1593–1596
107. Mosso L, Carvajal C, Gonzalez A, Barraza A, Avila F, Montero J, Huete A, Gederlini A, Fardella CE (2003) Primary aldosteronism and hypertensive disease. Hypertension 42:161–165

108. Hannemann A, Friedrich N, Ludemann J, Volzke H, Rettig R, Peters J, Reincke M, Doring A, Nauck M, Wallaschofski H (2010) Reference intervals for aldosterone, renin, and the aldosterone-to-renin ratio in the population-based study of health in pomerania (ship-1). Horm Metab Res 42:392–399
109. Fardella CE, Mosso L, Gomez-Sanchez C, Cortes P, Soto J, Gomez L, Pinto M, Huete A, Oestreicher E, Foradori A, Montero J (2000) Primary hyperaldosteronism in essential hypertensives: prevalence, biochemical profile, and molecular biology. J Clin Endocrinol Metab 85:1863–1867
110. Olivieri O, Ciacciarelli A, Signorelli D, Pizzolo F, Guarini P, Pavan C, Corgnati A, Falcone S, Corrocher R, Micchi A, Cressoni C, Blengio G (2004) Aldosterone to renin ratio in a primary care setting: the bussolengo study. J Clin Endocrinol Metab 89:4221–4226
111. Mulatero P, Stowasser M, Loh KC, Fardella CE, Gordon RD, Mosso L, Gomez-Sanchez CE, Veglio F, Young WF Jr (2004) Increased diagnosis of primary aldosteronism, including surgically correctable forms, in centers from five continents. J Clin Endocrinol Metab 89:1045–1050
112. Calhoun DA, Nishizaka MK, Zaman MA, Thakkar RB, Weissmann P (2002) Hyperaldosteronism among black and white subjects with resistant hypertension. Hypertension 40:892–896
113. Rossi GP, Bernini G, Caliumi C, Desideri G, Fabris B, Ferri C, Ganzaroli C, Giacchetti G, Letizia C, Maccario M, Mallamaci F, Mannelli M, Mattarello MJ, Moretti A, Palumbo G, Parenti G, Porteri E, Semplicini A, Rizzoni D, Rossi E, Boscaro M, Pessina AC, Mantero F, Investigators PS (2006) A prospective study of the prevalence of primary aldosteronism in 1,125 hypertensive patients. J Am Coll Cardiol 48:2293–2300
114. Calhoun DA (2007) Is there an unrecognized epidemic of primary aldosteronism? Pro Hypertension 50:447–453, discussion 447–453
115. Kaplan NM (2007) Is there an unrecognized epidemic of primary aldosteronism? Con Hypertension 50:454–458, discussion 454–458
116. Kaplan NM (2008) Deja vu for primary aldosteronism. Lancet 371:1890–1891
117. Adlin EV, Braitman LE, Vasan RS (2013) Bimodal aldosterone distribution in low-renin hypertension. Am J Hypertens 26:1076–1085
118. Eide IK, Torjesen PA, Drolsum A, Babovic A, Lilledahl NP (2004) Low-renin status in therapy-resistant hypertension: a clue to efficient treatment. J Hypertens 22:2217–2226
119. Fisher ND, Hurwitz S, Ferri C, Jeunemaitre X, Hollenberg NK, Williams GH (1999) Altered adrenal sensitivity to angiotensin II in low-renin essential hypertension. Hypertension 34:388–394
120. Lim PO, Struthers AD, MacDonald TM (2002) The neurohormonal natural history of essential hypertension: towards primary or tertiary aldosteronism? J Hypertens 20:11–15
121. Warnock DG (1999) Low-renin and nonmodulating essential hypertension. Hypertension 34:395–397
122. Newton-Cheh C, Guo CY, Gona P, Larson MG, Benjamin EJ, Wang TJ, Kathiresan S, O'Donnell CJ, Musone SL, Camargo AL, Drake JA, Levy D, Hirschhorn JN, Vasan RS (2007) Clinical and genetic correlates of aldosterone-to-renin ratio and relations to blood pressure in a community sample. Hypertension 49:846–856
123. Tomaschitz A, Maerz W, Pilz S, Ritz E, Scharnagl H, Renner W, Boehm BO, Fahrleitner-Pammer A, Weihrauch G, Dobnig H (2010) Aldosterone/renin ratio determines peripheral and central blood pressure values over a broad range. J Am Coll Cardiol 55:2171–2180
124. Meneton P, Galan P, Bertrais S, Heudes D, Hercberg S, Menard J (2008) High plasma aldosterone and low renin predict blood pressure increase and hypertension in middle-aged caucasian populations. J Hum Hypertens 22:550–558
125. Makhanova N, Hagaman J, Kim HS, Smithies O (2008) Salt-sensitive blood pressure in mice with increased expression of aldosterone synthase. Hypertension 51:134–140
126. Connell JM, MacKenzie SM, Freel EM, Fraser R, Davies E (2008) A lifetime of aldosterone excess: long-term consequences of altered regulation of aldosterone production for cardiovascular function. Endocr Rev 29:133–154

127. Hood SJ, Taylor KP, Ashby MJ, Brown MJ (2007) The spironolactone, amiloride, losartan, and thiazide (salt) double-blind crossover trial in patients with low-renin hypertension and elevated aldosterone-renin ratio. Circulation 116:268–275
128. Nishizaka MK, Zaman MA, Calhoun DA (2003) Efficacy of low-dose spironolactone in subjects with resistant hypertension. Am J Hypertens 16:925–930
129. Lane DA, Shah S, Beevers DG (2007) Low-dose spironolactone in the management of resistant hypertension: a surveillance study. J Hypertens 25:891–894
130. Chapman N, Dobson J, Wilson S, Dahlof B, Sever PS, Wedel H, Poulter NR (2007) Anglo-Scandinavian cardiac outcomes trial I. Effect of spironolactone on blood pressure in subjects with resistant hypertension. Hypertension 49:839–845
131. Saruta T, Kageyama S, Ogihara T, Hiwada K, Ogawa M, Tawara K, Gatlin M, Garthwaite S, Bittman R, Patrick J (2004) Efficacy and safety of the selective aldosterone blocker eplerenone in Japanese patients with hypertension: a randomized, double-blind, placebo-controlled, dose-ranging study. J Clin Hypertens 6:175–183, quiz 184–175
132. Weinberger MH, Roniker B, Krause SL, Weiss RJ (2002) Eplerenone, a selective aldosterone blocker, in mild-to-moderate hypertension. Am J Hypertens 15:709–716
133. Mancia G, Fagard R, Narkiewicz K, Redon J, Zanchetti A, Bohm M, Christiaens T, Cifkova R, De Backer G, Dominiczak A, Galderisi M, Grobbee DE, Jaarsma T, Kirchhof P, Kjeldsen SE, Laurent S, Manolis AJ, Nilsson PM, Ruilope LM, Schmieder RE, Sirnes PA, Sleight P, Viigimaa M, Waeber B, Zannad F, Redon J, Dominiczak A, Narkiewicz K, Nilsson PM, Burnier M, Viigimaa M, Ambrosioni E, Caufield M, Coca A, Olsen MH, Schmieder RE, Tsioufis C, van de Borne P, Zamorano JL, Achenbach S, Baumgartner H, Bax JJ, Bueno H, Dean V, Deaton C, Erol C, Fagard R, Ferrari R, Hasdai D, Hoes AW, Kirchhof P, Knuuti J, Kolh P, Lancellotti P, Linhart A, Nihoyannopoulos P, Piepoli MF, Ponikowski P, Sirnes PA, Tamargo JL, Tendera M, Torbicki A, Wijns W, Windecker S, Clement DL, Coca A, Gillebert TC, Tendera M, Rosei EA, Ambrosioni E, Anker SD, Bauersachs J, Hitij JB, Caulfield M, De Buyzere M, De Geest S, Derumeaux GA, Erdine S, Farsang C, Funck-Brentano C, Gerc V, Germano G, Gielen S, Haller H, Hoes AW, Jordan J, Kahan T, Komajda M, Lovic D, Mahrholdt H, Olsen MH, Ostergren J, Parati G, Perk J, Polonia J, Popescu BA, Reiner Z, Ryden L, Sirenko Y, Stanton A, Struijker-Boudier H, Tsioufis C, van de Borne P, Vlachopoulos C, Volpe M, Wood DA (2013) 2013 esh/esc guidelines for the management of arterial hypertension: the task force for the management of arterial hypertension of the European Society of Hypertension (ESH) and of the European Society of Cardiology (ESC). Eur Heart J 34:2159–2219
134. Pratt JH (2005) Central role for enac in development of hypertension. J Am Soc Nephrol 16:3154–3159
135. McDougall I, Brown FH, Fleagle JG (2005) Stratigraphic placement and age of modern humans from Kibish, Ethiopia. Nature 433:733–736
136. Fournier D, Luft FC, Bader M, Ganten D, Andrade-Navarro MA (2012) Emergence and evolution of the renin-angiotensin-aldosterone system. J Mol Med 90:495–508
137. Nowaczynski W, Oliver WJ, Neel JV (1985) Serum aldosterone and protein-binding variables in Yanomama Indians: a no-salt culture as compared to partially acculturated Guaymi Indians. Clin Physiol Biochem 3:289–306
138. Oki K, Gomez-Sanchez EP, Gomez-Sanchez CE (2012) Role of mineralocorticoid action in the brain in salt-sensitive hypertension. Clin Exp Pharmacol Physiol 39:90–95
139. Libianto R, Jerums G, Lam Q, Chen A, Baqar S, Pyrlis F, Macisaac RJ, Moran J, Ekinci EI (2014) Relationship between urinary sodium excretion and serum aldosterone in patients with diabetes in the presence and absence of modifiers of the renin-angiotensin-aldosterone system. Clin Sci 126:147–154
140. Alderman MH, Cohen HW (2012) Dietary sodium intake and cardiovascular mortality: controversy resolved? Curr Hypertens Rep 14:193–201
141. Wehling M, Spes CH, Win N, Janson CP, Schmidt BM, Theisen K, Christ M (1998) Rapid cardiovascular action of aldosterone in man. J Clin Endocrinol Metab 83:3517–3522

142. Farquharson CA, Struthers AD (2000) Spironolactone increases nitric oxide bioactivity, improves endothelial vasodilator dysfunction, and suppresses vascular angiotensin I/angiotensin II conversion in patients with chronic heart failure. Circulation 101:594–597
143. Lieb W, Larson MG, Benjamin EJ, Yin X, Tofler GH, Selhub J, Jacques PF, Wang TJ, Vita JA, Levy D, Vasan RS, Mitchell GF (2009) Multimarker approach to evaluate correlates of vascular stiffness: the Framingham Heart Study. Circulation 119:37–43
144. Savoia C, Touyz RM, Amiri F, Schiffrin EL (2008) Selective mineralocorticoid receptor blocker eplerenone reduces resistance artery stiffness in hypertensive patients. Hypertension 51:432–439
145. Oberleithner H, Ludwig T, Riethmuller C, Hillebrand U, Albermann L, Schafer C, Shahin V, Schillers H (2004) Human endothelium: target for aldosterone. Hypertension 43:952–956
146. Kusche-Vihrog K, Urbanova K, Blanque A, Wilhelmi M, Schillers H, Kliche K, Pavenstadt H, Brand E, Oberleithner H (2011) C-reactive protein makes human endothelium stiff and tight. Hypertension 57:231–237
147. Druppel V, Kusche-Vihrog K, Grossmann C, Gekle M, Kasprzak B, Brand E, Pavenstadt H, Oberleithner H, Kliche K (2013) Long-term application of the aldosterone antagonist spironolactone prevents stiff endothelial cell syndrome. FASEB J 27:3652–3659
148. Nagata K, Obata K, Xu J, Ichihara S, Noda A, Kimata H, Kato T, Izawa H, Murohara T, Yokota M (2006) Mineralocorticoid receptor antagonism attenuates cardiac hypertrophy and failure in low-aldosterone hypertensive rats. Hypertension 47:656–664
149. Sanz-Rosa D, Oubina MP, Cediel E, DelasHeras N, Aragoncillo P, Balfagon G, Cachofeiro V, Lahera V (2005) Eplerenone reduces oxidative stress and enhances eNOS in SHR: vascular functional and structural consequences. Antioxid Redox Signal 7:1294–1301
150. Park JB, Schiffrin EL (2001) Et(a) receptor antagonist prevents blood pressure elevation and vascular remodeling in aldosterone-infused rats. Hypertension 37:1444–1449
151. Keidar S, Hayek T, Kaplan M, Pavlotzky E, Hamoud S, Coleman R, Aviram M (2003) Effect of eplerenone, a selective aldosterone blocker, on blood pressure, serum and macrophage oxidative stress, and atherosclerosis in apolipoprotein e-deficient mice. J Cardiovasc Pharmacol 41:955–963
152. Wehling M, Ulsenheimer A, Schneider M, Neylon C, Christ M (1994) Rapid effects of aldosterone on free intracellular calcium in vascular smooth muscle and endothelial cells: subcellular localization of calcium elevations by single cell imaging. Biochem Biophys Res Commun 204:475–481
153. Liu SL, Schmuck S, Chorazcyzewski JZ, Gros R, Feldman RD (2003) Aldosterone regulates vascular reactivity: short-term effects mediated by phosphatidylinositol 3-kinase-dependent nitric oxide synthase activation. Circulation 108:2400–2406
154. Krug AW, Grossmann C, Schuster C, Freudinger R, Mildenberger S, Govindan MV, Gekle M (2003) Aldosterone stimulates epidermal growth factor receptor expression. J Biol Chem 278:43060–43066
155. Callera GE, Touyz RM, Tostes RC, Yogi A, He Y, Malkinson S, Schiffrin EL (2005) Aldosterone activates vascular p38MAP kinase and NADPH oxidase via c-Src. Hypertension 45:773–779
156. Grossmann C, Gekle M (2007) Non-classical actions of the mineralocorticoid receptor: misuse of EGF receptors? Mol Cell Endocrinol 277:6–12
157. Caprio M, Newfell BG, la Sala A, Baur W, Fabbri A, Rosano G, Mendelsohn ME, Jaffe IZ (2008) Functional mineralocorticoid receptors in human vascular endothelial cells regulate intercellular adhesion molecule-1 expression and promote leukocyte adhesion. Circ Res 102:1359–1367
158. Kasal DA, Barhoumi T, Li MW, Yamamoto N, Zdanovich E, Rehman A, Neves MF, Laurant P, Paradis P, Schiffrin EL (2012) T regulatory lymphocytes prevent aldosterone-induced vascular injury. Hypertension 59:324–330
159. Swedberg K, Eneroth P, Kjekshus J, Wilhelmsen L (1990) Hormones regulating cardiovascular function in patients with severe congestive heart failure and their relation to mortality. Consensus trial study group. Circulation 82:1730–1736

160. Vantrimpont P, Rouleau JL, Ciampi A, Harel F, de Champlain J, Bichet D, Moye LA, Pfeffer M (1998) Two-year time course and significance of neurohumoral activation in the survival and ventricular enlargement (save) study. Eur Heart J 19:1552–1563
161. Beygui F, Collet JP, Benoliel JJ, Vignolles N, Dumaine R, Barthelemy O, Montalescot G (2006) High plasma aldosterone levels on admission are associated with death in patients presenting with acute ST-elevation myocardial infarction. Circulation 114:2604–2610
162. Palmer BR, Pilbrow AP, Frampton CM, Yandle TG, Skelton L, Nicholls MG, Richards AM (2008) Plasma aldosterone levels during hospitalization are predictive of survival post-myocardial infarction. Eur Heart J 29:2489–2496
163. Mignano A, Pitruzzella V, Arnone G, Arnone MT, Rotolo A, Assennato P, Novo G, Corrado E, Novo S (2013) Prognostic role of aldosterone in patients with acute coronary syndrome: short and medium term follow-up. J Cardiovasc Med (Hagerstown)
164. Girerd N, Pang PS, Swedberg K, Fought A, Kwasny MJ, Subacius H, Konstam MA, Maggioni A, Gheorghiade M, Zannad F (2013) Serum aldosterone is associated with mortality and re-hospitalization in patients with reduced ejection fraction hospitalized for acute heart failure: analysis from the EVEREST trial. Eur J Heart Fail 15:1228–1235
165. de Resende MM, Kauser K, Mill JG (2006) Regulation of cardiac and renal mineralocorticoid receptor expression by captopril following myocardial infarction in rats. Life Sci 78:3066–3073
166. Velagaleti RS, Gona P, Levy D, Aragam J, Larson MG, Tofler GH, Lieb W, Wang TJ, Benjamin EJ, Vasan RS (2008) Relations of biomarkers representing distinct biological pathways to left ventricular geometry. Circulation 118:2252–2258, 2255p following 2258
167. Edelmann F, Tomaschitz A, Wachter R, Gelbrich G, Knoke M, Dungen HD, Pilz S, Binder L, Stahrenberg R, Schmidt A, Marz W, Pieske B (2012) Serum aldosterone and its relationship to left ventricular structure and geometry in patients with preserved left ventricular ejection fraction. Eur Heart J 33:203–212
168. Iraqi W, Rossignol P, Angioi M, Fay R, Nuee J, Ketelslegers JM, Vincent J, Pitt B, Zannad F (2009) Extracellular cardiac matrix biomarkers in patients with acute myocardial infarction complicated by left ventricular dysfunction and heart failure: insights from the eplerenone post-acute myocardial infarction heart failure efficacy and survival study (EPHESUS) study. Circulation 119:2471–2479
169. Pitt B, Reichek N, Willenbrock R, Zannad F, Phillips RA, Roniker B, Kleiman J, Krause S, Burns D, Williams GH (2003) Effects of eplerenone, enalapril, and eplerenone/enalapril in patients with essential hypertension and left ventricular hypertrophy: the 4E-left ventricular hypertrophy study. Circulation 108:1831–1838
170. McMurray JJ, Adamopoulos S, Anker SD, Auricchio A, Bohm M, Dickstein K, Falk V, Filippatos G, Fonseca C, Gomez-Sanchez MA, Jaarsma T, Kober L, Lip GY, Maggioni AP, Parkhomenko A, Pieske BM, Popescu BA, Ronnevik PK, Rutten FH, Schwitter J, Seferovic P, Stepinska J, Trindade PT, Voors AA, Zannad F, Zeiher A, Task Force for the Diagnosis and Treatment of Acute and Chronic Heart Failure 2012 of the European Society of Cardiology, Bax JJ, Baumgartner H, Ceconi C, Dean V, Deaton C, Fagard R, Funck-Brentano C, Hasdai D, Hoes A, Kirchhof P, Knuuti J, Kolh P, McDonagh T, Moulin C, Popescu BA, Reiner Z, Sechtem U, Sirnes PA, Tendera M, Torbicki A, Vahanian A, Windecker S, McDonagh T, Sechtem U, Bonet LA, Avraamides P, Ben Lamin HA, Brignole M, Coca A, Cowburn P, Dargie H, Elliott P, Flachskampf FA, Guida GF, Hardman S, Iung B, Merkely B, Mueller C, Nanas JN, Nielsen OW, Orn S, Parissis JT, Ponikowski P (2012) Guidelines ESCCfP. ESC guidelines for the diagnosis and treatment of acute and chronic heart failure 2012: The task force for the diagnosis and treatment of acute and chronic heart failure 2012 of the European Society of Cardiology. Developed in collaboration with the heart failure association (HFA) of the ESC. European journal of heart failure 14:803–869
171. Pitt B, Anker SD, Bushinsky DA, Kitzman DW, Zannad F, Huang IZ, Investigators P-H (2011) Evaluation of the efficacy and safety of RLY5016, a polymeric potassium binder, in a double-blind, placebo-controlled study in patients with chronic heart failure (the PEARL-HF) trial. Eur Heart J 32:820–828

172. Mohammed SF, Ohtani T, Korinek J, Lam CS, Larsen K, Simari RD, Valencik ML, Burnett JC Jr, Redfield MM (2010) Mineralocorticoid accelerates transition to heart failure with preserved ejection fraction via "nongenomic effects". Circulation 122:370–378
173. Edelmann F, Wachter R, Schmidt AG, Kraigher-Krainer E, Colantonio C, Kamke W, Duvinage A, Stahrenberg R, Durstewitz K, Loffler M, Dungen HD, Tschope C, Herrmann-Lingen C, Halle M, Hasenfuss G, Gelbrich G, Pieske B, Aldo DHFI (2013) Effect of spironolactone on diastolic function and exercise capacity in patients with heart failure with preserved ejection fraction: the Aldo-DHF randomized controlled trial. JAMA 309:781–791
174. Desai AS, Lewis EF, Li R, Solomon SD, Assmann SF, Boineau R, Clausell N, Diaz R, Fleg JL, Gordeev I, McKinlay S, O'Meara E, Shaburishvili T, Pitt B, Pfeffer MA (2011) Rationale and design of the treatment of preserved cardiac function heart failure with an aldosterone antagonist trial: a randomized, controlled study of spironolactone in patients with symptomatic heart failure and preserved ejection fraction. Am Heart J 162:966–972e910
175. Qin W, Rudolph AE, Bond BR, Rocha R, Blomme EA, Goellner JJ, Funder JW, McMahon EG (2003) Transgenic model of aldosterone-driven cardiac hypertrophy and heart failure. Circ Res 93:69–76
176. Gekle M, Grossmann C (2009) Actions of aldosterone in the cardiovascular system: the good, the bad, and the ugly? Pflugers Arch 458:231–246
177. He BJ, Joiner ML, Singh MV, Luczak ED, Swaminathan PD, Koval OM, Kutschke W, Allamargot C, Yang J, Guan X, Zimmerman K, Grumbach IM, Weiss RM, Spitz DR, Sigmund CD, Blankesteijn WM, Heymans S, Mohler PJ, Anderson ME (2011) Oxidation of CaMKII determines the cardiotoxic effects of aldosterone. Nat Med 17:1610–1618
178. De Giusti VC, Nolly MB, Yeves AM, Caldiz CI, Villa-Abrille MC, Chiappe de Cingolani GE, Ennis IL, Cingolani HE, Aiello EA (2011) Aldosterone stimulates the cardiac na(+)/h(+) exchanger via transactivation of the epidermal growth factor receptor. Hypertension 58:912–919
179. Brown NJ, Kim KS, Chen YQ, Blevins LS, Nadeau JH, Meranze SG, Vaughan DE (2000) Synergistic effect of adrenal steroids and angiotensin II on plasminogen activator inhibitor-1 production. J Clin Endocrinol Metab 85:336–344
180. Latouche C, Sainte-Marie Y, Steenman M, Castro Chaves P, Naray-Fejes-Toth A, Fejes-Toth G, Farman N, Jaisser F (2010) Molecular signature of mineralocorticoid receptor signaling in cardiomyocytes: from cultured cells to mouse heart. Endocrinology 151:4467–4476
181. Chu PY, Zatta A, Kiriazis H, Chin-Dusting J, Du XJ, Marshall T, Kaye DM (2011) CXCR4 antagonism attenuates the cardiorenal consequences of mineralocorticoid excess. Circ Heart Fail 4:651–658
182. Fraccarollo D, Galuppo P, Schraut S, Kneitz S, van Rooijen N, Ertl G, Bauersachs J (2008) Immediate mineralocorticoid receptor blockade improves myocardial infarct healing by modulation of the inflammatory response. Hypertension 51:905–914
183. Usher MG, Duan SZ, Ivaschenko CY, Frieler RA, Berger S, Schutz G, Lumeng CN, Mortensen RM (2010) Myeloid mineralocorticoid receptor controls macrophage polarization and cardiovascular hypertrophy and remodeling in mice. J Clin Invest 120:3350–3364
184. Brilla CG, Pick R, Tan LB, Janicki JS, Weber KT (1990) Remodeling of the rat right and left ventricles in experimental hypertension. Circ Res 67:1355–1364
185. Weber KT, Brilla CG (1991) Pathological hypertrophy and cardiac interstitium. Fibrosis and renin-angiotensin-aldosterone system. Circulation 83:1849–1865
186. Brilla CG, Matsubara LS, Weber KT (1993) Anti-aldosterone treatment and the prevention of myocardial fibrosis in primary and secondary hyperaldosteronism. J Mol Cell Cardiol 25:563–575
187. White PC (2003) Aldosterone: direct effects on and production by the heart. J Clin Endocrinol Metab 88:2376–2383
188. Fraccarollo D, Berger S, Galuppo P, Kneitz S, Hein L, Schutz G, Frantz S, Ertl G, Bauersachs J (2011) Deletion of cardiomyocyte mineralocorticoid receptor ameliorates adverse remodeling after myocardial infarction. Circulation 123:400–408

189. Ambroisine ML, Favre J, Oliviero P, Rodriguez C, Gao J, Thuillez C, Samuel JL, Richard V, Delcayre C (2007) Aldosterone-induced coronary dysfunction in transgenic mice involves the calcium-activated potassium (BKCa) channels of vascular smooth muscle cells. Circulation 116:2435–2443
190. Hayashi M, Tsutamoto T, Wada A, Maeda K, Mabuchi N, Tsutsui T, Matsui T, Fujii M, Matsumoto T, Yamamoto T, Horie H, Ohnishi M, Kinoshita M (2001) Relationship between transcardiac extraction of aldosterone and left ventricular remodeling in patients with first acute myocardial infarction: extracting aldosterone through the heart promotes ventricular remodeling after acute myocardial infarction. J Am Coll Cardiol 38:1375–1382
191. Chai W, Hofland J, Jansen PM, Garrelds IM, de Vries R, van den Bogaerdt AJ, Feelders RA, de Jong FH, Danser AH (2010) Steroidogenesis vs. steroid uptake in the heart: do corticosteroids mediate effects via cardiac mineralocorticoid receptors? J Hypertens 28:1044–1053
192. Pilz S, Tomaschitz A, Marz W, Cavalier E, Ritz E (2010) Aldosterone and parathyroid hormone: a complex and clinically relevant relationship. Calcified Tissue Int 87:373–374
193. Tomaschitz A, Ritz E, Pieske B, Rus-Machan J, Kienreich K, Verheyen N, Gaksch M, Grübler M, Fahrleitner-Pammer A, Mrak P, Toplak H, Kraigher-Krainer E, März W, Pilz S (2013) Aldosterone and parathyroid hormone interactions as mediators of metabolic and cardiovascular disease. Metabolism 63:20–31
194. Pilz S, Kienreich K, Drechsler C, Ritz E, Fahrleitner-Pammer A, Gaksch M, Meinitzer A, Marz W, Pieber TR, Tomaschitz A (2012) Hyperparathyroidism in patients with primary aldosteronism: cross-sectional and interventional data from the gecoh study. J Clin Endocrinol Metab 97:E75–E79
195. Kovacs L, Goth MI, Szabolcs I, Dohan O, Ferencz A, Szilagyi G (1998) The effect of surgical treatment on secondary hyperaldosteronism and relative hyperinsulinemia in primary hyperparathyroidism. Eur J Endocrinol 138:543–547
196. Maniero C, Fassina A, Guzzardo V, Lenzini L, Amadori G, Pelizzo MR, Gomez-Sanchez C, Rossi GP (2011) Primary hyperparathyroidism with concurrent primary aldosteronism. Hypertension 58:341–346
197. Salcuni AS, Palmieri S, Carnevale V, Morelli V, Battista C, Guarnieri V, Guglielmi G, Desina G, Eller-Vainicher C, Beck-Peccoz P, Scillitani A, Chiodini I (2012) Bone involvement in aldosteronism. J Bone Miner Res 27:2217–2222
198. Chhokar VS, Sun Y, Bhattacharya SK, Ahokas RA, Myers LK, Xing Z, Smith RA, Gerling IC, Weber KT (2005) Hyperparathyroidism and the calcium paradox of aldosteronism. Circulation 111:871–878
199. Tomaschitz A, Fahrleitner-Pammer A, Pieske B, Verheyen N, Amrein K, Ritz E, Kienreich K, Horina JH, Schmidt A, Kraigher-Krainer E, Colantonio C, Meinitzer A, Pilz S (2012) Effect of eplerenone on parathyroid hormone levels in patients with primary hyperparathyroidism: a randomized, double-blind, placebo-controlled trial. BMC Endocr Disord 12:19
200. Menard J, Gonzalez MF, Guyene TT, Bissery A (2006) Investigation of aldosterone-synthase inhibition in rats. J Hypertens 24:1147–1155
201. Mulder P, Mellin V, Favre J, Vercauteren M, Remy-Jouet I, Monteil C, Richard V, Renet S, Henry JP, Jeng AY, Webb RL, Thuillez C (2008) Aldosterone synthase inhibition improves cardiovascular function and structure in rats with heart failure: a comparison with spironolactone. Eur Heart J 29:2171–2179
202. Calhoun DA, White WB, Krum H, Guo W, Bermann G, Trapani A, Lefkowitz MP, Menard J (2011) Effects of a novel aldosterone synthase inhibitor for treatment of primary hypertension: results of a randomized, double-blind, placebo- and active-controlled phase 2 trial. Circulation 124:1945–1955
203. Lalevee N, Rebsamen MC, Barrere-Lemaire S, Perrier E, Nargeot J, Benitah JP, Rossier MF (2005) Aldosterone increases t-type calcium channel expression and in vitro beating frequency in neonatal rat cardiomyocytes. Cardiovasc Res 67:216–224

204. Ouvrard-Pascaud A, Sainte-Marie Y, Benitah JP, Perrier R, Soukaseum C, Nguyen Dinh Cat A, Royer A, Le Quang K, Charpentier F, Demolombe S, Mechta-Grigoriou F, Beggah AT, Maison-Blanche P, Oblin ME, Delcayre C, Fishman GI, Farman N, Escoubet B, Jaisser F (2005) Conditional mineralocorticoid receptor expression in the heart leads to life-threatening arrhythmias. Circulation 111:3025–3033
205. Perrier R, Richard S, Sainte-Marie Y, Rossier BC, Jaisser F, Hummler E, Benitah JP (2005) A direct relationship between plasma aldosterone and cardiac L-type Ca^{2+} current in mice. J Physiol 569:153–162
206. Gomez AM, Rueda A, Sainte-Marie Y, Pereira L, Zissimopoulos S, Zhu X, Schaub R, Perrier E, Perrier R, Latouche C, Richard S, Picot MC, Jaisser F, Lai FA, Valdivia HH, Benitah JP (2009) Mineralocorticoid modulation of cardiac ryanodine receptor activity is associated with downregulation of FK506-binding proteins. Circulation 119:2179–2187
207. Dartsch T, Fischer R, Gapelyuk A, Weiergraeber M, Ladage D, Schneider T, Schirdewan A, Reuter H, Mueller-Ehmsen J, Zobel C (2013) Aldosterone induces electrical remodeling independent of hypertension. Int J Cardiol 164:170–178
208. Yee KM, Pringle SD, Struthers AD (2001) Circadian variation in the effects of aldosterone blockade on heart rate variability and qt dispersion in congestive heart failure. J Am Coll Cardiol 37:1800–1807
209. Reil JC, Hohl M, Selejan S, Lipp P, Drautz F, Kazakow A, Munz BM, Muller P, Steendijk P, Reil GH, Allessie MA, Bohm M, Neuberger HR (2012) Aldosterone promotes atrial fibrillation. Eur Heart J 33:2098–2108
210. Goette A, Hoffmanns P, Enayati W, Meltendorf U, Geller JC, Klein HU (2001) Effect of successful electrical cardioversion on serum aldosterone in patients with persistent atrial fibrillation. Am J Cardiol 88:906–909, A908
211. Tsai CT, Chiang FT, Tseng CD, Hwang JJ, Kuo KT, Wu CK, Yu CC, Wang YC, Lai LP, Lin JL (2010) Increased expression of mineralocorticoid receptor in human atrial fibrillation and a cellular model of atrial fibrillation. J Am Coll Cardiol 55:758–770
212. Li YY, Zhou CW, Xu J, Qian Y, Wang B (2012) CYP11B2 T-344C gene polymorphism and atrial fibrillation: a meta-analysis of 2,758 subjects. PLoS One 7:e50910
213. Zhao J, Li J, Li W, Li Y, Shan H, Gong Y, Yang B (2010) Effects of spironolactone on atrial structural remodelling in a canine model of atrial fibrillation produced by prolonged atrial pacing. Br J Pharmacol 159:1584–1594
214. Ito Y, Yamasaki H, Naruse Y, Yoshida K, Kaneshiro T, Murakoshi N, Igarashi M, Kuroki K, Machino T, Xu D, Kunugita F, Sekiguchi Y, Sato A, Tada H, Aonuma K (2013) Effect of eplerenone on maintenance of sinus rhythm after catheter ablation in patients with long-standing persistent atrial fibrillation. Am J Cardiol 111:1012–1018
215. Swedberg K, Zannad F, McMurray JJ, Krum H, van Veldhuisen DJ, Shi H, Vincent J, Pitt B, Investigators E-HS (2012) Eplerenone and atrial fibrillation in mild systolic heart failure: results from the emphasis-hf (eplerenone in mild patients hospitalization and survival study in heart failure) study. J Am Coll Cardiol 59:1598–1603
216. Perrier E, Kerfant BG, Lalevee N, Bideaux P, Rossier MF, Richard S, Gomez AM, Benitah JP (2004) Mineralocorticoid receptor antagonism prevents the electrical remodeling that precedes cellular hypertrophy after myocardial infarction. Circulation 110:776–783
217. Shah NC, Pringle SD, Donnan PT, Struthers AD (2007) Spironolactone has antiarrhythmic activity in ischaemic cardiac patients without cardiac failure. J Hypertens 25:2345–2351
218. Beygui F, Labbe JP, Cayla G, Ennezat PV, Motreff P, Roubille F, Silvain J, Barthelemy O, Delarche N, Van Belle E, Collet JP, Montalescot G (2013) Early mineralocorticoid receptor blockade in primary percutaneous coronary intervention for ST-elevation myocardial infarction is associated with a reduction of life-threatening ventricular arrhythmia. Int J Cardiol 167:73–79
219. Conn JW (1965) Hypertension, the potassium ion and impaired carbohydrate tolerance. N Engl J Med 273:1135–1143
220. Luther JM, Brown NJ (2011) The renin-angiotensin-aldosterone system and glucose homeostasis. Trends Pharmacol Sci 32:734–739

221. Colussi G, Catena C, Lapenna R, Nadalini E, Chiuch A, Sechi LA (2007) Insulin resistance and hyperinsulinemia are related to plasma aldosterone levels in hypertensive patients. Diabetes Care 30:2349–2354
222. Garg R, Hurwitz S, Williams GH, Hopkins PN, Adler GK (2010) Aldosterone production and insulin resistance in healthy adults. J Clin Endocrinol Metab 95:1986–1990
223. Fallo F, Veglio F, Bertello C, Sonino N, Della Mea P, Ermani M, Rabbia F, Federspil G, Mulatero P (2006) Prevalence and characteristics of the metabolic syndrome in primary aldosteronism. J Clin Endocrinol Metab 91:454–459
224. Fallo F, Della Mea P, Sonino N, Bertello C, Ermani M, Vettor R, Veglio F, Mulatero P (2007) Adiponectin and insulin sensitivity in primary aldosteronism. Am J Hypertens 20:855–861
225. Somloova Z, Widimsky J Jr, Rosa J, Wichterle D, Strauch B, Petrak O, Zelinka T, Vlkova J, Masek M, Dvorakova J, Holaj R (2010) The prevalence of metabolic syndrome and its components in two main types of primary aldosteronism. J Hum Hypertens 24:625–630
226. Ingelsson E, Pencina MJ, Tofler GH, Benjamin EJ, Lanier KJ, Jacques PF, Fox CS, Meigs JB, Levy D, Larson MG, Selhub J, D'Agostino RB Sr, Wang TJ, Vasan RS (2007) Multimarker approach to evaluate the incidence of the metabolic syndrome and longitudinal changes in metabolic risk factors: the Framingham Offspring Study. Circulation 116:984–992
227. Hannemann A, Meisinger C, Bidlingmaier M, Doring A, Thorand B, Heier M, Belcredi P, Ladwig KH, Wallaschofski H, Friedrich N, Schipf S, Ludemann J, Rettig R, Peters J, Volzke H, Seissler J, Beuschlein F, Nauck M, Reincke M (2011) Association of plasma aldosterone with the metabolic syndrome in two German populations. Eur J Endocrinol 164:751–758
228. Catena C, Lapenna R, Baroselli S, Nadalini E, Colussi G, Novello M, Favret G, Melis A, Cavarape A, Sechi LA (2006) Insulin sensitivity in patients with primary aldosteronism: a follow-up study. J Clin Endocrinol Metab 91:3457–3463
229. Shimamoto K, Shiiki M, Ise T, Miyazaki Y, Higashiura K, Fukuoka M, Hirata A, Masuda A, Nakagawa M, Iimura O (1994) Does insulin resistance participate in an impaired glucose tolerance in primary aldosteronism? J Hum Hypertens 8:755–759
230. Giacchetti G, Ronconi V, Turchi F, Agostinelli L, Mantero F, Rilli S, Boscaro M (2007) Aldosterone as a key mediator of the cardiometabolic syndrome in primary aldosteronism: an observational study. J Hypertens 25:177–186
231. Sindelka G, Widimsky J, Haas T, Prazny M, Hilgertova J, Skrha J (2000) Insulin action in primary hyperaldosteronism before and after surgical or pharmacological treatment. Exp Clin Endocrinol Diabetes 108:21–25
232. Skrha J, Haas T, Sindelka G, Prazny M, Widimsky J, Cibula D, Svacina S (2004) Comparison of the insulin action parameters from hyperinsulinemic clamps with homeostasis model assessment and QUICKI indexes in subjects with different endocrine disorders. J Clin Endocrinol Metab 89:135–141
233. Reincke M, Meisinger C, Holle R, Quinkler M, Hahner S, Beuschlein F, Bidlingmaier M, Seissler J, Endres S, Participants of the German Conn‘s R (2010) Is primary aldosteronism associated with diabetes mellitus? Results of the German Conn's Registry. Horm Metab Res 42:435–439
234. Matrozova J, Steichen O, Amar L, Zacharieva S, Jeunemaitre X, Plouin PF (2009) Fasting plasma glucose and serum lipids in patients with primary aldosteronism: a controlled cross-sectional study. Hypertension 53:605–610
235. Mosso LM, Carvajal CA, Maiz A, Ortiz EH, Castillo CR, Artigas RA, Fardella CE (2007) A possible association between primary aldosteronism and a lower beta-cell function. J Hypertens 25:2125–2130
236. Goodfriend TL, Calhoun DA (2004) Resistant hypertension, obesity, sleep apnea, and aldosterone: theory and therapy. Hypertension 43:518–524
237. Ronconi V, Turchi F, Bujalska IJ, Giacchetti G, Boscaro M (2008) Adipose cell-adrenal interactions: current knowledge and future perspectives. Trends Endocrinol Metab 19:100–103
238. Bentley-Lewis R, Adler GK, Perlstein T, Seely EW, Hopkins PN, Williams GH, Garg R (2007) Body mass index predicts aldosterone production in normotensive adults on a high-salt diet. J Clin Endocrinol Metab 92:4472–4475

239. Iacobellis G, Petramala L, Cotesta D, Pergolini M, Zinnamosca L, Cianci R, De Toma G, Sciomer S, Letizia C (2010) Adipokines and cardiometabolic profile in primary hyperaldosteronism. J Clin Endocrinol Metab 95:2391–2398
240. Ronconi V, Turchi F, Rilli S, Di Mattia D, Agostinelli L, Boscaro M, Giacchetti G (2010) Metabolic syndrome in primary aldosteronism and essential hypertension: relationship to adiponectin gene variants. Nutr Metab Cardiovasc Dis 20:93–100
241. O'Seaghdha CM, Hwang SJ, Vasan RS, Larson MG, Hoffmann U, Wang TJ, Fox CS (2012) Correlation of renin angiotensin and aldosterone system activity with subcutaneous and visceral adiposity: the framingham heart study. BMC Endocr Disord 12:3
242. Rossi GP, Belfiore A, Bernini G, Fabris B, Caridi G, Ferri C, Giacchetti G, Letizia C, Maccario M, Mannelli M, Palumbo G, Patalano A, Rizzoni D, Rossi E, Pessina AC, Mantero F (2008) Primary Aldosteronism Prevalence in hYpertension Study I. Body mass index predicts plasma aldosterone concentrations in overweight-obese primary hypertensive patients. J Clin Endocrinol Metab 93:2566–2571
243. Ishimori M, Takeda N, Okumura S, Murai T, Inouye H, Yasuda K (1994) Increased insulin sensitivity in patients with aldosterone producing adenoma. Clin Endocrinol (Oxf) 41:433–438
244. Fallo F, Pilon C, Urbanet R (2012) Primary aldosteronism and metabolic syndrome. Horm Metab Res 44:208–214
245. Campion J, Maestro B, Mata F, Davila N, Carranza MC, Calle C (1999) Inhibition by aldosterone of insulin receptor mrna levels and insulin binding in U-937 human promonocytic cells. J Steroid Biochem Mol Biol 70:211–218
246. Calle C, Campion J, Garcia-Arencibia M, Maestro B, Davila N (2003) Transcriptional inhibition of the human insulin receptor gene by aldosterone. J Steroid Biochem Mol Biol 84:543–553
247. Campion J, Lahera V, Cachofeiro V, Maestro B, Davila N, Carranza MC, Calle C (1998) In vivo tissue specific modulation of rat insulin receptor gene expression in an experimental model of mineralocorticoid excess. Mol Cell Biochem 185:177–182
248. Wada T, Ohshima S, Fujisawa E, Koya D, Tsuneki H, Sasaoka T (2009) Aldosterone inhibits insulin-induced glucose uptake by degradation of insulin receptor substrate (IRS) 1 and IRS2 via a reactive oxygen species-mediated pathway in 3T3-L1 adipocytes. Endocrinology 150:1662–1669
249. Lastra G, Whaley-Connell A, Manrique C, Habibi J, Gutweiler AA, Appesh L, Hayden MR, Wei Y, Ferrario C, Sowers JR (2008) Low-dose spironolactone reduces reactive oxygen species generation and improves insulin-stimulated glucose transport in skeletal muscle in the TG(mRen2)27 rat. Am J Physiol Endocrinol Metab 295:E110–E116
250. Kraus D, Jager J, Meier B, Fasshauer M, Klein J (2005) Aldosterone inhibits uncoupling protein-1, induces insulin resistance, and stimulates proinflammatory adipokines in adipocytes. Horm Metab Res 37:455–459
251. DeMarco VG, Johnson MS, Whaley-Connell AT, Sowers JR (2010) Cytokine abnormalities in the etiology of the cardiometabolic syndrome. Curr Hypertens Rep 12:93–98
252. Hoppmann J, Perwitz N, Meier B, Fasshauer M, Hadaschik D, Lehnert H, Klein J (2010) The balance between gluco- and mineralo-corticoid action critically determines inflammatory adipocyte responses. J endocrinol 204:153–164
253. Boscaro M, Giacchetti G, Ronconi V (2012) Visceral adipose tissue: emerging role of gluco- and mineralocorticoid hormones in the setting of cardiometabolic alterations. Ann N Y Acad Sci 1264:87–102
254. Krug AW, Ehrhart-Bornstein M (2008) Adrenocortical dysfunction in obesity and the metabolic syndrome. Horm Metab Res 40:515–517
255. Caprio M, Feve B, Claes A, Viengchareun S, Lombes M, Zennaro MC (2007) Pivotal role of the mineralocorticoid receptor in corticosteroid-induced adipogenesis. FASEB J 21: 2185–2194
256. Zennaro MC, Caprio M, Feve B (2009) Mineralocorticoid receptors in the metabolic syndrome. Trends Endocrinol Metab 20:444–451

257. Briones AM, Nguyen Dinh Cat A, Callera GE, Yogi A, Burger D, He Y, Correa JW, Gagnon AM, Gomez-Sanchez CE, Gomez-Sanchez EP, Sorisky A, Ooi TC, Ruzicka M, Burns KD, Touyz RM (2012) Adipocytes produce aldosterone through calcineurin-dependent signaling pathways: implications in diabetes mellitus-associated obesity and vascular dysfunction. Hypertension 59:1069–1078
258. Northcott CA, Fink GD, Garver H, Haywood JR, Laimon-Thomson EL, McClain JL, Pires PW, Rainey WE, Rigsby CS, Dorrance AM (2012) The development of hypertension and hyperaldosteronism in a rodent model of life-long obesity. Endocrinology 153:1764–1773
259. Flynn C, Bakris GL (2011) Interaction between adiponectin and aldosterone. Cardiorenal Med 1:96–101
260. Guo C, Ricchiuti V, Lian BQ, Yao TM, Coutinho P, Romero JR, Li J, Williams GH, Adler GK (2008) Mineralocorticoid receptor blockade reverses obesity-related changes in expression of adiponectin, peroxisome proliferator-activated receptor-gamma, and proinflammatory adipokines. Circulation 117:2253–2261
261. Hirata A, Maeda N, Hiuge A, Hibuse T, Fujita K, Okada T, Kihara S, Funahashi T, Shimomura I (2009) Blockade of mineralocorticoid receptor reverses adipocyte dysfunction and insulin resistance in obese mice. Cardiovasc Res 84:164–172
262. Selvaraj J, Muthusamy T, Srinivasan C, Balasubramanian K (2009) Impact of excess aldosterone on glucose homeostasis in adult male rat. Clin Chim Acta 407:51–57
263. Lastra G, Dhuper S, Johnson MS, Sowers JR (2010) Salt, aldosterone, and insulin resistance: impact on the cardiovascular system. Nat Rev Cardiol 7:577–584
264. Wada T, Kenmochi H, Miyashita Y, Sasaki M, Ojima M, Sasahara M, Koya D, Tsuneki H, Sasaoka T (2010) Spironolactone improves glucose and lipid metabolism by ameliorating hepatic steatosis and inflammation and suppressing enhanced gluconeogenesis induced by high-fat and high-fructose diet. Endocrinology 151:2040–2049
265. Swaminathan K, Davies J, George J, Rajendra NS, Morris AD, Struthers AD (2008) Spironolactone for poorly controlled hypertension in type 2 diabetes: conflicting effects on blood pressure, endothelial function, glycaemic control and hormonal profiles. Diabetologia 51:762–768
266. Tonelli M, Wiebe N, Culleton B, House A, Rabbat C, Fok M, McAlister F, Garg AX (2006) Chronic kidney disease and mortality risk: a systematic review. J Am Soc Nephrol 17:2034–2047
267. Ribstein J, Du Cailar G, Fesler P, Mimran A (2005) Relative glomerular hyperfiltration in primary aldosteronism. J Am Soc Nephrol 16:1320–1325
268. Reincke M, Rump LC, Quinkler M, Hahner S, Diederich S, Lorenz R, Seufert J, Schirpenbach C, Beuschlein F, Bidlingmaier M, Meisinger C, Holle R, Endres S, Participants of German Conn‘s R (2009) Risk factors associated with a low glomerular filtration rate in primary aldosteronism. J Clin Endocrinol Metab 94:869–875
269. Rossi GP, Bernini G, Desideri G, Fabris B, Ferri C, Giacchetti G, Letizia C, Maccario M, Mannelli M, Matterello MJ, Montemurro D, Palumbo G, Rizzoni D, Rossi E, Pessina AC, Mantero F, Participants PS (2006) Renal damage in primary aldosteronism: results of the PAPY study. Hypertension 48:232–238
270. Fourkiotis V, Vonend O, Diederich S, Fischer E, Lang K, Endres S, Beuschlein F, Willenberg HS, Rump LC, Allolio B, Reincke M, Quinkler M, Mephisto Study Group (2013) Effectiveness of eplerenone or spironolactone treatment in preserving renal function in primary aldosteronism. Eur J Endocrinol 168:75–81
271. Terata S, Kikuya M, Satoh M, Ohkubo T, Hashimoto T, Hara A, Hirose T, Obara T, Metoki H, Inoue R, Asayama K, Kanno A, Totsune K, Hoshi H, Satoh H, Sato H, Imai Y (2012) Plasma renin activity and the aldosterone-to-renin ratio are associated with the development of chronic kidney disease: the ohasama study. J Hypertens 30:1632–1638
272. Fox CS, Gona P, Larson MG, Selhub J, Tofler G, Hwang SJ, Meigs JB, Levy D, Wang TJ, Jacques PF, Benjamin EJ, Vasan RS (2010) A multi-marker approach to predict incident ckd and microalbuminuria. J Am Soc Nephrol 21:2143–2149

273. Boesby L, Elung-Jensen T, Klausen TW, Strandgaard S, Kamper AL (2011) Moderate antiproteinuric effect of add-on aldosterone blockade with eplerenone in non-diabetic chronic kidney disease. A randomized cross-over study. PLoS One 6:e26904
274. Nielsen SE, Persson F, Frandsen E, Sugaya T, Hess G, Zdunek D, Shjoedt KJ, Parving HH, Rossing P (2012) Spironolactone diminishes urinary albumin excretion in patients with type 1 diabetes and microalbuminuria: a randomized placebo-controlled crossover study. Diabet Med 29:e184–e190
275. Edwards NC, Steeds RP, Stewart PM, Ferro CJ, Townend JN (2009) Effect of spironolactone on left ventricular mass and aortic stiffness in early-stage chronic kidney disease: a randomized controlled trial. J Am Coll Cardiol 54:505–512
276. Quinkler M, Zehnder D, Eardley KS, Lepenies J, Howie AJ, Hughes SV, Cockwell P, Hewison M, Stewart PM (2005) Increased expression of mineralocorticoid effector mechanisms in kidney biopsies of patients with heavy proteinuria. Circulation 112:1435–1443
277. Terada Y, Ueda S, Hamada K, Shimamura Y, Ogata K, Inoue K, Taniguchi Y, Kagawa T, Horino T, Takao T (2012) Aldosterone stimulates nuclear factor-kappa B activity and transcription of intercellular adhesion molecule-1 and connective tissue growth factor in rat mesangial cells via serum- and glucocorticoid-inducible protein kinase-1. Clin Exp Nephrol 16:81–88
278. Xue C, Siragy HM (2005) Local renal aldosterone system and its regulation by salt, diabetes, and angiotensin II type 1 receptor. Hypertension 46:584–590
279. Lee SH, Yoo TH, Nam BY, Kim DK, Li JJ, Jung DS, Kwak SJ, Ryu DR, Han SH, Lee JE, Moon SJ, Han DS, Kang SW (2009) Activation of local aldosterone system within podocytes is involved in apoptosis under diabetic conditions. Am J Physiol Renal Physiol 297: F1381–F1390
280. Kawarazaki H, Ando K, Shibata S, Muraoka K, Fujita M, Kawarasaki C, Fujita T (2012) Mineralocorticoid receptor–Rac1 activation and oxidative stress play major roles in salt-induced hypertension and kidney injury in prepubertal rats. J Hypertens 30:1977–1985
281. Fu Y, Hall JE, Lu D, Lin L, Manning RD Jr, Cheng L, Gomez-Sanchez CE, Juncos LA, Liu R (2012) Aldosterone blunts tubuloglomerular feedback by activating macula densa mineralocorticoid receptors. Hypertension 59:599–606
282. Ritz E, Tomaschitz A (2009) Aldosterone, a vasculotoxic agent – novel functions for an old hormone. Nephrol Dial Transplant 24:2302–2305

Chapter 13
Quality-of-Life Aspects of Primary Aldosteronism

Michael Stowasser and Ashraf H. Ahmed

Abstract Evidence from case reports and group data suggest that primary aldosteronism (PA) is associated with a variety of mood disorders (including anxiety, irritability, and, to a lesser extent, depression) which contribute to reduced quality of life (QOL). Specific treatment (unilateral adrenalectomy for unilateral PA or aldosterone antagonist medications for bilateral PA) results in reversal of these adverse states, with benefits appearing to be more rapidly achieved and more complete with surgical versus medical therapy. Possible contributors to reduced QOL in PA include effects of hypertension, hypokalemia, medications, aldosterone-induced obstructive sleep apnea, and direct actions of aldosterone on the central nervous system (CNS), but how such putative direct central actions may come about remains speculative. As QOL is of paramount importance from the patient's perspective, these observations add to the weight of arguments supporting early detection of PA among hypertensive populations, careful differentiation of its subtypes, and institution of appropriate specific treatment.

Keywords Primary aldosteronism • Quality of life • Anxiety • Depression • Mood disorders • Effects of medical treatment • Effects of surgical treatment • Central effects

---

M. Stowasser, M.B.B.S., F.R.A.C.P., Ph.D. (✉) • A.H. Ahmed, M.B.B.S., M.Sc., Ph.D.
Endocrine Hypertension Research Centre, University of Queensland School of Medicine, Princess Alexandra Hospital, Ipswich Road, Woolloongabba, Brisbane, QLD 4102, Australia
e-mail: m.stowasser@uq.edu.au

P. Hellman (ed.), *Primary Aldosteronism: Molecular Genetics, Endocrinology, and Translational Medicine*, DOI 10.1007/978-1-4939-0509-6_13,

Introduction

Measurement of disease status alone, such as severity of hypertension, size of myocardial infarction, or tumor load, provides only partial insights into health status [36, 48]. Psychosocial factors such as pain, mood disturbance, restricted mobility, difficulty fulfilling personal and family responsibilities, and financial burden are also important as contributors to personal burden of illness [36] but are frequently ignored in clinical research. This may be at least partly because they are less easily defined and measured due to their relative complexity and subjectivity. Consequently, measurement of health-related quality of life, otherwise known as quality of life (QOL), has emerged as a major area of research development in the field of health status assessment [48].

Definition and Importance of QOL

The term QOL refers to the physical, psychological, and social domains of health, seen as distinct areas that are influenced by a person's experiences, beliefs, expectations, and perceptions [62]. QOL has been defined by the World Health Organization as "individual's perception of their position in life in the context of the culture and value systems in which they live in relation to their goals, expectations, standards and concerns" [48]. It is affected by the person's physical health, psychological state, personal beliefs, social relationships, and educational level [47]. Measurement of QOL considers the impact of the disease or its treatment from the patient's perspective [6] and determines the need for any support during illness including social, emotional, and physical support. To many patients, including those with primary aldosteronism (PA), this is likely to be at least as important (if not more so) as more objectively measured clinical parameters such as blood pressure level.

Evaluation of Health Burden and Treatment Response in PA: An Evolving Perspective

The decision whether to screen for, definitively diagnose, and then determine the subtype of a secondary form of hypertension such as PA is to a large extent dependent on the degree of benefit that the patient is likely to experience as a result of receiving specific treatment. Traditionally, this has meant the blood pressure response. In the case of PA, unilateral laparoscopic adrenalectomy leads to cure of hypertension in 50–60 % and improvement in virtually all remaining patients with unilateral forms [11, 35]. On the other hand, treatment with aldosterone antagonists usually brings about marked improvement in hypertension control in patients with bilateral forms [29, 56, 58]. More recently, attention has turned to the effects of treatment on other downstream consequences of PA after the emergence of growing evidence that long-term exposure to aldosterone excess causes damage to the cardiovascular [8, 10, 42] and renal [9, 21, 41] systems independently of its effects on blood pressure. This would help to explain why patients with PA have been reported to be at higher risk of cardiovascular events [34] and renal dysfunction [43] than subjects with "essential" hypertension matched for blood pressure levels. Most importantly, both surgical and specific medical treatment against PA have been reported to abrogate the excess in cardiovascular and renal morbidity that otherwise occurs when patients with PA are treated with nonspecific antihypertensive medications [46].

Psychosocial factors, and their response to specific treatment, have been less well explored in PA, but have received growing attention, particularly in recent years.

PA and Disorders of Psychological Functioning

Several case reports have described the association of PA with depression [2, 25, 30]. In a study conducted by Sonino and colleagues [50] to investigate the presence of psychiatric disorders and subclinical psychological syndromes in newly diagnosed PA patients, seven of ten patients were found to have anxiety disorder, with one also having major depression. Demoralization was reported in five cases. In this study, however, a chance association between these psychological disorders and PA could not be excluded because of the small sample size. Also, whether the psychological distress preceded or followed the onset of aldosteronism could not be determined. In a more recent study conducted by Sonino and colleagues [51], a series of interviews and questionnaires were used to assess psychological correlates in PA. Twelve (52 %) of 23 patients with PA suffered from an anxiety disorder compared with four (17.4 %) of 23 patients with essential hypertension and one (4.3 %) of 23 normotensive controls. Generalized anxiety disorder, but not depression, was more frequent in PA than in essential hypertensive patients and normotensive controls.

Anecdotally, observers (medical and nursing staff and patients' relatives) from the Endocrine Hypertension Research Centre (EHRC) at Greenslopes and Princess Alexandra Hospitals have suggested that PA patients appear to exhibit more anger, irritability, and emotionality than patients with hypertension from other causes. Verbal reports from patients or their spouses include statements such as "impatient," "cranky," "irritable" and "moody" with no obvious cause. Houlihan [23] described a 51-year-old male with a 4-month history of irritable mood and episodes of rage, in whom the presence of hypertension and hypokalemia, raised ARR and identification of a 1.5 cm left adrenal mass on computed tomography scanning led to laparoscopic left adrenalectomy. In the days following the procedure, not only did his hypertension improve markedly and plasma potassium levels return to normal, but his irritable mood and episodic rage also resolved without the need for psychotropic agents.

The above reports prompted us to attempt to quantify QOL in patients with PA and to assess responses to both surgical and medical treatment modalities.

Measurement of QOL: The SF36 Survey

Ware and colleagues developed The Medical Outcomes Study Short Form 36 General Health Survey (SF-36) in 1988–1989 [65]. Many researchers have preferred the use of the SF-36 to measure various aspects of QOL over other instruments because it is comprehensive, short, and relatively easy to score and interpret [17, 22, 27, 60, 63]. Validity and reliability tests from a number of worldwide studies have indicated that the SF-36 is psychometrically sound [4, 31–33].

The SF-36 is a multipurpose short form instrument [64]. It consists of 36 items with one item used to measure health transition and the remaining 35 items used to assess the following eight domains: limitation in physical activities because of health problems ("Physical Functioning"); limitations in social activities because of physical or emotional problems ("Social Functioning"); limitations in usual role activities because of physical health problems ("Role Physical"); bodily pain ("Bodily Pain"); general mental health ("Mental Health"); limitations in usual role activities because of emotional problems ("Role Emotional"); vitality ("Vitality"); and general health perceptions ("General Health").

For simplicity in monitoring disease cohorts and comparing with the normative general population, the above eight domains can be categorized into two summary measures: the Physical Component Summary (which includes Physical Functioning, Role Physical, Bodily Pain, and General Health scales) and the Mental Component Summary (includes Vitality, Social Functioning, Role Emotional, and Mental Health scales) [64]. Across the eight SF-36 scales, the Australian population norms are of similar value to those reported for the US and UK populations [54]. Comparing the data of a study with the national norms provides a way by which disease groups (such as patients with PA) may be characterized and their response to treatment assessed from a psychometric point of view.

QOL and Effects of Treatment in PA, as Measured by SF-36

We used the SF-36 form to assess 22 patients with unilateral PA before and after undergoing unilateral adrenalectomy. For each domain of QOL, the score was lower for PA patients than that reported for the Australian general population, and significantly so for Physical Functioning, Role Physical, General Health, and Vitality. In this study, QOL was significantly improved to normal levels within 3 months following unilateral adrenalectomy, with this improvement being maintained at 6 months [61]. A subsequent study in 21 patients with bilateral PA showed that the baseline scores were again significantly lower than that reported for the Australian general population, and in the same four domains as for patients with unilateral PA [1]. There was statistically significant improvement in these four domains of QOL after 6 months of starting medical treatment of bilateral PA with spironolactone and/or amiloride. These two studies suggest that treatment of PA has a positive impact

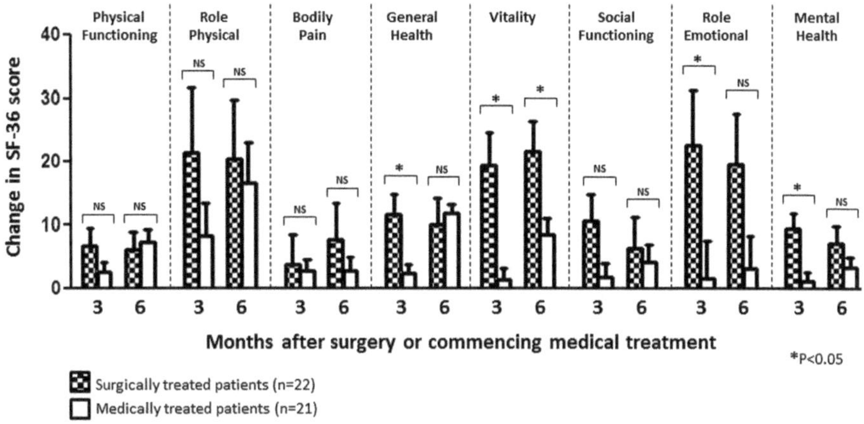

Fig. 13.1 Change in SF-36 scores from baseline at 3 and 6 months following unilateral adrenalectomy in patients with unilateral primary aldosteronism (*checkered bars*) or commencement of specific medical treatment (spironolactone and/or amiloride) in patients with bilateral primary aldosteronism (*open bars*). $*P<0.05$ for comparison of mean change in score for surgically versus medically treated patients

not only on blood pressure and biochemical parameters but also on QOL, further supporting the value of detecting and specifically treating PA early.

In medically treated patients, there were no significant changes observed in any domain of QOL 3 months after commencing medical treatment, whereas surgical treatment of patients with unilateral PA demonstrated significant, early QOL improvement, with scores in each of the eight domains rising to normal by 3 months after surgery. Hence, a faster and more profound effect on QOL was observed for surgical than medical treatment, with the differences in degree of improvement reaching significance at the 3-month mark for the domains of General Health, Vitality, Role Emotional, and Mental Health, and continuing out to 6 months for Vitality (Fig. 13.1).

There are a number of possible explanations for the more rapid and complete correction of reduced QOL scores seen with surgical compared with medical treatment of PA. Surgically removing the source of aldosterone excess is clearly faster and might, as well, be more absolute than attempted pharmacological reversal of excessive mineralocorticoid action. We tried to avoid inadequate dosage of aldosterone antagonist treatment in our study by monitoring renin levels, and these were not suppressed compared with the surgically treated patients. This would not, however, rule out the possibility that mineralocorticoid action was incompletely blocked at sites (including intracerebral) other than the distal renal tubule. We have previously reported that, whereas the majority of patients with unilateral PA who undergo unilateral adrenalectomy are cured of hypertension postoperatively without requiring antihypertensive agents become readily controlled with only one drug (mean 0.7 agents), those with bilateral PA, although experiencing a fall in blood pressure, do not experience a reduction in medication requirements (mean 2.4) by the addition of an aldosterone antagonist (when this is included as one drug) [57]. The ongoing need for medical treatment in the medically treated patients might bring with it reduced QOL through drug-related sides effects, medication costs, or disappointment at not being candidates for a surgical, potentially curative procedure which, in our experience, is the preferred option for the great majority of patients found to have PA.

More complete and/or rapid responses to surgical treatment have been described for other measured aldosterone-induced target organ effects. Strauch and colleagues [59] reported reduced arterial stiffness (measured as carotid-femoral pulse wave velocity and augmentation index) at approximately 1 year following unilateral adrenalectomy in 15 patients with unilateral PA but not after a year of spironolactone treatment in 14 other subjects with PA treated medically. Catena and coworkers [8] similarly found surgery ($n=24$) to be more effective than spironolactone ($n=30$) in reducing left ventricular mass (which was greater prior to treatment in the patients with PA than in matched essential hypertensives) after 1 year, with significant decreases only seen in the surgically treated group. Although subsequent changes were greater in the medically treated group so that by the end of the study (mean follow-up 6.4 years) the overall reduction from baseline was comparable in the two groups, it is quite possible that the apparent delay in response to medical treatment could equate to a less effective reduction in overall risk of cardiovascular events.

Possible Mechanisms for Reduced QOL in PA

Mechanisms by which QOL might be reduced in subjects with PA include nonspecific symptoms of hypertension, adverse effects of antihypertensive medications, and symptoms of aldosterone excess including those due to reduced potassium (palpitations, neuromuscular symptoms, and nocturia) and possibly obstructive sleep apnoea (reported to be more frequent in PA than in other forms of hypertension [18, 39]). Correction of these parameters following treatment of PA would at least partly explain how specific medical or surgical treatment can improve QOL. In addition to these classic effects, however, aldosterone excess may bring about disturbances in psychological function (including mood and anxiety disorders) through central mechanisms. Depression is associated with many symptoms which significantly affect QOL, including melancholic mood, loss of interest or pleasure, fatigue, sleep disturbances, and agitation [28]. Increased plasma aldosterone levels have been reported in patients with depression [13, 37] and there have been several case reports of PA presenting with depression [2, 25, 30]. Anxiety has a negative impact on QOL [66], and chronic treatment with aldosterone in rats caused anxiety-like behavior [20], while administration of eplerenone, a mineralocorticoid receptor blocker, was observed to exert anxiolytic effects [19]. Pharmacological blockade of the renin–angiotensin system by angiotensin II receptor blockers (ARB) or angiotensin converting enzyme inhibitors (ACEI), with reduction in aldosterone levels has been reported to improve mood and have anxiolytic effects in man [16, 44]. Treatment with ARBs in rats also has anxiolytic effects [24, 45, 53] and reduces plasma aldosterone [38]. Hence, considerable evidence from both clinical and experimental studies supports relationships between aldosterone and mood disorders with improvement when aldosterone effects are opposed by medications.

How may aldosterone exert such central effects to bring about these psychological disturbances? Aldosterone can stimulate activation of pro-inflammatory cytokines [14, 55]. Continuous intravenous infusion over 24 h of human tumor necrosis factor-α, a cytokine, was reported to induce depressive symptoms such as fatigue, malaise, lethargy, and irritability in human subjects [52]. Therapeutic administration of the cytokine interferon-a (IFN-a) for clinical treatment of malignant melanoma has been found to cause depression [7] but we are unaware of any studies examining effects of aldosterone excess on IFN-a levels. IFN-a-induced depression is responsive to treatment with standard antidepressants [7, 40]. Depressed patients have been found to have higher levels of pro-inflammatory cytokines [40]. Aldosterone also causes salt and water retention and salt-sensitive individuals have been shown to complain from increased levels of irritability, higher levels of anxiety, and lower levels of anger control [5, 12]. Aldosterone may also have direct central nervous system (CNS) actions. Injection of mineralocorticoid receptor antagonists into the brains of rats has been shown to induce anxiolytic effects [3, 26, 49]. However, consideration of direct CNS effects of aldosterone needs to be taken in the context of its very high reflection coefficient at the blood brain barrier and the very limited CNS expression of 11-beta hydroxysteroid dehydrogenase type II which, in other tissues where it is more abundant, serves to "protect" the mineralocorticoid receptor from binding by cortisol by converting this hormone into cortisone [15].

Conclusions

In conclusion, PA is associated with a variety of mood disorders, QOL scores appear to be lower in PA patients than reported for the general population, and both medical and surgical treatment are associated with a positive effect on mood and QOL. These findings support the view that early detection of PA is crucial, not only because treatment minimizes the cardiovascular and renal complications of long-term exposure to aldosterone excess and brings about marked improvement in hypertension control, but because it also improves QOL. Importantly, patients with unilateral PA treated surgically show a faster and more complete recovery of QOL than those with bilateral PA treated medically. That being the case, where a surgical option is desired by the patient, detection of PA should be followed by careful attempts at differentiating subtypes of PA so that optimal treatment options can be offered.

References

1. Ahmed AH, Gordon RD, Sukor N, Pimenta E, Stowasser M (2011) Quality of life in patients with bilateral primary aldosteronism before and during treatment with spironolactone and/or amiloride, including a comparison with our previously published results in those with unilateral disease treated surgically. J Clin Endocrinol Metab 96(9):2904–2911
2. Avery TL (1984) Primary hyperaldosteronism and depression. N Z Med J 97(761):537
3. Bitran D, Shiekh M, Dowd JA, Dugan MM, Renda P (1998) Corticosterone is permissive to the anxiolytic effect that results from the blockade of hippocampal mineralocorticoid receptors. Pharmacol Biochem Behav 60(4):879–887
4. Brazier JE, Harper R, Jones NM, O'Cathain A, Thomas KJ, Usherwood T, Westlake L (1992) Validating the SF-36 health survey questionnaire: new outcome measure for primary care. BMJ 305(6846):160–164
5. Buchholz K, Schorr U, Turan S, Sharma AM, Deter HC (1999) [Emotional irritability and anxiety in salt-sensitive persons at risk for essential hypertension]. Psychother Psychosom Med Psychol 49(8):284–289
6. Canavarro MC, Serra AV, Simoes MR, Rijo D, Pereira M, Gameiro S, Quartilho MJ, Quintais L, Carona C, Paredes T (2009) Development and psychometric properties of the World Health Organization Quality of Life Assessment Instrument (WHOQOL-100) in Portugal. Int J Behav Med 16(2):116–124
7. Capuron L, Miller AH (2004) Cytokines and psychopathology: lessons from interferon-alpha. Biol Psychiatry 56(11):819–824
8. Catena C, Colussi G, Lapenna R, Nadalini E, Chiuch A, Gianfagna P, Sechi LA (2007) Long-term cardiac effects of adrenalectomy or mineralocorticoid antagonists in patients with primary aldosteronism. Hypertension 50(5):911–918
9. Catena C, Colussi G, Nadalini E, Chiuch A, Baroselli S, Lapenna R, Sechi LA (2007) Relationships of plasma renin levels with renal function in patients with primary aldosteronism. Clin J Am Soc Nephrol 2(4):722–731
10. Catena C, Colussi G, Nadalini E, Chiuch A, Baroselli S, Lapenna R, Sechi LA (2008) Cardiovascular outcomes in patients with primary aldosteronism after treatment. Arch Intern Med 168(1):80–85
11. Clarke D, Wilkinson R, Johnston ID, Hacking PM, Haggith JW (1979) Severe hypertension in primary aldosteronism and good response to surgery. Lancet 1(8114):482–485
12. Deter HC, Buchholz K, Schorr U, Schachinger H, Turan S, Sharma AM (1997) Psychophysiological reactivity of salt-sensitive normotensive subjects. J Hypertens 15(8):839–844
13. Emanuele E, Geroldi D, Minoretti P, Coen E, Politi P (2005) Increased plasma aldosterone in patients with clinical depression. Arch Med Res 36(5):544–548
14. Francis J, Beltz T, Johnson AK, Felder RB (2003) Mineralocorticoids act centrally to regulate blood-borne tumor necrosis factor-alpha in normal rats. Am J Physiol Regul Integr Comp Physiol 285(6):R1402–R1409
15. Funder JW (2004) Aldosterone, mineralocorticoid receptors and vascular inflammation. Mol Cell Endocrinol 217(1–2):263–269
16. Gard PR (2004) Angiotensin as a target for the treatment of Alzheimer's disease, anxiety and depression. Expert Opin Ther Targets 8(1):7–14
17. Gliklich RE, Hilinski JM (1995) Longitudinal sensitivity of generic and specific health measures in chronic sinusitis. Qual Life Res 4(1):27–32
18. Gonzaga CC, Gaddam KK, Ahmed MI, Pimenta E, Thomas SJ, Harding SM, Oparil S, Cofield SS, Calhoun DA (2010) Severity of obstructive sleep apnea is related to aldosterone status in subjects with resistant hypertension. J Clin Sleep Med 6(4):363–368
19. Hlavacova N, Bakos J, Jezova D (2010) Eplerenone, a selective mineralocorticoid receptor blocker, exerts anxiolytic effects accompanied by changes in stress hormone release. J Psychopharmacol 24(5):779–786
20. Hlavacova N, Jezova D (2008) Chronic treatment with the mineralocorticoid hormone aldosterone results in increased anxiety-like behavior. Horm Behav 54(1):90–97

21. Hollenberg NK (2004) Aldosterone in the development and progression of renal injury. Kidney Int 66(1):1–9
22. Hollingworth W, Mackenzie R, Todd CJ, Dixon AK (1995) Measuring changes in quality of life following magnetic resonance imaging of the knee: SF-36, EuroQol or Rosser index? Qual Life Res 4(4):325–334
23. Houlihan DJ (2011) Episodic rage associated with primary aldosteronism resolved with adrenalectomy. Psychother Psychosom 80(5):306–307
24. Kaiser FC, Palmer GC, Wallace AV, Carr RD, Fraser-Rae L, Hallam C (1992) Antianxiety properties of the angiotensin II antagonist, DUP 753, in the rat using the elevated plus-maze. Neuroreport 3(10):922–924
25. Khurshid KA, Weaver ME (2005) Conn's syndrome presenting as depression. Am J Psychiatry 162(6):1226
26. Korte SM, de Boer SF, de Kloet ER, Bohus B (1995) Anxiolytic-like effects of selective mineralocorticoid and glucocorticoid antagonists on fear-enhanced behavior in the elevated plus-maze. Psychoneuroendocrinology 20(4):385–394
27. Kurtin PS, Davies AR, Meyer KB, DeGiacomo JM, Kantz ME (1992) Patient-based health status measures in outpatient dialysis. Early experiences in developing an outcomes assessment program. Med Care 30(5 Suppl):MS136–MS149
28. Lichtenberg P, Belmaker RH (2010) Subtyping major depressive disorder. Psychother Psychosom 79(3):131–135
29. Lim PO, Young WF, MacDonald TM (2001) A review of the medical treatment of primary aldosteronism. J Hypertens 19(3):353–361
30. Malinow KC, Lion JR (1979) Hyperaldosteronism (Conn's disease) presenting as depression. J Clin Psychiatry 40(8):358–359
31. McCallum J (1995) The SF-36 in an Australian sample: validating a new, generic health status measure. Aust J Public Health 19(2):160–166
32. McHorney CA, Ware JE Jr, Lu JF, Sherbourne CD (1994) The MOS 36-item Short-Form Health Survey (SF-36): III. Tests of data quality, scaling assumptions, and reliability across diverse patient groups. Med Care 32(1):40–66
33. McHorney CA, Ware JE Jr, Raczek AE (1993) The MOS 36-Item Short-Form Health Survey (SF-36): II. Psychometric and clinical tests of validity in measuring physical and mental health constructs. Med Care 31(3):247–263
34. Milliez P, Girerd X, Plouin P-F, Blacher J, Safar ME, Mourad J-J (2005) Evidence for an increased rate of cardiovascular events in patients with primary aldosteronism. J Am Coll Cardiol 45(8):1243–1248
35. Milsom SR, Espiner EA, Nicholls MG, Gwynne J, Perry EG (1986) The blood pressure response to unilateral adrenalectomy in primary aldosteronism. Q J Med 61(236):1141–1151
36. Muldoon MF, Barger SD, Flory JD, Manuck SB (1998) What are quality of life measurements measuring? BMJ 316(7130):542–545
37. Murck H, Held K, Ziegenbein M, Kunzel H, Koch K, Steiger A (2003) The renin-angiotensin-aldosterone system in patients with depression compared to controls—a sleep endocrine study. BMC Psychiatry 3:15
38. Naruse M, Tanabe A, Sato A, Takagi S, Tsuchiya K, Imaki T, Takano K (2002) Aldosterone breakthrough during angiotensin II receptor antagonist therapy in stroke-prone spontaneously hypertensive rats. Hypertension 40(1):28–33
39. Pimenta E, Calhoun DA, Oparil S (2009) Sleep apnea, aldosterone, and resistant hypertension. Prog Cardiovasc Dis 51(5):371–380
40. Raison CL, Capuron L, Miller AH (2006) Cytokines sing the blues: inflammation and the pathogenesis of depression. Trends Immunol 27(1):24–31
41. Reincke M, Rump LC, Quinkler M, Hahner S, Diederich S, Lorenz R, Seufert J, Schirpenbach C, Beuschlein F, Bidlingmaier M, Meisinger C, Holle R, Endres S (2009) Risk factors associated with a low glomerular filtration rate in primary aldosteronism. J Clin Endocrinol Metab 94(3):869–875
42. Rossi G, Boscaro M, Ronconi V, Funder JW (2005) Aldosterone as a cardiovascular risk factor. Trends Endocrinol Metab 16(3):104–107

43. Rossi GP, Bernini G, Desideri G, Fabris B, Ferri C, Giacchetti G, Letizia C, Maccario M, Mannelli M, Matterello MJ, Montemurro D, Palumbo G, Rizzoni D, Rossi E, Pessina AC, Mantero F (2006) Renal damage in primary aldosteronism: results of the PAPY Study. Hypertension 48(2):232–238
44. Saavedra JM, Ando H, Armando I, Baiardi G, Bregonzio C, Juorio A, Macova M (2005) Anti-stress and anti-anxiety effects of centrally acting angiotensin II AT1 receptor antagonists. Regul Pept 128(3):227–238
45. Saavedra JM, Armando I, Bregonzio C, Juorio A, Macova M, Pavel J, Sanchez-Lemus E (2006) A centrally acting, anxiolytic angiotensin II AT1 receptor antagonist prevents the isolation stress-induced decrease in cortical CRF1 receptor and benzodiazepine binding. Neuropsychopharmacology 31(6):1123–1134
46. Sechi LA, Colussi G, Di Fabio A, Catena C (2010) Cardiovascular and renal damage in primary aldosteronism: outcomes after treatment. Am J Hypertens 23(12):1253–1260
47. Skevington SM (2010) Qualities of life, educational level and human development: an international investigation of health. Soc Psychiatry Psychiatr Epidemiol 45(10):999–1009
48. Skevington SM, Lotfy M, O'Connell KA (2004) The World Health Organization's WHOQOL-BREF quality of life assessment: psychometric properties and results of the international field trial. A report from the WHOQOL group. Qual Life Res 13(2):299–310
49. Smythe JW, Murphy D, Timothy C, Costall B (1997) Hippocampal mineralocorticoid, but not glucocorticoid, receptors modulate anxiety-like behavior in rats. Pharmacol Biochem Behav 56(3):507–513
50. Sonino N, Fallo F, Fava GA (2006) Psychological aspects of primary aldosteronism. Psychother Psychosom 75(5):327–330
51. Sonino N, Tomba E, Genesia ML, Bertello C, Mulatero P, Veglio F, Fava GA, Fallo F (2011) Psychological assessment of primary aldosteronism: a controlled study. J Clin Endocrinol Metab 96(6):E878–E883
52. Spriggs DR, Sherman ML, Michie H, Arthur KA, Imamura K, Wilmore D, Frei E 3rd, Kufe DW (1988) Recombinant human tumor necrosis factor administered as a 24-hour intravenous infusion. A phase I and pharmacologic study. J Natl Cancer Inst 80(13):1039–1044
53. Srinivasan J, Suresh B, Ramanathan M (2003) Differential anxiolytic effect of enalapril and losartan in normotensive and renal hypertensive rats. Physiol Behav 78(4–5):585–591
54. Stevenson C (1996) SF-36: interim norms for Australian data. Australian Institute of Health and Welfare, Canberra
55. Stier CT Jr, Chander PN, Rocha R (2002) Aldosterone as a mediator in cardiovascular injury. Cardiol Rev 10(2):97–107
56. Stowasser M, Gordon RD (2004) Primary aldosteronism—careful investigation is essential and rewarding. Mol Cell Endocrinol 217(1–2):33–39
57. Stowasser M, Gordon RD, Gunasekera TG, Cowley DC, Ward G, Archibald C, Smithers BM (2003) High rate of detection of primary aldosteronism, including surgically treatable forms, after 'non-selective' screening of hypertensive patients. J Hypertens 21(11):2149–2157
58. Stowasser M, Gordon RD, Rutherford JC, Nikwan NZ, Daunt N, Slater GJ (2001) Diagnosis and management of primary aldosteronism. J Renin Angiotensin Aldosterone Syst 2(3):156–169
59. Strauch B, Petrak O, Zelinka T, Wichterle D, Holaj R, Kasalicky M, Safarik L, Rosa J, Widimsky J Jr (2008) Adrenalectomy improves arterial stiffness in primary aldosteronism. Am J Hypertens 21(10):1086–1092
60. Stucki G, Liang MH, Phillips C, Katz JN (1995) The Short Form-36 is preferable to the SIP as a generic health status measure in patients undergoing elective total hip arthroplasty. Arthritis Care Res 8(3):174–181
61. Sukor N, Kogovsek C, Gordon RD, Robson D, Stowasser M (2010) Improved quality of life, blood pressure, and biochemical status following laparoscopic adrenalectomy for unilateral primary aldosteronism. J Clin Endocrinol Metab 95(3):1360–1364
62. Testa MA, Simonson DC (1996) Assesment of quality-of-life outcomes. N Engl J Med 334(13):835–840

63. VanderZee KI, Sanderman R, Heyink J (1996) A comparison of two multidimensional measures of health status: the Nottingham Health Profile and the RAND 36-Item Health Survey 1.0. Qual Life Res 5(1):165–174
64. Ware JE Jr (2000) SF-36 health survey update. Spine (Phila Pa 1976) 25(24):3130–3139
65. Ware JE Jr, Sherbourne CD (1992) The MOS 36-item short-form health survey (SF-36). I. Conceptual framework and item selection. Med Care 30(6):473–483
66. Wyrwich KW, Harnam N, Revicki DA, Locklear JC, Svedsater H, Endicott J (2011) Assessment of quality of life enjoyment and satisfaction questionnaire-short form responder thresholds in generalized anxiety disorder and bipolar disorder studies. Int Clin Psychopharmacol 26(3):121–129

Chapter 14
Medical Treatment of Primary Aldosteronism

Yoshiyu Takeda, Masashi Demura, and Takashi Yoneda

Abstract Primary aldosteronism (PA) is an important cause of secondary hypertension, and therefore, efficient diagnostic procedures and effective treatment are of increasing importance due to the severe cardiovascular and renal complications associated with disorder. Eplerenone, a specific mineralocorticoid receptor antagonist and spironolactone are effective drugs for improving blood pressure and cardiovascular and renal injuries in patients with idiopathic hyperaldosteronism (IHA) or aldosterone-producing adenoma (APA). No significant differences in prognosis have been reported between medical treatment and adrenalectomy in patients with APA. The remission rate of PA is 5–8 % with spironolactone or eplerenone, which represents a beneficial effect of medical treatment. The cause of remission of PA remains unknown, although it is possible that epigenetic control of the *CYP11B2* gene may be responsible. As the prevalence of subclinical PA is approximately 10 % in pre-hypertensive patients, there is a need to determine effective treatment for subclinical PA.

Keywords Primary aldosteronism • Aldosterone-producing adenoma • Idiopathic hyperaldosteronism • Eplerenone • Spironolactone • Remission • Epigenetics • *CYP11B2*

Introduction

Until the 1990s the primary aldosteronism (PA) syndrome was characterized by hypertension with excessive production of aldosterone, potassium loss, and suppression of the renin–angiotensin system. In those days, clinicians did not consider

Y. Takeda, M.D. (✉) • M. Demura, M.D. • T. Yoneda, M.D.
Division of Endocrinology and Hypertension, Department of Internal Medicine, Graduate School of Medical Science, Kanazawa University, 13-1 Takara-machi, Kanazawa 920-8641, Japan
e-mail: takeday@med.kanazawa-u.ac.jp

P. Hellman (ed.), *Primary Aldosteronism: Molecular Genetics, Endocrinology, and Translational Medicine*, DOI 10.1007/978-1-4939-0509-6_14,

a diagnosis of PA unless the patient presented with spontaneous hypokalemia. The reported prevalence rate of the disorder was therefore less than 1 %. During the past two decades it has become increasingly recognized that PA is more common in patients with secondary hypertension with an estimated prevalence of 5–15 % in all hypertensive patients. Aldosterone excess has adverse cardiovascular and renal consequences not only in patients with hypertension but also in those with diabetes mellitus or chronic renal disease [18]. We have reported previously that PA patients have a higher incidence of cardiovascular complications than age- and sex-matched patients with essential hypertension [17]. Numerous studies have also shown that PA is common in patients with resistant hypertension with a prevalence of approximately 20 %, and is associated with a significant increase in risk for end-organ damage and cardiovascular events compared with more easily controlled hypertension [23].

Patients with a documented aldosterone-producing adenoma (APA) or unilateral adrenal hyperplasia are often treated with unilateral laparoscopic adrenalectomy. Although surgical removal of APA improves hypertension by up to 30–50 % [16], there are no data to show adrenalectomy is superior to the medical treatment. Spironolactone and eplerenone, which both antagonize the mineralocorticoid receptor (MR) directly, are the most appropriate choice of therapeutic agents in these patients. Spironolactone has been used widely for the treatment of PA, but its use is limited by adverse effects such as gynecomastia, mastodynia, menstrual abnormalities, and impotence due to its agonist activity of the androgen receptor. Eplerenone is a specific MR antagonist and possesses very few side effects.

Pharmacology of Eplerenone

Eplerenone exerts the selective aldosterone blockade that is specific for the MR. Its chemical structure differs from that of the non-selective aldosterone antagonist, spironolactone, in that the 17 thioacetyl group is replaced by a carbomethoxy group. For example, in rats the IC_{50} of eplerenone for the aldosterone receptor is 360 nmol/L, whereas the IC_{50} values for the androgen, progesterone, and estrogen receptors is >10,000 nmol/L. Eplerenone is cleared primarily via metabolism by CYP4503A4 to inactive metabolites, and has an elimination half-life of 4–6 h. Studies in humans have shown that eplerenone is 50–75 % as potent as spironolactone [2].

Aldosterone Blockade Therapy in Patients with Primary Aldosteronism

IHA is the most common subtype of PA accounting for 40–60 % of cases, and should therefore be treated medically. In addition to their use in IHA, spironolactone and eplerenone are administered to patients with bilateral APA and APA in whom surgical excision of the adrenal is not possible. Spironolactone has been used successfully for more than four decades as either as monotherapy or in combination with other antihypertensive drugs. In recent years, lower doses of spironolactone (25–50 mg/day) have been shown to reduce the need for antihypertensive drugs, and achieved normal blood pressure levels nearly one-half of treated patients. As mentioned previously, the major side effect of spironolactone in males is gynecomastia. In patients with a glomerular filtration rate <60 mL/min, spironolactone should be used with caution due to the risk of hyperkalemia. Potassium levels often respond quickly to spironolactone therapy, whereas reduction in blood pressure is seen after a few weeks [13].

Eplerenone is approved for the treatment of essential hypertension in the USA and Japan, but not in Europe. There is only limited data on the effects of eplerenone in patients with PA. We treated 33 patients with IHA (who were diagnosed finally by AVS and CT) with either spironolactone (25–50 mg/day) ($n = 18$) or eplerenone (50–100 mg/day) ($n = 15$) for 36 weeks. Systolic (SBP) and diastolic blood pressure (DBP) decreased significantly in both groups ($p < 0.05$): eplerenone 156 ± 14 to 128 ± 10 mmHg (SBP) and 98 ± 9 to 77 ± 9 mmHg (DBP). Spironolactone was associated with significant increases in serum potassium from 3.4 ± 0.3 to 4.1 ± 0.3 mEq/L ($p < 0.05$). Treatment with eplerenone has been reported to cause identical elevations [20]. Karagiannis et al. [14] showed that after 16 weeks of treatment, the percentage of patients with BP<140/90 mmHg was 76.5 % with spironolactone therapy and 82.4 % with eplerenone treatment. Systolic BP decreased more rapidly with eplerenone and serum potassium levels were normalized (>3.5 mmol/L) in all patients. Treatment with eplerenone also reduced the frequency of sex-hormone-related adverse effects compared with spironolactone. In that report, two patients who received spironolactone developed painful bilateral gynecomastia that resolved completely when they were switched to eplerenone. No cases of gynecomastia were observed in patients treated with eplerenone. Parthasarathy et al. [15] showed that DBP was lower with eplerenone (100 mg/day) than with spironolactone (75 mg/day) in treatment of PA, and that spironolactone caused development of male gynecomastia and female mastodynia. Hyperkalemia occurred in one eplerenone patient and seven spironolactone patients. Fourkiotis et al. [10] reported that medical therapies with spironolactone or eplerenone were as effective as adrenalectomy on renal function and blood pressure control.

Recent studies have suggested that aldosterone and MR may be involved in adipocyte biology, given the high binding affinity of these receptors for both mineralocorticoids and glucocorticoids. There is also evidence a study by Caprio et al. [4] that aldosterone promotes maturation of pre-adipocytes to adipocytes cells in a time-, dose-, and MR-dependent manner. Fallo et al. [8] also reported the prevalence of metabolic syndrome was higher in primary aldosteronism than in essential hypertension. Distribution of single components of the metabolic syndrome other than hypertension showed a higher prevalence of hyperglycemia in primary aldosteronism than in essential hypertension. There is only limited data on the effects of MR antagonists in patients with PA. We found no beneficial effects of spironolactone or eplerenone on glucose and lipids levels in patients with PA, although MR antagonists significantly decreased abdominal visceral adipose tissue area measured by CT and Fat Scan software (93.3 ± 45.9 cm^2 vs 88.2 ± 47.8 cm^2, $p < 0.05$) independent of body weight. The pleiotropic effects of MR antagonists in PA therefore need to be investigated in greater detail.

Catena et al. [5] reported that the long-term cardiac effects of adrenalectomy and mineralocorticoid antagonists were similar in patients with PA. We also observed elevated PRA and PAC in patients with IHA treated with spironolactone or eplerenone. Increased activity of the renin–angiotensin–aldosterone system in the circulation or tissues causes cardiovascular and renal injuries independently of increases in blood pressure [19]. Several non-genomic effects of aldosterone cannot be prevented by MR antagonists and therefore the differences in long-term effects of aldosterone blockade and adrenalectomy need to be studied further.

Calcium channel blockers (CCBs) may reduce aldosterone secretion and BP in patients with PA by blocking the influx of calcium into adrenal glomerulosa cells [1]. Several CCBs possess mineralocorticoid receptor antagonistic effects in vitro [7] and there is evidence ACEIs and ARBs also have a moderate BP-lowering effect in patients with IHA [11]. These agents may therefore be useful in combination with aldosterone blockers.

Aldosterone synthase inhibitors may be beneficial in the treatment of PA. Calhoun et al. [3] reported that LCI699, a novel inhibitor of aldosterone synthase lowered BP in hypertensive patients to the same extent as eplerenone. Its effects may differ from those of other MR antagonists, as they also inhibit any extra-adrenal synthesis of aldosterone and do not activate the renin–angiotensin system. Additional research to evaluate the use of aldosterone synthase inhibition in PA is therefore necessary.

Remission of PA After Long-Term Treatment with MR Antagonist

Treatment with potassium canrenoate or spironolctone is known to produce remission of IHA. The prevalence of remission with spironolactone treatment was reported to be 5.4 % [9]. We have reported previously a case of unilateral PA with spontaneous remission and reduction of cardiac hypertrophy after long-term spironolactone therapy [22]. However, there is no report of the remission of PA using eplerenone. We treated 45 patients of PA with eplerenone for 3.1 years and achieved partial remission in 4 patients (8 %). The causes of sporadic IHA have yet to be determined. Several factors have been implicated such as genetic predisposition leading to increased sensitivity to angiotensin II or potassium chloride, production of stimulating factors, and direct inhibition of spironolactone in aldosterone synthesis [21]. DNA methylation at the 5′-cytosine of CpG dinucleotides is a major epigenetic modification in eukaryotic genomes and is related to the pathophysiology of tumorigenesis, hypertension and diabetes mellitus. Ad1/CRE and Ad5 contain CpG dinucleotides, which are target sites for DNA methylation, leading to the hypothesis that CpG dinucleotide methylation may regulate *CYP11B2* gene expression.

We have reported that there is a relationship between the methylation status of the *CYP11B2* prompter region and aldosterone synthesis [6]. Long-term treatment with MR antagonists may therefore influence methylation status and normalize the aldosterone synthase activity.

Should Subclinical PA Be Treated?

We have reported previously that the prevalence of primary aldosteronism is at least 6.8 % in prehypertensive patients and 3.3 % in stage 1 hypertensive patients. Hypertension was staged according to the JNC 7: prehypertension, 120–139/80–89 mmHg and stage 1 hypertension, 140–159/90–99 mmHg [12]. Normotensive individuals that are at increased risk for primary aldosteronism should be screened for subclinical forms of the disease in order to initiate early diagnosis and treatment and prevent the cardiovascular events associated with hyperaldosteronism. Future studies should address whether hypertension develops later or the blood pressure remains at normotensive levels. These adverse effects of hyperaldosteronemia should be investigated in normotensive patients with PA. Comparative trials are also needed on therapeutic interventions aimed at preventing cardiovascular complications in these patients.

Conclusion

Medical treatment with spironolactone or eplerenone improves not only blood pressure but also the cardiovascular and renal complications of PA. Spironolactone has a higher incidence of side effects than eplerenone, but is the less expensive of the two drugs. No significant differences in prognosis between medical treatment and adrenalectomy have been noted in patients with APA. The remission rate of PA during treatment with spironolactone or eplerenone is between 5 and 8 %. This represents an additional beneficial effect of MR antagonists.

References

1. Akizuki O, Inayoshi A, Kitayama T et al (2008) Blockade of T-type voltage-dependent Ca^{2+} channels by benidipine, a dihydropyridine calcium channel blocker, inhibits aldosterone production in human adrenocortical cell line NCI-H295R. Eur J Pharmacol 28:424–434
2. Brown NJ (2003) Eplerenone, cardiovascular protection. Circulation 107:2512–2518
3. Calhoun DA, White WB, Krum H et al (2011) Effects of novel aldosterone synthase inhibitor for treatment of primary hypertension. Circulation 124:1945–1955
4. Caprio M, Fève B, Claës A et al (2007) Pivotal role of the mineralocorticoid receptor in corticosteroid-induced adipogenesis. FASEB J 21:2185–2194

5. Catena C, Colussi GL, Marzano L et al (2012) Predictive factors of left ventricular mass changes after treatment of primary aldosteronism. Horm Metab Res 44:188–193
6. Demura M, Wang F, Yoneda T et al (2012) Differential DNA methylation of the CYP11B1 and CYP11B2 genes in association with human adrenal zonation. Endocrine Abstracts 29: P35
7. Dietz JD, Du S, Bolten CW et al (2008) A number of marketed dihydropyridine calcium channel blockers have mineralocorticoid receptor antagonist activity. Hypertension 51: 742–748
8. Fallo F, Veglio F, Bertello C et al (2006) Prevalence and characteristics of the metabolic syndrome in primary aldosteronism. J Clin Endocrinol Metab 91:454–459
9. Fischer E, Beuschlein F, Degenhart C et al (2012) Spontaneously remission of idiopathic aldosternism after long-term treatment with spironolactone: results from the German Conn's Registry. Clin Endocrinol 76:437–477
10. Fourkiotis VG, Vonend O, Diederich S et al (2012) Effectiveness of eplerenone or spironolactone treatment in preserving renal function in primary aldosteronism. Eur J Endocrinol. doi:10.1530/EJE-12-0631
11. Griffing GT, Melby JC (1985) The therapeutic effect of a new angiotensin-converting enzyme inhibitor, enalapril maleate, in idiopathic hyperaldosteronism. J Clin Hypertens 1:265–276
12. Ito Y, Takeda R, Karashima S et al (2011) Prevalence of primary aldosteronism among prehypertensive and stage 1 hypertensive subjects. Hypertens Res 34:98–102
13. Karagiannis A (2011) Treatment of primary aldosteronism: where are we now? Rev Endocr Metab Disord 12:15–20
14. Karagiannis A, Tziomalos K, Kahafika A et al (2008) Medical treatment as an alternative to adrenalectomy in patients with aldosterone-producing adenomas. Endocr Relat Cancer 15: 693–700
15. Parthaasarathy HK, Menard J, White WB et al (2011) A double-blind, randomized study comparing the antihypertensive effect of eplerenone and spironolactone in patients with hypertension and evidence of primary aldosteronism. J Hypertens 29:980–990
16. Quinkler M, Stewart PM (2010) Treatment of primary aldosteronism. Best Pract Res Clin Endocrinol Metab 24:923–932
17. Takeda R, Matsubara T, Miyamori I et al (1995) Vascular complications in patients with aldosterone producing adenoma in Japan: comparative study with essential hypertension. J Endocrinol Invest 18:370–373
18. Takeda Y (2004) Pleiotropic actions of aldosterone and the effects of eplerenone, a selective mineralocorticoid receptor antagonist. Hypertens Res 27:781–789
19. Takeda Y (2009) Effects of eplerenone, a selective mineralocorticoid receptor antagonist, on clinical and experimental salt-sensitive hypertension. Hypertens Res 32:321–324
20. Takeda Y, Karashima S, Yoneda T (2011) Primary aldosteronism, diagnosis and treatment in Japan. Rev Endocr Metab Disord 12:21–25
21. Ye P, Yamashita T, Pollock DM et al (2009) Contrasting effects of eplerenone and spironolactone on adrenal cell steroidogenesis. Horm Metab Res 41:35–39
22. Yoneda T, Demura M, Takata H et al (2012) Unilateral primary aldosteronism with spontaneous remission after long-term spironolactone therapy. J Clin Endocrinol Metab 97:1109–1113
23. Young WF (2007) Primary aldosteronism: renaissance of a syndrome. Clin Endocrinol 66: 607–618

Chapter 15
Surgical Treatment of Unilateral Excessive Aldosterone Production

Peter Stålberg and Per Hellman

Abstract Adrenal surgery today is safe and if performed laparoscopically or retroperitoneoscopically comparably easy for the patient with short hospital stays. Larger lesions suspected for being malignant should preferably be operated with an open technique. The outcome is usually excellent, with no needs for potassium replacement and reduction in the number of hypertensive drugs, as well as usual normalization of blood pressure. Also cases with nodular hyperplasia may be operated if lateralization of aldosterone excess is found.

Keywords Surgery • Laparoscopy • Retroperitoneoscopy • Outcome

In this chapter, surgery and surgical outcomes are purely discussed in the setting of aldosterone producing lesions. Regardless of the cause of unilateral excessive aldosterone production, the treatment of choice is unilateral adrenalectomy. The diagnosis of unilateral disease should be confirmed with adrenal venous sampling (AVS). The patient should be made normokalemic before any surgical intervention to reduce surgical risks. The optimal surgical approach is laparoscopic adrenalectomy. There are a vast number of studies describing the advantages of laparoscopic surgery over open adrenalectomy. These advantages include less blood loss, shorter operating time, less need of analgesics, earlier recovery, and, of course, smaller wound with less hernia complications [1–5].

Laparoscopic surgery was introduced in 1992, and today most published series of adrenalectomy for excessive aldosterone production are done by either of the laparoscopic techniques described (see below). The exception is pure excessive

P. Stålberg, M.D., Ph.D. (✉) • P. Hellman, M.D., Ph.D.
Department of Surgical Sciences, Uppsala University, Akademiska sjukhuset ing 70 1 tr, Uppsala 751 85, Sweden
e-mail: Peter.Stalberg@surgsci.uu.se

P. Hellman (ed.), *Primary Aldosteronism: Molecular Genetics, Endocrinology, and Translational Medicine*, DOI 10.1007/978-1-4939-0509-6_15,

aldosterone production from an adrenocortical cancer (ACC) (extremely rare, accounts for <1 % of all ACC) since the evidence points out that for oncological reasons all ACCs should probably be performed using an open approach [6].

There are basically two techniques for laparoscopic adrenalectomy, the lateral transabdominal approach and the posterior retroperitoneal approach. These can be performed by traditional techniques or using a robotic approach; however, the surgical dissection is basically the same in both approaches.

Adrenalectomy with the Laparoscopic Transabdominal Approach

Surgical Techniques and Postoperative Care

Advantages of this approach include a familiar anatomy and the ability to perform a general abdominal exploration. The patient is placed in the lateral decubitus position, which provides the best exposure to the adrenals since gravity helps retraction of the liver on the right and the pancreas and spleen on the left. On the right, retraction and dissection of the liver to get medial rotation is necessary to expose the adrenal and the inferior caval vein (IVC). The adrenal vein and any accessory veins are usually drained into the IVC and can be cautiously dealt with using any of the modern instruments such as the LigaSure (Covidien) or Harmonic scalpel (Johnson & Johnson). For unusually large veins clips can be necessary. On the left, dissection in the plane between the spleen/tail of pancreas and the retroperitoneum creates a situation sometimes denoted as an open book, where gravity retracts the spleen/pancreas medially. On the left side the adrenal vein drains into the renal vein and can be dealt with in a similar fashion as on the right side. Caution should be taken to not divide any suprarenal artery, which may lead to devascularization of the upper pole of the kidney. On the left side an inferior phrenic vein can be seen medial to the adrenal, and may be sharing the same drainage as the adrenal vein. This vein can be safely divided if necessary.

Adrenalectomy with the Laparoscopic Retroperitoneal Approach

This technique was described in 1995 [7] and has been refined ever since by a number of authors [8–10]. The patient is placed in a prone, jack-knife position with a 90° angle at the hip joints and the knees. This opens up the space between the inferior costal margin and the iliac crest (Fig. 15.1). The retroperitoneum is

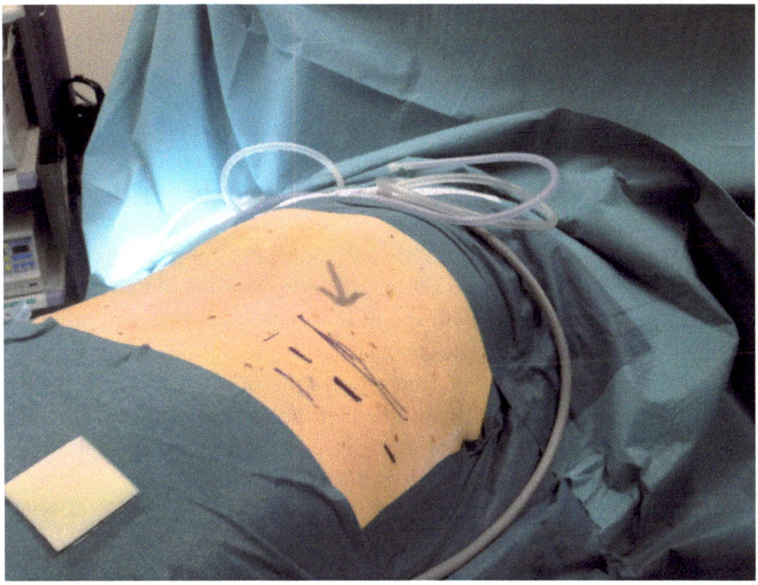

Fig. 15.1 Port placement in a retroperitoneoscopic adrenalectomy. The retroperitoneum is entered below the 12th rib

then entered in this space. Compared to the transabdominal approach, a higher pressure of 25–30 mmHg is used for insufflation. Identification of the kidney surface and the paraspinous muscles are crucial for anatomical orientation. On the right side the posterior surface of the liver is visible through the peritoneum. Traction of the kidney and careful dissection along the IVC will expose the adrenal vein. The left side traction of the kidney and having the superior attachments of the periadrenal fat in place help in dissection of the adrenal vein and inferior phrenic vein.

Advantages with this approach include less postoperative pain, no bowel paralysis, and avoidance of adhesions from previous abdominal surgery.

Disadvantages may be the limitations in creating enough space in the morbidly obese patients (BMI>45) and CO_2 retention in patients with severe COPD.

Complications

Complications are uncommon and occur in less than 1 % of patients, and if present include postoperative bleeding, port-site infection, incisional hernia, and pneumothorax. Approximately 8 % of patients will experience hypoesthesia and/or abdominal wall laxity; however, these are usually temporary findings.

Postoperative Care (Correction of Potassium and Hypertensives)

Postoperative care is routine, with pain control and early ambulation. General diet should be routine immediately postoperatively as tolerated for both approaches. Patients undergoing the posterior approach may generally be discharged earlier than patients undergoing the lateral approach.

Spironolactone should be discontinued and potassium levels checked the morning after surgery. As a rule of thumb, if the patient is on high doses of potassium preoperatively, half of this dose can be administered the day after surgery. In the outpatient setting blood pressure (BP) and potassium levels are checked. Potassium levels need to be monitored closely the first week and doses adjusted accordingly. Most patients can discontinue their potassium supplementation within the first week. BP needs monitoring on a weekly basis with special attention to hypotensive symptoms and medications adjusted accordingly.

Postoperative Outcomes

Histopathology Related to Outcomes

Several reports have shown that in supposedly unilateral adenomas (APAs) there is often a presence of hyperplasia and/or nodular hyperplasia on histopathologic examination of the specimen (Figs. 15.2 and 15.3) [11–13].

In a recent series by Weisbrod et al. [14], 95 patients underwent adrenalectomy for unilateral overproduction of aldosterone based on AVS. Of these, 66 patients had an aldosterone-producing cortical adenoma, and 14 patients demonstrated an aldosterone-producing adenoma with diffuse adrenal hyperplasia. Histopathology of the remaining 15 patients showed diffuse cortical hyperplasia without evidence of a cortical adenoma. For these 15 patients, the diagnosis manifested as multinodular hyperplasia in 10 patients and non-nodular hyperplasia in 5 patients. Interestingly, there was no significant difference between these groups in terms of age at diagnosis, gender distribution, BMI, duration of hypertension, number of preoperative antihypertensive medications, or preoperative aldosterone or renin level. Additionally, there was no significant difference in the clinical and laboratory features associated with patient outcome by histologic groups. This report is highly relevant in the discussion of whom to offer surgical intervention in primary aldosteronism (Fig. 15.4).

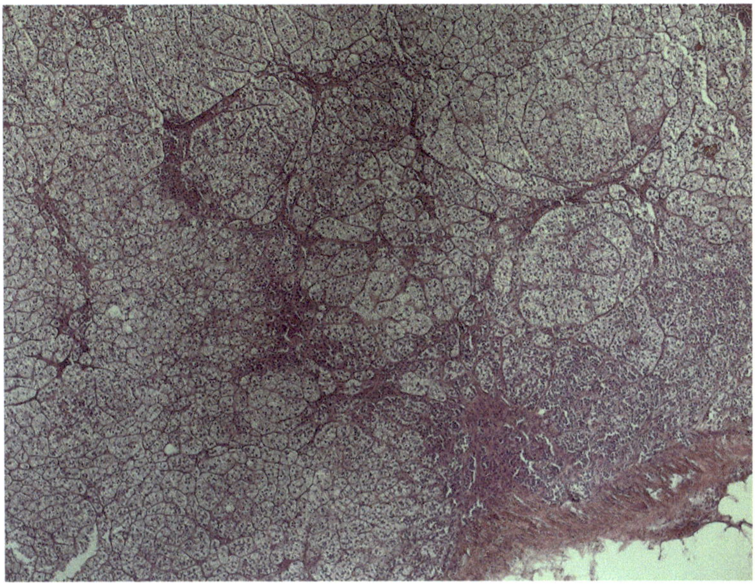

Fig. 15.2 Hematoxylin–Eosin staining of an adrenocortical hyperplasia

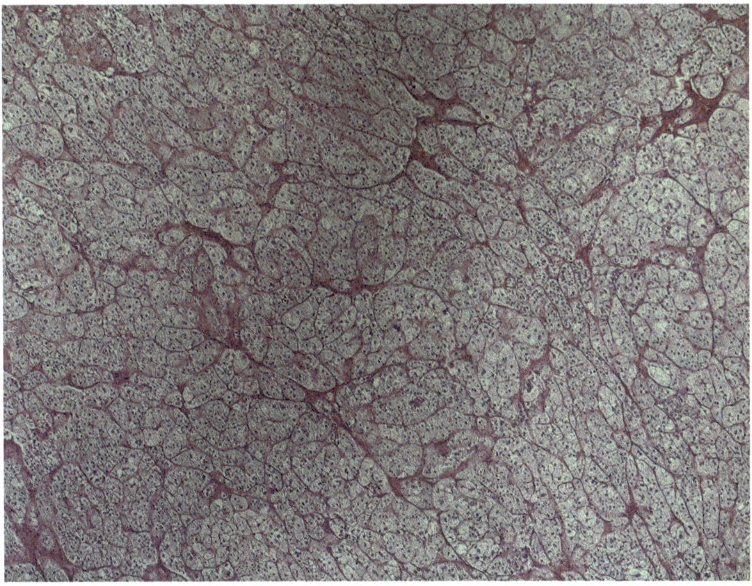

Fig. 15.3 Hematoxylin–Eosin staining of an adrenocortical adenoma

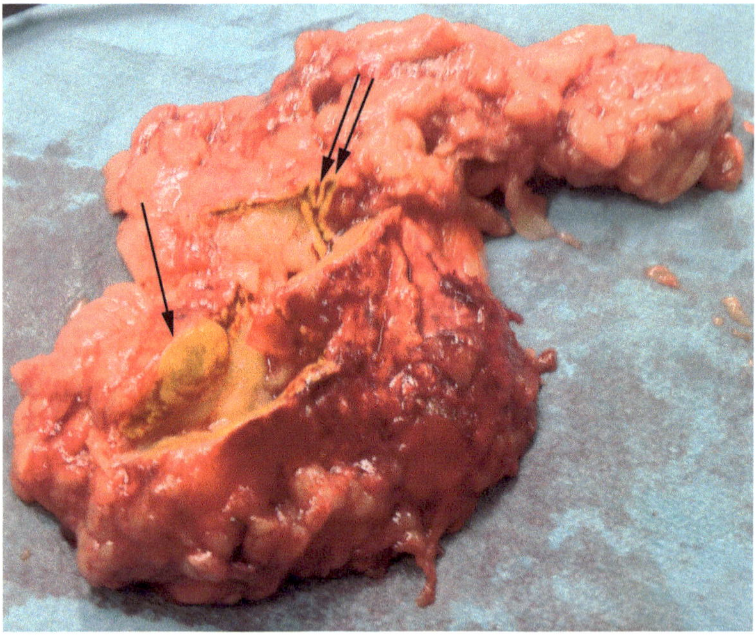

Fig. 15.4 Typical aldosterone-producing adenoma (*single arrow*), diameter 10 mm, in an otherwise normal-appearing adrenal gland (*double arrow*)

Potassium Requirements

Following adrenalectomy, normalization of potassium levels is achieved in close to 100 % of patients [11, 12, 15].

Hypertension

Published reports describing outcomes of patients undergoing adrenalectomy for presumed single adenomas (open or laparoscopic) for hyperaldosteronism show cure rates between 30 and 60 % [11, 12, 16–20]. A study by Meyer et al. on open adrenalectomy with a long mean follow-up duration of 86 months showed a cure rate of 33 % [20]. In terms of studies on laparoscopic adrenalectomy alone, a large series by Meria et al. with 212 cases showed a cure rate of 58 % after a mean follow-up of 44 months, with the remainder having improved BP control [21].

A significant proportion of patients show improved hypertension control but not cure when defined as normotension and without needing any medication. In published series improved BP control can be achieved in >90 % of patients, including the patients cured from disease [11, 12, 16–20]. We believe this represents an important favorable outcome for patients as a result of decrease in circulating aldosterone concentrations. We consider the important end-points in the management of hyperaldosteronism to be BP parameters and normalization of blood aldosterone levels. High aldosterone level itself has a vascular remodelling effect independent of hypertension and may impair both cardiac and renal functions [22, 23].

As mentioned, similar results as for APAs, have been shown for lateralized disease (using AVS) for hyperplasia and nodular disease as well [14]. Walz and colleagues have shown similar results as the present NIH series [19]. When investigating a Norwegian population, tumors with a KCNJ5 mutation was related to better postoperative BP control [24].

The cause of hypertension at postoperative follow-up is not known. With multivariable analysis, different studies have found independent negative predictors of outcome in terms of age and gland size [12]. Other researchers have also found age to be a predictor of persistent hypertension postoperatively [16, 17, 25]. A component of this may be because of essential hypertension, which is more common with advancing age, and the hypertension that remains may simply be a reflection of this. Indeed, Sawka et al. found that persistence of hypertension after adrenalectomy was associated independently with a presence of family history [26]. The vascular remodelling effects of prolonged untreated hypertension and hyperaldosteronism have also been suggested as a possible cause [18, 20, 27]. Fukudome et al. have found that recurrent hypertension in patients (16 of 34 patients initially cured of hypertension) after a mean follow-up period of 12.2 years was related only to serum creatinine and not family history, age, or known duration of hypertension [28]. Regarding gland size as a prognostic indicator in different series, it may be that this difference in size reflects a greater degree of underlying cortical hyperplasia which has not been detected in histological assessment. If this is the case, then the partial cure often seen in these patients may reflect an element of background hyperplasia but with a dominant presenting nodule that, when removed, gives amelioration of hypertension. In a study by Pang et al., all patients had a definite diagnosis of either hyperplasia or adenoma made by the pathologist, a closer examination of pathology reports showed that a significant proportion had an adenoma on a background of hyperplasia (15/52, 29 %) or hyperplasia with discrete nodules/micronodules (3/8, 38 %). The presence of these multiple space-occupying lesions in addition to the main APA was also noted in 27 % (17/63) of adrenal specimens by Ishidoya et al. [12, 13].

Conclusion

Lateralized hyperaldosteronism on the basis of AVS offers patients a significant chance of cure or better BP control by having an adrenalectomy performed on the lateralized side. This should be done by laparoscopy performed by a surgeon familiar with any of the two dominating techniques. The results are encouraging, potassium replenishments can be ceased in nearly 100 % of cases, 30–50 % of patients are cured from disease, and the remaining 50–70 % of patients will have improved BP control. On the basis of available data as of today, partial adrenalectomy cannot generally be recommended for APAs since there is often a background of nodular or diffuse hyperplasia on closer examination.

References

1. Brunt LM, Doherty GM, Norton JA, Soper NJ, Quasebarth MA, Moley JF (1996) Laparoscopic adrenalectomy compared to open adrenalectomy for benign adrenal neoplasms. J Am Coll Surg 183(1):1–10, Epub 1996/07/01
2. Gagner M, Pomp A, Heniford BT, Pharand D, Lacroix A (1997) Laparoscopic adrenalectomy: lessons learned from 100 consecutive procedures. Ann Surg 226(3):238–246, discussion 46–7. Epub 1997/10/27
3. Prager G, Heinz-Peer G, Passler C, Kaczirek K, Scheuba C, Niederle B (2004) Applicability of laparoscopic adrenalectomy in a prospective study in 150 consecutive patients. Arch Surg 139(1):46–49, Epub 2004/01/14
4. Thompson GB, Grant CS, van Heerden JA, Schlinkert RT, Young WF Jr, Farley DR et al (1997) Laparoscopic versus open posterior adrenalectomy: a case-control study of 100 patients. Surgery 122(6):1132–1136, Epub 1998/01/14
5. Winfield HN, Hamilton BD, Bravo EL, Novick AC (1998) Laparoscopic adrenalectomy: the preferred choice? A comparison to open adrenalectomy. J Urol 160(2):325–329, Epub 1998/07/29
6. Porpiglia F, Miller BS, Manfredi M, Fiori C, Doherty GM (2011) A debate on laparoscopic versus open adrenalectomy for adrenocortical carcinoma. Horm Cancer 2(6):372–377, Epub 2011/11/30
7. Mercan S, Seven R, Ozarmagan S, Tezelman S (1995) Endoscopic retroperitoneal adrenalectomy. Surgery 118(6):1071–1075, discussion 5–6. Epub 1995/12/01
8. Siperstein AE, Berber E, Engle KL, Duh QY, Clark OH (2000) Laparoscopic posterior adrenalectomy: technical considerations. Arch Surg 135(8):967–971, Epub 2000/08/02
9. Walz MK, Alesina PF, Wenger FA, Deligiannis A, Szuczik E, Petersenn S et al (2006) Posterior retroperitoneoscopic adrenalectomy–results of 560 procedures in 520 patients. Surgery 140(6):943–948, discussion 8–50. Epub 2006/12/26
10. Walz MK, Peitgen K, Hoermann R, Giebler RM, Mann K, Eigler FW (1996) Posterior retroperitoneoscopy as a new minimally invasive approach for adrenalectomy: results of 30 adrenalectomies in 27 patients. World J Surg 20(7):769–774, Epub 1996/09/01
11. Hennings J, Andreasson S, Botling J, Hagg A, Sundin A, Hellman P (2010) Long-term effects of surgical correction of adrenal hyperplasia and adenoma causing primary aldosteronism. Langenbecks Arch Surg 395(2):133–137, Epub 2009/05/07
12. Pang TC, Bambach C, Monaghan JC, Sidhu SB, Bune A, Delbridge LW et al (2007) Outcomes of laparoscopic adrenalectomy for hyperaldosteronism. ANZ J Surg 77(9):768–773, Epub 2007/08/10
13. Ishidoya S, Ito A, Sakai K, Satoh M, Chiba Y, Sato F et al (2005) Laparoscopic partial versus total adrenalectomy for aldosterone producing adenoma. J Urol 174(1):40–43, Epub 2005/06/11
14. Weisbrod AB, Webb RC, Mathur A, Barak S, Abraham SB, Nilubol N et al (2013) Adrenal histologic findings show no difference in clinical presentation and outcome in primary hyperaldosteronism. Ann Surg Oncol 20(3):753–758, Epub 2012/10/24
15. Gockel I, Heintz A, Polta M, Junginger T (2007) Long-term results of endoscopic adrenalectomy for Conn's syndrome. Am Surg 73(2):174–180, Epub 2007/02/20

16. Goh BK, Tan YH, Yip SK, Eng PH, Cheng CW (2004) Outcome of patients undergoing laparoscopic adrenalectomy for primary hyperaldosteronism. JSLS 8(4):320–325, Epub 2004/11/24
17. Harris DA, Au-Yong I, Basnyat PS, Sadler GP, Wheeler MH (2003) Review of surgical management of aldosterone secreting tumours of the adrenal cortex. Eur J Surg Oncol 29(5):467–474, Epub 2003/06/12
18. Rossi H, Kim A, Prinz RA (2002) Primary hyperaldosteronism in the era of laparoscopic adrenalectomy. Am Surg 68(3):253–256, discussion 6–7. Epub 2002/03/15
19. Walz MK, Gwosdz R, Levin SL, Alesina PF, Suttorp AC, Metz KA et al (2008) Retroperitoneoscopic adrenalectomy in Conn's syndrome caused by adrenal adenomas or nodular hyperplasia. World J Surg 32(5):847–853, Epub 2008/03/18
20. Meyer A, Brabant G, Behrend M (2005) Long-term follow-up after adrenalectomy for primary aldosteronism. World J Surg 29(2):155–159, Epub 2005/01/15
21. Meria P, Kempf BF, Hermieu JF, Plouin PF, Duclos JM (2003) Laparoscopic management of primary hyperaldosteronism: clinical experience with 212 cases. J Urol 169(1):32–35, Epub 2002/12/13
22. Sechi LA, Novello M, Lapenna R, Baroselli S, Nadalini E, Colussi GL et al (2006) Long-term renal outcomes in patients with primary aldosteronism. JAMA 295(22):2638–2645, Epub 2006/06/15
23. Young WF Jr (2003) Minireview: primary aldosteronism–changing concepts in diagnosis and treatment. Endocrinology 144(6):2208–2213, Epub 2003/05/15
24. Arnesen T, Glomnes N, Stromsoy S, Knappskog S, Heie A, Akslen LA et al (2013) Outcome after surgery for primary hyperaldosteronism may depend on KCNJ5 tumor mutation status: a population-based study from Western Norway. Langenbecks Arch Surg 398(6):869–874, Epub 2013/06/20
25. Lo CY, Tam PC, Kung AW, Lam KS, Wong J (1996) Primary aldosteronism. Results of surgical treatment. Ann Surg 224(2):125–130, Epub 1996/08/01
26. Sawka AM, Young WF, Thompson GB, Grant CS, Farley DR, Leibson C et al (2001) Primary aldosteronism: factors associated with normalization of blood pressure after surgery. Ann Intern Med 135(4):258–261, Epub 2001/08/21
27. Rossi GP, Cesari M, Cuspidi C, Maiolino G, Cicala MV, Bisogni V et al (2013) Long-term control of arterial hypertension and regression of left ventricular hypertrophy with treatment of primary aldosteronism. Hypertension 62(1):62–69, Epub 2013/05/08
28. Fukudome Y, Fujii K, Arima H, Ohya Y, Tsuchihashi T, Abe I et al (2002) Discriminating factors for recurrent hypertension in patients with primary aldosteronism after adrenalectomy. Hypertens Res 25(1):11–18, Epub 2002/04/02

Index

P. Hellman (ed.), *Primary Aldosteronism: Molecular Genetics, Endocrinology, and Translational Medicine*, DOI 10.1007/978-1-4939-0509-6,

D

G

H

MIX
Papier aus verantwortungsvollen Quellen
Paper from responsible sources
FSC® C105338

If you have any concerns about our products,
you can contact us on
ProductSafety@springernature.com

In case Publisher is established outside the EU,
the EU authorized representative is:
Springer Nature Customer Service Center GmbH
Europaplatz 3, 69115 Heidelberg, Germany

Printed by Libri Plureos GmbH
in Hamburg, Germany